POLYMERS *for* VASCULAR *and* UROGENITAL APPLICATIONS

Advances in Polymeric Biomaterials

Series Editor: Shalaby W. Shalaby

Published Titles:

Absorbable and Biodegradable Polymers
Shalaby W. Shalaby; Karen J.L. Burg

Polymers for Dental and Orthopedic Applications
Editors: Shalaby W. Shalaby and Ulrich Salz

Polymers for Vascular and Urogenital Applications
Editors: Shalaby W. Shalaby, Karen J.L. Burg, and Waleed Shalaby

POLYMERS *for* VASCULAR *and* UROGENITAL APPLICATIONS

Edited by

SHALABY W. SHALABY
KAREN J.L. BURG
WALEED SHALABY

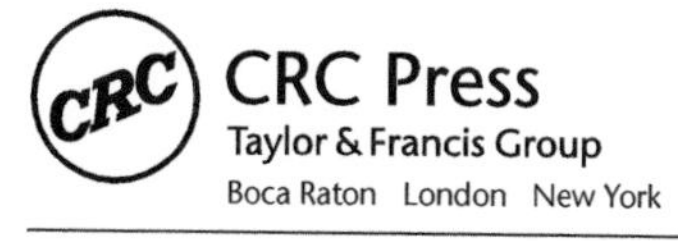

CRC Press is an imprint of the
Taylor & Francis Group, an **informa** business

CRC Press
Taylor & Francis Group
6000 Broken Sound Parkway NW, Suite 300
Boca Raton, FL 33487-2742

First issued in paperback 2017

Version Date: 20120313

ISBN 13: 978-1-138-07745-4 (pbk)
ISBN 13: 978-1-4200-7694-3 (hbk)

Library of Congress Cataloging-in-Publication Data

Polymers for vascular and urogenital applications / editors, Shalaby W. Shalaby, Karen J.L. Burg, Waleed Shalaby.
p. cm. -- (Advances in polymeric biomaterials)
Includes bibliographical references and index.
ISBN 978-1-4200-7694-3 (hardback)
1. Polymers in medicine. 2. Genitourinary organs--Diseases--Treatment--Equipment and supplies--Materials. 3. Cardiovascular system--Diseases--Treatment--Equipment and supplies--Materials. I. Shalaby, Shalaby W. II. Burg, Karen J. L. III. Shalaby, Waleed.

R857.P6P6226 2012
547'.7--dc23 2012005185

Visit the Taylor & Francis Web site at
http://www.taylorandfrancis.com

and the CRC Press Web site at
http://www.crcpress.com

Dedication

This book was inspired by Dr. Shalaby W. Shalaby, President and Director of Research and Development at Poly-Med Incorporated and Adjunct Professor of Bioengineering at Clemson University and is dedicated to his memory. His unending passion for knowledge is reflected in the chapters of this volume and in this monograph series. His innovative spirit continues at a resounding level through his many collaborators and mentees.

Contents

Contents

Preface

This monograph is the third volume in the series addressing advances in polymeric biomaterials. The first volume was dedicated to the general areas of absorbable and biodegradable polymers and discussed the technological and clinical significance of this family of highly significant class of biomaterials. The second volume, like the first, was prepared in an evolutionary format, with the first chapter providing the significance and rationale for use of polymers in dental and orthopedic applications. The second volume integrated discussion of the technological advances with the clinical drivers for polymers of orthopedic and dental application. This, the third volume, focuses on polymeric materials for vascular and urogenital applications. This monograph not only attempts to integrate the clinical needs with current and future research responses but also provides a comprehensive overview to foster future innovation. The volume is divided into three major areas, each with supportive chapters. The first section identifies the clinical paradigms specific to vascular applications, while the second section focuses on issues specific to urogenital applications. The third section provides biomaterial innovations specific to both areas. The underlying theme of this third installment illustrates how two important and dissimilar areas in medicine can be interrelated by shared biomaterials, yet the clinical paradigm establishes the driving force for innovation.

Acknowledgments

The editors express their gratitude to Dr. Joanne E. Shalaby of Poly-Med Incorporated for her assistance and patience with the initial planning and launch of the book, and to Mrs. Victoria Artigliere of the Institute for Biological Interfaces of Engineering at Clemson University for her tireless patience and dedication in working with authors to compile and integrate the chapters.

We also express our gratitude to the many contributing authors for taking the time to thoughtfully compile the following chapters. We thank Allison Shatkin and Amy Blalock of CRC Press/Taylor & Francis for their gracious persistence in moving this writing project to a successful close.

About the Editors

Shalaby W. Shalaby (deceased) served as President and Director of Research and Development (R&D) at Poly-Med Incorporated, Anderson, South Carolina, from 1994 to 2010. After completing his undergraduate training in chemistry and botany as well as pharmacy in Egypt at Ain Shams University and Cairo University, he enrolled at the University of Massachusetts at Lowell to complete his graduate studies toward an MS degree in textiles, a PhD in chemistry, and a second PhD in polymer science. Following the completion of his graduate training, 2 years of teaching, and a postdoctoral assignment, Dr. Shalaby spent 4 years as a senior research chemist at Allied Signal, Polymer Research Group. Subsequently, he joined Ethicon/Johnson & Johnson to start an exploratory group on polymers for biomedical applications, with some focus on new absorbable and radiation-sterilizable polymers. Before joining Clemson University in the summer of 1990, Dr. Shalaby headed the Johnson & Johnson Polymer Technology Center. Dr. Shalaby's previous research activities pertained to the molecular design of polymeric systems, with a major focus on biomedical and pharmaceutical applications. At Clemson University, Dr. Shalaby's research activities addressed primarily the molecular and engineering design of bioabsorbable systems, high-performance composites, radiostabilization of polymers, and new aspects of radiation processing. He supervised or co-supervised 30 MS and PhD thesis projects. After joining United States Surgical Corporation in 1993 as a corporate research scientist/senior director, Dr. Shalaby directed his efforts toward the establishment of new R&D programs pertinent to surgical and allied products and assessment of new product opportunities through technology acquisition. In late 1994, Shalaby directed his industrial efforts, as President of Poly-Med, toward focused R&D of polymeric materials for biomedical and pharmaceutical applications. Since 1994, he was an adjunct or visiting professor at four universities. He is the inventor of record for over 100 patents and the author of 250 publications, including eight books.

Karen J. L. Burg earned a BS in chemical engineering with a minor in biochemical engineering from North Carolina State University in 1990, an MS in bioengineering from Clemson University in 1992, and a PhD in bioengineering with a minor in experimental statistics from Clemson University in 1996. She completed a tissue engineering postdoctoral research fellowship in 1998 at Carolinas Medical Center in Charlotte, North Carolina, and is currently Hunter Endowed Chair of Bioengineering and Director of the Institute for Biological Interfaces of Engineering at Clemson University. Karen served as the President of the Society for Biomaterials from 2011 to 2012 and was a member of the Tissue Engineering and Regenerative Medicine International

Society North American Council from 2009 to 2011. Honors to Dr. Burg include the 2001 National Science Foundation Faculty Early Career Award and 2001 Presidential Early Career Award for Scientists and Engineers; she is an American Council on Education Fellow and a Fellow of the American Institute for Medical and Biological Engineering. Among her research interests are the optimization of absorbable biomaterials processing for tissue engineering applications and the development of three-dimensional tissue-engineered benchtop systems for diagnostic and discovery applications.

Waleed S. W. Shalaby earned his BS in chemistry and a PhD in pharmaceutical sciences from Purdue University in 1988 and 1992, respectively. He later obtained an MD from the Medical University of South Carolina in 1996. After medical school, he went on to complete a residency in obstetrics/gynecology and then a fellowship in gynecologic oncology at the University of Pennsylvania Medical Center in 2003. His research interests are grounded in the novel development of biomaterials for surgical and pharmaceutical applications. Clinically, Dr. Shalaby has extensive experience performing radical abdominal and pelvic surgical procedures as well as minimally invasive laparoscopic and robotic-assisted surgeries for gynecologic malignancies, benign gynecology, and pelvic reconstruction.

Dr. Shalaby has been involved in clinical and translational research related to biomaterials for over 20 years. He is the coauthor of *Biodegradable Hydrogels for Drug Delivery*, (Technomic, 1993) has authored 15 book chapters and three review articles, holds two patents, and has coauthored over 60 scientific publications and extended abstracts. He assumed the position of Chief Science Officer of Poly-Med Incorporated, Anderson, South Carolina in 2011.

Contributors

Frank Alexis
Department of Bioengineering
and
Institute for Biological Interfaces of Engineering
Clemson University
Clemson, South Carolina

Ben H. Chew
Department of Urological Sciences
University of British Columbia
Vancouver, British Columbia, Canada

George Fercana
Biocompatibility and Tissue Regeneration Laboratories
Department of Bioengineering
Clemson University
Clemson, South Carolina
and
Laboratory for Regenerative Medicine
Patewood/CU Bioengineering Translational Research Center
Greenville Hospital System
Greenville, South Carolina

Georgios T. Hilas
Poly-Med Incorporated
Anderson, South Carolina

Yingying Huang
School of Materials Science and Engineering
Nanyang Technological University
Singapore

Kevin Keith
Department of Bioengineering
Clemson University
Clemson, South Carolina

David M. Kwartowitz
Department of Bioengineering
Clemson University
Clemson, South Carolina
and
Medical University of South Carolina
Department of Pediatrics
Charleston, South Carolina

Dirk Lange
Department of Urological Sciences
University of British Columbia
Vancouver, British Columbia, Canada

Elizabeth A. Lipke
Department of Chemical Engineering
Auburn University
Auburn, Alabama

Jiro Nagatomi
Department of Bioengineering
Clemson University
Clemson, South Carolina

Jason Olbrich
Poly-Med Incorporated
Anderson, South Carolina

Ryan F. Paterson
Department of Urological Sciences
University of British Columbia
Vancouver, British Columbia, Canada

Shawn J. Peniston
Poly-Med Incorporated
Anderson, South Carolina

Yitzhak Rosen
Superior NanoBioSystems LLC
Washington, District of Columbia

Waleed S. W. Shalaby
Poly-Med Incorporated
Anderson, South Carolina

Dan Simionescu
Department of Bioengineering
Clemson University
Clemson, South Carolina
and
Patewood/CU Bioengineering Translational Research Center
Greenville Hospital System
Greenville, South Carolina
and
Department of Anatomy
University of Medicine and Pharmacy
Tirgu Mures, Romania

Srikanth Sivaraman
Department of Bioengineering
Clemson University
Clemson, South Carolina

Terry W. J. Steele
School of Materials Science and Engineering
Nanyang Technological University
Singapore

Lakeshia J. Taite
School of Chemical & Biomolecular Engineering
Georgia Institute of Technology
Atlanta, Georgia

M. Scott Taylor
Poly-Med Incorporated
Anderson, South Carolina

G. Lawrence Thatcher
TESco Associates Incorporated
Tyngsborough, Massachusetts

Subbu Venkatraman
School of Materials Science and Engineering
Nanyang Technological University
Singapore

Jennifer L. West
Department of Bioengineering
Rice University
Houston, Texas

1

Introductory Notes

The traditional mode of thought is to design a biomedical solution to a particular application, thus inspiring "silos" of thought and rationale that are specific to a particular device. Innovation, however, occurs at the boundaries of disciplines (Burg, *Biomaterials Forum*, 29(1):2; 2007); hence, one can think of a polymeric material as the platform that connects different applications. That is, the very same polymeric material can be tailored to suit a particular application, as inspired by the clinical application. The polymers can be the same but can be combined or modified to obtain an array of different properties that meet the clinical needs for successful application. Despite the apparent silos between vascular and urogenital applications of biomaterials, their connectivity is the polymeric platforms that possess shared criteria for success. Controversy and U.S. Food and Drug Administration scrutiny surrounding polypropylene transvaginal mesh and slings highlights the continued disconnect between the technical limitations of nonabsorbable polymeric implants and the clinical understanding of the limitations. Media attention to this issue (*Boston Globe*, July 14, 2011) also highlights the need to provide enhanced opportunities for clinician-scientist interactions and for public dissemination of scientific and clinical information.

Over time, it has become increasingly apparent that the successful incorporation of novel biomaterials in clinical medicine may require a fundamental breakdown of the pervasive silos to more fundamental constituents. While the definitions of biomaterials and biocompatibility have evolved and expanded, there continues to be a disproportionate number of "novel biomaterials" without demonstrable clinical functionality. The evolving concept and definition of translational medical research were theoretically designed to bridge perceived silos. Unfortunately, even successful innovations in this arena can be superseded by practicality and cost and limited to small, select patient populations. Therefore the first step in breaking down pervasive silos is to begin with identifying a surmountable, yet important clinical shortcoming in patient care. The next step is assembling a multidisciplinary team to address the following:

- The relevant clinical venue by which the need arises
- The historical and current predicate in terms of materials or relevant surgical procedures

- The specific biomaterial innovation and possibly medical/surgical approach that could be disruptive, yet beneficial to both the patient and the clinician
- The cost effectiveness and relative adoptability in clinical medicine
- The overall feasibility, timeline requirements, and necessary resources

While this "blueprint" is regularly a topic of discussion, it is the silos described that limit practical biomaterial innovation and often lead to unforeseen expense and time required for "re-engineering." There is no question that vascular and urogenital medicine (urology and gynecology) are vastly different fields. However, they both share clinical needs that can be addressed by innovative biomaterials. Interestingly, the successful incorporation of novel biomaterials in either venue begins with defining a surmountable patient-centered need. The technology developed thereafter (e.g., those discussed in this monograph) could lead to a "suite" of technologies that may be effectively adopted for future vascular and urogenital applications.

The chapters in this monograph cover three areas: polymers for vascular applications, polymers for urogenital applications, and polymers for devices of common use. The final chapter highlights contemporary enabling technologies for improved applications. Common and specific functional requirements for vascular and urogenital applications are highlighted throughout. A thorough analysis is presented of polymers for specific vascular applications, including those associated with vascular grafts, endovascular stents, device components for angioplasty and vascular assist devices, hemostatic systems, and tissue engineering of blood vessels. One chapter is dedicated to local and systemic administration of cardiovascular drugs using polymeric drug delivery technologies. In particular, a description is given of preclinical and clinical results of epicardial drug delivery systems, drug-eluting metallic stents, drug-eluting biodegradable stents, drug-eluting balloons, and nanoparticle drug delivery systems. A discussion of the advantages and disadvantages of these technologies is included to guide the engineering of delivery systems. Tissue engineering of vascular grafts using naturally derived polymers is discussed, with particular respect to small-diameter application, and is contrasted against the full range of polymeric materials used in vascular grafts. Absorbable endovascular grafts are overviewed; complementary to these topics is the subject of nitric oxide delivery from a variety of polymeric devices, including stent coatings, perivascular delivery depots, or coatings applied to the luminal surface of the damaged vessel wall.

In the second part of the book, attention is given to specific urogenital applications, including those pertaining to urethral/ureteral stents, organ repair and mechanical support devices, controlled-release systems for bioactive agents, and polymer-based tissue engineering of the bladder. Clinical uses and applications of ureteral stents and their limitations are discussed. Current examples of intravaginal drug delivery are also reviewed, with particular intent to highlight areas for future investigation.

The final chapters in the book highlight polymers for devices of common use in vascular and urogenital applications, such as components of dialysis systems, sutures, tissue adhesives, blocking agents, sealants, and catheters. Vascular and urogenital sealants and blocks share a common goal of preventing the leakage of bodily fluids from the vasculature and urogenital conduits to the abdominal space, so it is interesting to consider the similarities and differences in design for both applications. Simulation and validation are examples of contemporary enabling technology for improving the applications of vascular and urogenital devices, allowing the clinician the opportunity to experience the clinical issues prior to handling a device in an operating room setting. The success of this technology relies on efficient selection of polymeric materials and development of new processing methods. All chapters emphasize that a multidisciplinary approach yields the most innovative, efficient, yet practical results.

2

Drug Delivery Systems for Vascular Disease Therapy

Subbu Venkatraman, Kevin Keith, Yitzhak Rosen, Yingying Huang, Terry W. J. Steele, and Frank Alexis

CONTENTS

Introduction

Drug delivery systems have been shown to have an impact on the treatment of cardiovascular diseases (CVDs), and this early success resulted in numerous technologies. Drug delivery systems offer the ability to maximize the therapeutic index of a drug, increase the tissue concentration of the drug, release the drug in a controlled manner for optimal dosing, and reduce side effects. This chapter describes local and systemic administration of cardiovascular drugs using polymeric drug delivery technologies. In particular, we describe preclinical and clinical results of epicardial drug delivery systems, drug-eluting metallic stents, drug-eluting biodegradable stents, drug-eluting balloons (DEBs), and nanoparticle drug delivery systems. A discussion of the advantages and disadvantages of these technologies is included to provide a guide for the engineering of delivery systems.

CVDs can result in numerous forms of life-threatening events, such as coronary obstructions, spasms, rhythm disturbances, infections, acquired valve deformities, congenital malformations, and more, with atherosclerosis and stroke remaining the leading cause of death in the United States. When evaluating the success rate of cardiovascular procedures, the type of vascular lesion needs to be kept in mind. Table 2.1 provides one of the most widely used classifications of lesion types accepted by the American Heart Association along with the treatment success rates for each type.

Although CVD death rates have declined, there remains a severe medical problem to address (Roger et al. 2011). According to a report by the American Heart Association in 2011, each year an estimated 785,000 Americans will have a new coronary attack, and more than 50% will have a recurrent attack. In addition, it has been estimated that 195,000 patients will suffer from silent first myocardial infarctions each year. It has been approximated that every 25 seconds, an American will have a coronary event, and every minute, someone will die of one (Roger et al. 2011). Despite considerable clinical developments of new drugs from Atherogenics/AstraZeneca, Merck & Company,

TABLE 2.1

Lesion Types and Treatment Success Rates

Type A	Type B	Type C
Discrete: Less than 10 mm long	Tubular: 10–20 mm long	Diffuse: More than 20 mm long
Little calcification	Moderate calcification	Significant calcification
No thrombus	Some thrombus formation	Some thrombus formation
85% success rate, low risk (1987)	60–85% success rate, moderate risk (1987)	<60% success rate, high risk (1987)
97% success rate (1997)	95% success rate (1997)	84% success rate (1997)

Note: 1987 rates from angioplasty procedures only; 1997 rates from a combination of stenting/angioplasty; success rates do not take restenosis rates into account.

Sanofi-Aventis, GlaxoSmithKline, Millennium Pharmaceuticals, and others, little therapeutic or prevention advancement has occurred since the Food and Drug Administration (FDA) approved statin drugs.

Generally, cardiovascular drugs are administered orally, which results in low bioavailability and low drug concentration in the diseased tissue due to (a) poor adsorption by the intestine; (b) rapid degradation in the gut and in the blood; (c) rapid excretion time; (d) distribution into the entire body; (e) poor solubility; and (f) side effects. The drug discovery and development industry related to CVDs was seriously damaged in 2006 after Pfizer's $800 million investment failure with torcetrapib, and it was speculated that it will take a decade or more to recover and stimulate more research to develop successful new drugs (Opar 2007). Pfizer's torcetrapib clinical trial phase III, enrolling 15,000 patients, was terminated after 82 patients treated with the drug died compared to 51 patients in the control group. This race to bring to the market new drugs is mostly motivated by the patent expiration of atorvastatin in 2011 and the production of generics ("Learning Lessons" 2011). Therefore the need for long-term clinical trials with a large number of patients and the difficulties of demonstrating a better prognosis than current treatments is making the discovery of new cardiovascular drugs much less profitable (Karlberg 2008). Despite this failure and difficulties, Merck and Roche continued the development of their leading cardiovascular drugs, but it is estimated that the delay will be about 5 years due to strategy changes.

While there is much optimism for these drugs to be efficient and safe, it is not guaranteed that any will become a leading drug in the market; due to the delay of development, it is expected that the pharmaceutical companies will still need to invest in innovation and expand their programs to look at other diseases (Plump 2010). One way to expand the life of the drugs is to manufacture formulations with drug combinations to improve patient compliance when taking multiple drugs. Another approach could be to develop drug delivery systems to increase the life of new drugs or rescue old drugs that have failed. There are numerous drug delivery systems on the market for CVDs, and the clinical benefits are as follows:

1. Decreased side effects because the drug is released over a prolonged period of time in a therapeutic window lower than the toxic concentration.
2. Increased patient compliance because it reduces a drug's schedule.
3. Increased efficacy because the drug concentration reaches a therapeutic level in the diseased tissue.

More important, most drug delivery systems are not suitable for the production of generics due to their high cost and complicated compositions. Numerous startup companies are developing drug delivery technologies for CVDs, and it is expected that pharmaceutical companies will acquire the most successful ones or initiate specific drug delivery programs. For example, Johnson & Johnson and Abbott are the leading pharmaceutical companies developing drug delivery systems for CVDs. Also, Merck is developing a prolonged-release system for niacin approved by the FDA to decrease its side effects. The major advantage of niacin is its low cost compared to any blockbuster drug. Niacin is currently part of about 28 clinical trials in the United States (http://www.clinicaltrials.gov).

Because there are already multiple drug delivery systems for CVDs approved by the FDA and numerous new technologies in preclinical or clinical stages, this chapter describes both the localized and systemic approaches to deliver drugs to treat CVDs with the focus on technologies and clinical benefits.

Drug Delivery Systems for Localized Administration

Epicardial Drug Delivery

The logic of implementing epicardial drug delivery for preventing postoperative atrial fibrillation is to minimize vulnerability to atrial tachyarrhythmias by minimizing ventricular and plasma drug concentrations. This may allow the expansion of the current patient population, which is limited only to high-risk patients, for prophylactic amiodarone therapy. Bolderman and coworkers used the right atrial epicardia of goats fitted with electrodes and a bilayered patch (poly[ethylene glycol]-based matrix and poly[lactide-*co*-caprolactone] backing layer loaded with amiodarone to test the feasibility of such delivery. Delivery was local to the tissue using this patch with amiodarone, which was sutured to the right atrial lateral wall; electrophysiological measurements were made to assess the activity of this delivery. The patches contained 9.9 ± 0.4 mg of amiodarone. The results showed a persistently higher drug concentration in the right atrium than in the left atrium, ventricles, and extracardiac tissues by two to four orders of magnitude. Furthermore, the following were demonstrated: (a) atrial effective refractory period; (b) conduction time increased; and (c) rapid atrial response inducibility decreased significantly during the 1-month follow-up when compared to animals treated with drug-free patches. Finally, a key objective of having amiodarone concentrations in plasma undetectably low (<10 ng/mL) was achieved (Bolderman et al. 2010).

Preventing Cardiac Adhesions Using Local Delivery

Preventing cardiac adhesions, particularly when repeated sternotomy takes place, is an important clinical objective as serious complications may occur

(Chorny et al. 2006). In general, adhesions have been considered part of the inflammatory process that involves mast cells and the enzyme chymase (Yao et al. 2000; Liebman et al. 1993). Soga and coworkers demonstrated that the use of a chymase inhibitor can suppress cardiac chymase activity and the level of transforming growth factor b1 and can result in a reduction in postoperative cardiac adhesions in a hamster model (Soga et al. 2004). A dexamethasone-loaded biodegradable poly(lactide)-poly(ethyleneglycol) copolymer film for site-specific drug delivery was tested in a rabbit model with postoperative cardiac adhesions. A biphasic dexamethasone release in the serum with 69% drug released after 72 hours was used, with the drug-releasing surface facing the epicardium. The matrices were implanted in rabbits between the epicardium and the sternum following a variety of procedures, which included sternotomy, pericardiectomy, and epicardium abrasion. The adhesion formation was significantly reduced, with a preservation of anatomy shown using this matrix when examined 21 days after the procedure (Chorny et al. 2006).

Clinical Studies of Paclitaxel and Sirolimus-Eluting Metallic Stents

The earliest drug-eluting stents (DESs) to obtain FDA approval were Cypher® and TAXUS®; hence they have the longest clinical follow-ups. In the first "real-world" testing of sirolimus-eluting stents (SESs) by the Rotterdam group, 508 patients with various lesion types were stented with SESs and 450 patients with a bare metal stent (BMS) (Lemos et al. 2004). This study had target lesion revascularization (TLR) as one of the end points; typically, this procedure is carried out when the diameter of stenosis is greater than 70%. TLR rates were significantly lower in the SES group (9.8%) compared to the BMS group (14.8%).

Similar differentials have been reported for paclitaxel-eluting stents (PESs) versus BMSs in the real world; e.g., a second-generation DES based on a different stent design, the TAXUS LIBERTE®, appears to show improved outcomes. For example, in a 1-year study comparing TAXUS LIBERTE 2.25 mm in small vessels and in long lesions (38 mm), it was found that the thinner strut LIBERTE stent design reduced the rate of both 9-month angiographic restenosis (18.5% vs. 32.7%) and 12-month TLR (6.1% vs. 16.9%) in small vessels while lowering 12-month myocardial infarction rates for those with long lesions. Longer-term studies (>12 months) have consistently confirmed the reduction in TLR rates for SES and PES in comparison to BMS, as discussed in a thorough review (Garg et al. 2010). There are currently four drug-eluting metallic stent brands available, which differ by design, drug, coating, drug loading drug release kinetics, and composition. Table 2.2 shows all the

TABLE 2.2

Features of Metallic Stent Products

Stent Brand	Construction	Features
CYPHER®; SES	BxVelocity SS stent; 12.6-μm[a] biostable coating; 3 layers	80% sirolimus elutes in 30 days, completely elutes over 90 days
TAXUS®; PES	Express 316 SS stent; 16-μm[a] biostable coating	Most of the paclitaxel eluted over 90 days
Endeavor®; ZES	Driver Co-Cr stent (91 μm) with 4.6-μm[a] "biocompatible" coating	Elutes zotarolimus over 21 days
Xience®; EES	ML vision Co-Cr[b] stent (81 μm) with 7.6-μm[a] biostable coating	Elutes everolimus (80% release over 30 days)

[a] Polymer coating thickness.

[b] Cobalt-chrome alloy stents are stronger and more radiopaque than 316L stainless steel (SS), so thinner struts are possible compared to 100- to 140-mm 316L SS stents. Thinner struts may reduce the degree of restenosis as well.

approved stents in this category; drugs include sirolimus and limus derivatives as well as paclitaxel.

Of all revascularization procedures, 90% in 2005 involved DES deployment; yet in 2010, DES deployment in the same revascularization procedures had dropped to 75% or less. In the same period, new and improved DESs were introduced and approved by the FDA (see Table 2.1), yet the overall share of revascularization procedures still decreased for *all* DESs. What caused this drop in DES use?

The drop in DES usage must be traced to a drop in cardiologists' confidence and increased caution following reports of late-stage thrombosis in DES-stented patients. The first report (McFadden et al. 2004) involved four patients, two with Cypher and the other two with TAXUS stents, who were reported to have angiographic thrombosis in the stented segments. Three of the four patients had antiplatelet therapy stopped prior to another surgery and shortly thereafter suffered occlusion of the stented segment in the DES. They were all treated with percutaneous intervention and recovered. The inference is that incomplete endothelialization was responsible for the occlusion after stoppage of antiplatelet therapy. This inference was reinforced in the fourth patient, who also had two vessels with BMSs that did not occlude. This late-stage thrombus formation has been definitively attributed to incomplete endothelial cell coverage of stent struts, using pig studies of SESs (total area of uncovered struts ~ 3 μm^2) and PESs (total area of uncovered struts ~ 3.5 μm^2) versus BMSs (total area of uncovered struts ~ 0.12 mm^2) (Joner, Nakazawa et al. 2008).

Clinical trials have demonstrated the influence of the coating on the rate of endothelialization. Using the newly available optical coherence tomography (OCT) technique, as adapted for vessel visualization, Guagliumi and coworkers (2010a) found a newer DES (zotarolimus-eluting stent [ZES] based on Co-Cr [91-μm strut] with a 4.6-μm coating of phosphotadylcholine) had virtually no exposed strut area at 6 months and was comparable to a similar BMS (Co-Cr, Driver® stent). This is a significant finding, perhaps indicating the importance of a biocompatible coating. In another study (Guagliumi et al. 2010b), however, the same group also found that the latest version (termed JACTAX) of TAXUS LIBERTE, which incorporated paclitaxel in "biodegradable microdots" deposited entirely on the abluminal surface, did not show any statistical improvement over the older coated LIBERTE. The JACTAX low dose showed about 4.6% of uncovered strut area, while the TAXUS LIBERTE coated stent showed about 5.4%.

These two studies raised some important questions: Does strut thickness make a difference? Or, are the differences due mainly to the coating itself? The LIBERTE is made of stainless steel and has struts that are approximately 132 μm thick. The Endeavor stent is made of Co-Cr with a strut thickness of approximately 91 μm. The coating thicknesses are 16 μm and 4.6 μm, respectively, for the LIBERTE and Endeavor stents. One might also be tempted to attribute the differences between PESs and ZESs to duration of exhaustion of the drug, which is 90 days and 21 days, respectively. However, the ESA is also higher for the bare LIBERTE stent compared to the bare Driver stent. Clearly, more OCT studies need to be carried out to answer these important questions.

Nevertheless, thinner struts and faster exhaustion of the drug may be important factors that influence the rate of endothelialization of the DES. Delayed endothelialization has two important consequences: late-stage thrombosis and longer use of dual antiplatelet therapy (DAPT) for all DESs, regardless of drug type. The FDA has mandated a minimum of 12-month DAPT for all DES-stented patients, with some data supporting a correlation of cessation of DAPT to stent thrombosis (Slottow and Waksman, 2006). This has cost and clinical implications for the patient (Venkataraman and Boey, 2007).

To address this delayed endothelialization issue with all DESs, researchers have proposed to pursue two novel concepts to eliminate the permanent presence of metal in the vessel: fully degradable stents eluting antiproliferatives, and DEBs.

Preclinical and Clinical Studies of Fully Degradable Stents

The concept of fully degradable stents is attractive for various reasons: (a) There is no permanent presence of "foreign" material in the blood vessel (or at least contacting blood); and (b) for at least 6–9 months, the stent offers protection against vessel recoil. Numerous fully biodegradable stents are currently undergoing preclinical and clinical trials, as summarized in Table 2.3, and are discussed next.

Following work by Duke University researchers (Stack et al. 1988), the Igaki-Tamai stent was tested successfully in humans in 2000 (Tamai et al. 2000). The degradable stent was prepared by knitting extruded monofilaments

TABLE 2.3
Features of Fully Degradable Stent Products

Fully Degradable Stents	Polymer Composition	Absorption Time	Advantages and Disadvantages
Igaki-Tamai stent	PLLA braided design	2 years	Human trials showed about 19% restenosis rates without drug; late lumen loss is significant.
IDEAL stent (Bioabsorbable Therapeutics Inc.)	Poly(anhydride ester) polymer	Stent decreased in strut thickness from 0.25 mm to 0.19 mm in 6 months, but with no change thereafter to 9 months (pig study)	The first-in-human trial of 11 patients did not show sufficient neointimal suppression.
REVA stent (REVA Medical)	Tyrosine-derived polycarbonate polymer	2 years	Tunable degradation rates; the tyrosine ring is also easily iodinated to yield inherently radiopaque polymers. Polymer embrittlement was noted as degradation proceeded, leading to a high TLR of 66.7% at the 4- to 6-month follow-up.
ReZolve stent (second-generation REVA stent)	Tyrosine-derived polycarbonate polymer	2 years	Braided design could overcome embrittlement.
Abbott Vascular's Xience bioabsorbable vascular stent	Poly(D-L-lactide) coating with everolimus on PLLA core laser-cut design	This stent lost 30% mass in 12 months and 60% in 18 months in porcine model; 35% of the stent struts had disappeared by month 24 in humans	At 2 years, the BVS stent showed no thrombosis and had only 19% stenosis. It is speculated that complete bioabsorption had indeed occurred at 2 years.

of poly(L-lactide) (PLLA). The knitted device contained no drug, yet the 6-month restenosis results were better than BMSs at 19% in a 1-year follow-up (Tsuji et al. 2001). These initially encouraging results with PLLA spurred considerable activity in fully biodegradable stents.

Other versions were developed with different designs and capabilities, including the controlled release of therapeutic drugs. The leader in this field is clearly Abbott Vascular's Xience® bioabsorbable vascular stent (BVS) made from PLLA with everolimus-encapsulated drug in a poly(D-L-lactide) coating. PLLA is extruded into a tube and then cut into the strut pattern using femtosecond lasers. The *in vivo* results (porcine model) showed that the stent lost 30% mass in 12 months and 60% in 18 months (Ormiston et al.

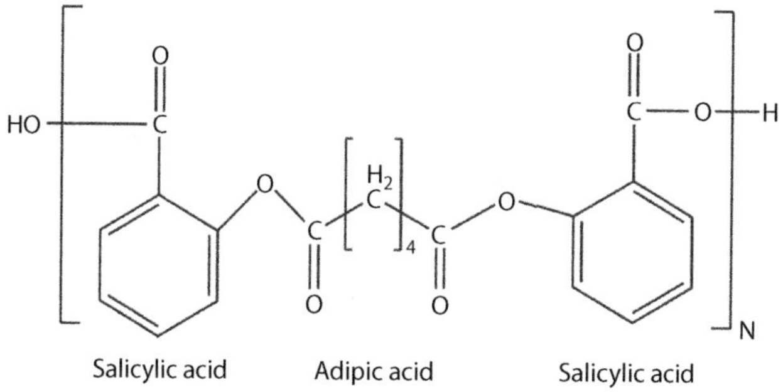

Salicylic acid Adipic acid Salicylic acid

FIGURE 2.1
Different polymer compositions were used in the IDEAL stent, which is based on a poly(anhydride ester) polymer.

2008). Using imaging techniques such as OCT, it was found that 35% of the stent struts had disappeared by month 24 in humans; however, it is speculated that complete bioabsorption had indeed occurred at 2 years. The drug elutes 80% of its loading (98 μg in a 12-mm stent) in 28 days. At 2 years, in 29 patients the BVS stent showed no thrombosis and had only 19% stenosis (Serruys, Ormiston et al. 2009). Some scaffold shrinkage was observed at 6 months, and a newer version of BVS has been developed by changing the manufacturing process as well as the design; it is currently being evaluated in a 101-patient trial (Onuma et al. 2011).

Different polymer compositions were used in the IDEAL stent (Figure 2.1), which is based on a poly(anhydride ester) polymer. These polymers have been presented (Jabara et al. 2008, 2009) as degrading into acceptable by-products, similar to PLLA.

In a porcine implantation study, this stent decreased in strut thickness from 0.25 to 0.19 mm in 6 months. No changes were observed for 6 to 9 months; no local reactions were observed during this period (Matsumoto et al. 2010). Despite encouraging results from coated metallic stents (using the salicylate polymer coating and sirolimus), the first-in-human trial of 11 patients failed to show sufficient neointimal suppression.

Another fully degradable stent, the REVA stent, made use of a proprietary slide-and-lock mechanism; this necessitated the use of a fairly rigid polymer (Figure 2.2), developed by Joachim Kohn's group at Rutgers. It is a novel tyrosine-derived polycarbonate with tunable degradation rates (through change of the R group) and glass transition temperatures. The tyrosine ring is also easily iodinated to yield inherently radiopaque polymers for imaging.

Nevertheless, the earlier design (slide and lock) for the REVA stent seems to have been abandoned because of unfavorable results in the first-in-human study conducted in 2007. Polymer embrittlement was noted as degradation proceeded, leading to a high TLR of 66.7% at the 4- to 6-month follow-up (Onuma et al. 2011). To overcome a high TLR at 6-month follow-up, a better design named ReZolve was developed, and the construct appears similar to a

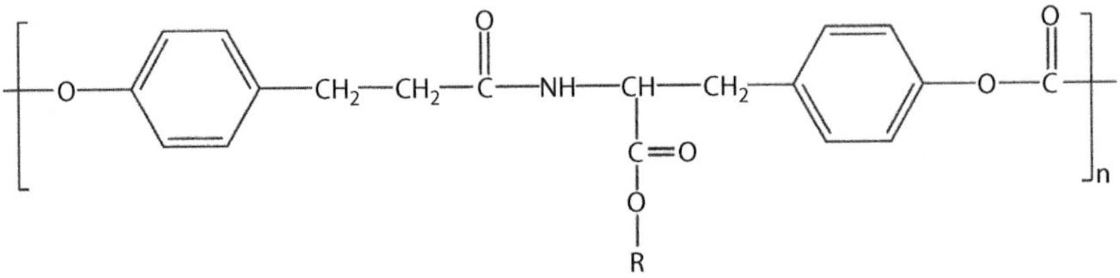

FIGURE 2.2
The REVA stent is another fully degradable stent, and it has made use of a proprietary slide-and-lock mechanism; this necessitated the use of a fairly rigid polymer developed by Joachim Kohn's group at Rutgers University.

spiral knitted design, resembling the earlier Igaki-Tamai stent (2011). ReZolve is currently in preclinical testing; a drug-eluting version using a limus derivative is also in early-stage testing. Other companies developing bioabsorbable stents include Arterial Remodeling Technologies (http://www.art-stent.com), which is developing a bioabsorbable stent based on a copolymer of L- and D-lactides, and Amaranth Medical (http://www.amaranthmedical.com/), which is basing its stents on PLLA with a high molar mass.

The future of DESs may rest with the possible success of biodegradable scaffolds, which have yet to reach the clinic. Although the most promising degradable prototypes to replace BMSs in humans with restenosis have been based on PLLA and human trials, there is still much more clinical data to be acquired, especially with respect to when dual antiplatelet therapy can be stopped. This might well be the deciding factor for preferring bioabsorbable stents to BMSs. In addition, the regulatory hurdles are considerably higher than for biostable stents due to contact with blood; not only must inflammatory reactions be manageable during bioabsorption, but also evidence of complete absorption may need to be provided. With fully polymeric stents, stent relaxation or creep is a major issue that needs to be minimized; in addition, postdeployment shrinkage is possible, particularly for a semicrystalline scaffold polymer. Peripheral stents are subject to considerable tension, compression, and bending deformations. Moreover, these stresses tend to be repetitive; hence fatigue strength is the most important criterion for stent survival in the long term. In spite of years of use, metallic stents continue to have fractures, particularly when employed in the superficial femoral artery (SFA). To date, most peripheral stents are metallic, with nitinol stents dominating over stainless steel (SS) because of the perceived higher elasticity of nitinol. Nevertheless, no studies to date have shown conclusively that nitinol stents suffer fewer fractures compared to SS stents.

In this context, introduction of a fully polymeric stent is also problematic, and such stents are not expected to be superior to metallic ones in terms of fatigue resistance. Of course, the failure modes may be altered, but long-term stent survival will likely not be improved. Therefore new technologies such as DEBs may ultimately offer the best option for peripheral vascular disease.

Drug-Eluting Balloon

This section focuses on several emerging technologies related to DEB drug delivery. The DEB is an emerging technology for interventional cardiologists that has been gaining attention. While long-term data are limited concerning the efficacy of DEBs, it has been suggested that the use of DEBs especially for the treatment of diffuse in-stent restenosis (ISR) can prevent the implantation of future stents. In fact, it has been suggested that the most appealing indication for paclitaxel-eluting balloons would be before the treatment of in-stent restenosis (Waksman and Pakala 2009).

Background

Treatment of coronary vessel stenosis underwent a radical change with balloon angioplasty in the 1970s. The first coronary angioplasty procedure was performed in 1977 by Dr. Andreas Gruntzig in Switzerland. This procedure was successful in treating a few lesion types, but did suffer from vessel collapse following the procedure in a sizable percentage of the cases; it was also not useful for calcified lesions. The latest exciting entry in the interventional market is the DEB, which promises to compete with both the BMS and the DES for certain lesion types in the coronary vasculature and likely surpasses stent use in the peripheral vasculature.

It has been indicated that the FDA perspective on DEB, presented at Cardiovascular Research Technologies 2006 in Washington, D.C., considers the DEB to be a hybrid product of balloon and drug. The DEB is considered a class III device that will be regulated by the Center for Devices and Radiological Health (CDRH) along with the Center for Drug Evaluation and Research (CDER). Drug dose, drug release profiles, absorption into various tissues, balloon coating and polymers, balloon sizes, and clinical indications are among the necessary characterization issues (Waksman and Pakala 2009).

The DEB can have a variety of components, including strands and lumen. For example, the balloon, which is subject to high pressures during inflation, can be enhanced by reinforcing strands between the inside surface of the balloon and the outside of the elongating member. Various materials may be used to construct the DEB strands; for example, polymer blends, metal alloy, or laminar or composite construction may all be used for the strands. In particular, some of the materials that can be used to construct balloons and elongated members include polytetrafluoroethylenes, polyethylenes, polypropylenes, polyurethanes, nylons, and polyesters, which include polyalkylene terephthalate polymers and copolymers (Holman et al. 2009).

The DEB has a lumen between the inner surface of the balloon and the outer surface of the elongated member when the balloon is not collapsed.

Flexible hollow members can be disposed in the lumen. These members have an external surface and internal cavity, which can contain the therapeutic agent. In addition, a channel can connect the outer surface of the balloon to the internal cavity to administer the drug. There is a variety of therapeutic candidates that can be used for treatment of restenosis: sirolimus, tacrolimus, everolimus, cyclosporine, steroids such as dexamethasone, paclitaxel, actinomycin, geldanamycin, cilostazole, methotrexate, vincristine, mitomycin, and others (Holman et al. 2009).

DEB Technologies

Several companies have developed DEBs; the drug of choice is paclitaxel since its tissue residence time (and hence duration of action) is longer than sirolimus. The main challenge in DEBs is to transfer a predictable dose of paclitaxel as uniformly as possible from the balloon to the lesion surface. The coating techniques employed should ensure that the drug is retained on the balloon while deployed percutaneously but is quickly transferred when the balloon is expanded. These challenges have been met to varying degrees with different technologies. Although sometimes confusing due to frequent licensing and sublicensing agreements, it is possible to differentiate the technologies, as discussed next.

Bayer Schering Pharma owns the trademark and the patent rights to Paccocath® technology. It has licensed this technology to a Bayer subsidiary, MEDRAD, for use on its Cotavance DEBs for peripheral artery treatment; the same technology is also used by B. Braun in its Sequent® Please DEB line (coronary) and by Invatec for its In.Pact platform (now named In.Pact Amphirion after acquisition by Medtronic). The first-generation Paccocath technology basically involved cocrystallizing paclitaxel with a component of contrast medium, iopromide 370 (trade name Ultravist). Apparently dissolving the paclitaxel in iopromide 370 allows for better transfer of paclitaxel from a coating of the two components. This is attributed to a finite solubility of paclitaxel in the contrast medium (Scheller et al. 2003) and the ability of the iopromide 370 to "adhere" to the blood vessel wall, at least for a few seconds, to facilitate the "transfer" of paclitaxel from the coating. The second-generation Paccocath improved on the first by replacing the iopromide with urea, which is a more hydrophilic small molecule. Urea presumably allows even faster transfer of the paclitaxel by adhering to the vessel wall in a more homogeneous method. This second-generation version is now being evaluated in the coronary and peripheral (above and below the knee) vasculature, with many lesion types, including bifurcations.

Another DEB technology developed by Eurocor in Germany is based on a microporous balloon surface that may be "coated" with paclitaxel. The DEB is called DIOR®. A schematic depiction of its mode of operation is shown in Figure 2.3. This design necessitates a thrice-folded balloon to protect the

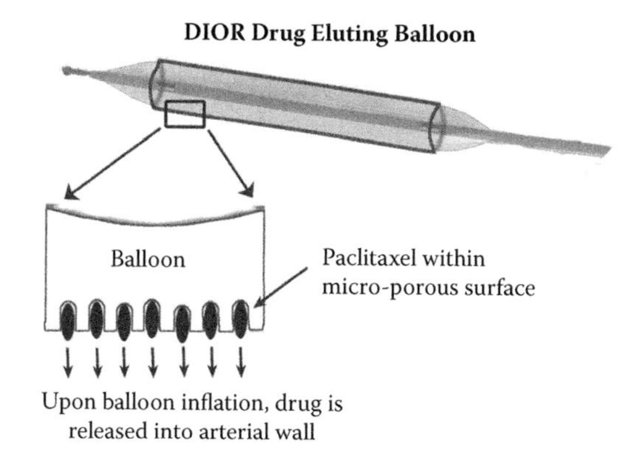

FIGURE 2.3
Shown here is a schematic depiction of DEB technology developed by Eurocor in Germany; the technology is based on a microporous balloon surface that may be "coated" with paclitaxel. The DEB is called DIOR®.

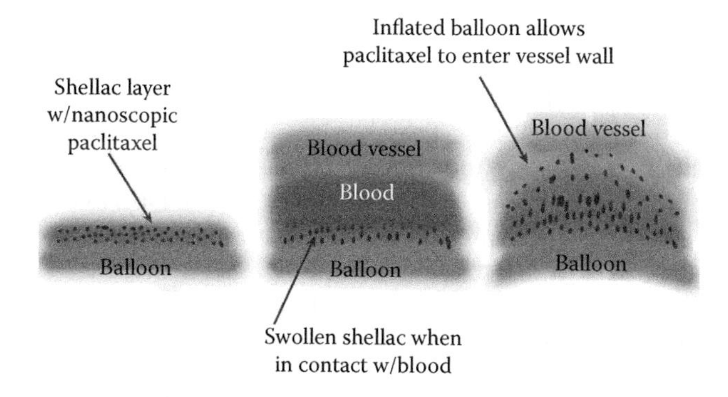

FIGURE 2.4
This resin is shellac (shelloic and alleuritic acids) and is mixed in a 1:1 ratio with paclitaxel and coated on a standard balloon catheter.

trapped drug from being washed away during deployment (De Labriolle et al. 2009). The drug transfer is "controlled" by the time of inflation: 20 seconds for partial transfer, 60 seconds for full transfer. The second-generation DIOR product uses a natural resin to encapsulate paclitaxel and transfer it to the blood vessel wall (Figure 2.4). This resin is shellac (shelloic and alleuritic acids) and is mixed in a 1:1 ratio with paclitaxel and coated on a standard balloon catheter. Schematically, the DEB works as shown in Figure 2.4 (DIOR 2011).

The shellac simply protects the paclitaxel during deployment, swells on inflation or just before inflation, and releases the paclitaxel into the tissue. A combination of Eurocor's cobalt-chromium stent (Genius MAGIC® stent) and the DIOR DEB has been approved for use in India under the name MAGICAL System.

Clinical Considerations and Rationale

The limitations of DESs have provided the impetus for the rationale of developing DEBs. DEBs may be implemented where DESs may not be delivered or underperform in a variety of locations, including tortuous vessels, small vessels, or long diffuse calcified lesions or where the scaffolding may cause obstructions in areas, such as major branches or bifurcated areas. DESs in these locations may also result in stent fracture. In addition, since sustained drug release is not required for the antiproliferative effect of paclitaxel and its uptake by smooth muscle cells (SMCs) is rapid and can be retained for 1 week, local delivery such as that seen by a DEB can be a logical approach (Waksman and Pakala 2009). Axel and coworkers indicated that continuous paclitaxel exposure for 24 hours or even 20 minutes with 0.1 to 10.0 μmol/L caused complete and prolonged inhibition of human arterial SMC growth up to day 14 with a half-maximal inhibitory concentration (IC_{50}) of 2.0 nmol/L (Axel et al. 1997). The DEB has therefore been suggested for ISR (Waksman and Pakala 2009). Waksman and Pakala noted several important potential advantages for DEBs. These include homogeneous drug transfer to the entire vessel wall along with rapid release of high concentrations of the drug sustained in the vessel wall for about a week. The drug dose mentioned is usually 300 to 600 mg, with balloon surface homogeneous distribution. Such delivery has little impact on long-term healing. For example, it has been mentioned that the absence of polymer may decrease chronic inflammation and the trigger for late thrombosis. In addition, the use of a DEB avoids the problem associated with placing a stent in bifurcations or small vessels, thereby minimizing the appearance of abnormal flow patterns that could occur with a stent. Finally, an overdependence on antiplatelet therapy could be minimized with local drug delivery (Waksman and Pakala 2009).

Preclinical Studies

Several preclinical studies have been used to support the rationale for DEB technologies. These include the use of paclitaxel to prevent the proliferation of human smooth muscle cells in the vessels where the stent is located. For example, Mori and coworkers have shown paclitaxel is retained up to 6 days when cells are exposed to paclitaxel. In this study, the paclitaxel concentration was quantified in cervical cells pretreated with 10 ng/mL of paclitaxel and in the tissue of cervical cancer patients treated weekly with 60 mg/m^2. *In vitro* paclitaxel remained in the cell lines tested for 24 hours after its removal (Mori et al. 2006).

Scheller and coworkers showed with a porcine model that most of the drug was released after a 60-second balloon dilation, with 10–15% of the drug detected in the vessel wall 40–60 minutes later as well. This study demonstrated rapid transfer of the drug from the balloon to the targeted tissue and accumulated in the tissue for a substantial amount of time. The study by Scheller and colleagues also indicated that treatment of paclitaxel resulted in a dose-dependent reduction of up to 63% of the neointimal stent area without any effect on the re-endothelialization of the stent struts. The procedure was carried out using acetone as a solvent to deliver two different concentrations of paclitaxel: a low and a high dose, respectively 1.3 and 2.5 mg/mm^2. The low dose of paclitaxel coating led to a reduction of the neointimal area by 42% and the typical dose coating by 63%. The conventional uncoated balloons and three different types of paclitaxel-coated percutaneous transluminal coronary angioplasty balloons used in this study had contact with the vessel wall for 1 minute (Scheller et al. 2004).

Cremers and colleagues evaluated the influence of two critical parameters of DEBs, inflation time and increased dose due to overlapping balloons. In their study, 56 stainless steel stents were implanted in the left anterior descending and circumflex coronary arteries of 28 domestic pigs using a 1.2:1.0 overstretch ratio. The stents were mounted on conventional uncoated balloons and paclitaxel-coated angioplasty balloon catheters. A marked reduction of neointimal proliferation along with endothelialization of stent struts in all samples was observed. The treatments ranged from short (i.e., 10 seconds with one DEB) to long (60 seconds treatment with two DEBs). The dose used was 5 µg paclitaxel per square millimeter of balloon surface, and the results showed a lumen loss of 0.37 ± 0.28 mm for 10-second inflation time and a loss of 0.30 ± 0.19 mm for the segment treated by two coated balloons for 60 seconds each. Cremers and colleagues demonstrated that DEBs effectively reduced neointimal proliferation regardless of inflation time and dose within the tested range after 28-day follow-up. Finally, no adverse reactions were observed even though the dose was increased to more than three times the clinically tested dose (Cremers et al. 2009).

Nakamura and coworkers used a porcine model to evaluate endothelial function after dilation of BMSs with paclitaxel-coated balloons and non-drug-coated balloons. The authors indicated that impaired endothelial function associated with DESs could also occur with DEBs. The results demonstrated that postdilation of BMSs with paclitaxel-coated balloons was associated with impaired vasodilatory response to acetylcholine distal to the treated segments. This was in contrast to the vasodilatory response after postdilation with non-drug-coated balloons, which was similar to control arteries. Nakamura and coworkers indicated that while the mechanisms of endothelial functional impairment are unknown, inflammatory mechanisms and mediators could diffuse and therefore could play a role into distal vasculature (Nakamura et al. 2011; Gossl et al. 2003).

Clinical Studies

A current prospective single-blind randomized trial conducted by Habara investigated the efficacy of a paclitaxel-eluting balloon for the treatment of SES ISR, a common phenomenon of DESs. This trial was conducted in 50 patients with SES restenosis; the patients were randomly assigned to either a paclitaxel group ($n = 25$) or a conventional balloon angioplasty group ($n = 25$). The study showed an incidence of recurrent restenosis of 8.7% for the DEB group versus 62.5% for the conventional balloon angioplasty group, with $p = 0.0001$ after a 6-month follow-up. TLR was 4.3% for the DEB versus 41.7% for the conventional balloon angioplasty, with $p = 0.003$. The cumulative major adverse cardiac event-free survival demonstrated a significantly better result for the DEB group (96%) than in the balloon angioplasty group (60%), with $p = 0.005$. It has been concluded by Habara and colleagues that the DEB provided significantly better clinical angiographic results than conventional balloon angioplasty for patients with SES restenosis (Habara et al. 2011).

Scheller and coworkers enrolled 52 patients in the randomized, double-blind, multicenter Paclitaxel-Coated Balloon Catheter for In-Stent Restenosis trial Paccocath ISR I. The patients selected showed clinical evidence of a single restenotic lesion in a stented coronary artery. The primary end point of this study was angiographic late lumen loss in-segment, while the secondary end points included binary restenosis and major adverse cardiovascular events (MACEs). The patients of this study were randomly assigned to either paclitaxel-coated balloon (3 $\mu g/mm^2$) or uncoated catheter. At 6 months, the results of this study indicated that in-segment late lumen loss was significantly less in the coated balloon group, with $p = 0.002$. In addition, the study demonstrated a coated balloon group with 5% binary restenosis and 4% MACEs compared with 43% binary stenosis and 31% MACEs in the uncoated balloon group (Waksman and Pakala 2009; Scheller et al. 2006). In an extension of this first study by enrollment of an additional 56 patients (Scheller et al. 2008), it was found that at 2 years, 20 (of 108, or 37%) required TLR in the coated balloon group, while three (or 6%) required TLR in the paclitaxel eluting balloon (PEB) group. These results were path breaking and led to other technologies being developed for DEBs. Paclitaxel continued to be the drug of choice due to its lipid solubility, which translated to long tissue residence times following what is essentially a local bolus "injection."

In an interesting trial (Valentine Trial I), in which 250 patients were studied over an 8-month period, the DIOR DEB was employed to treat ISR following BMS or DES implantation. Following the second intervention using a DEB, TLR rates were 5.9% for BMSs and 9.8% for DESs. This was better than either brachytherapy or a second DES for treating ISR (10–20% TLR). Clearly, DEBs are emerging as the interventional tool of choice in treating ISR.

Conclusions

The progression of treatment modalities for vascular stenosis may be highlighted by five mini-revolutions. The first was the use of balloon angioplasty, which decreased the number of coronary artery bypass graft (CABG) surgeries. The second was the use of the BMS following balloon angioplasty, which reduced failure rates with balloon angioplasty; the third was the DES, which further reduced restenosis rates. The fourth mini-revolution was indeed the clinical use of fully degradable stents, which required the longest development times and faced the highest regulatory hurdles. Finally, the DEB could revolutionize treatment by encroaching on territory considered sacred to stenting. It has been suggested that a combination of DEB and BMS should become the standard, while DEB might become an important tool for peripheral artery treatment.

Drug Delivery Systems for Systemic Administration

Background

Recent advancements in the field of nanotechnology may lead to systemic delivery of drugs to treat CVDs (Zhang et al. 2008). Nanotechnology, in its most general terms, may be simply defined as the engineering of devices at the nano- (molecular) scale (Jayagopal et al. 2010). One major advantage of a nanoparticle drug delivery system is the ability to improve a drug's internalization into cells and extend the protection of the drug. Although nanocarrier drug delivery systems have been used in the clinic for more than 30 years, no generic nanoparticle drug delivery systems have ever been approved, and it is expected that generic companies will not be able to develop such complex systems in the near future due to the difficulties in demonstrating bioequivalence (Burgess et al. 2010).

The application of nanotechnology to the clinical management of disease, by either diagnostic or treatment modalities, has led to the subfield of nanomedicine. Nanomedicine is an emerging field that utilizes the properties of a wide range of nanocarriers (liposomes, carbon nanotubes, micelles, etc.) to cross biological barriers, thus increasing the efficacy of a drug's action (Venkataraman et al. 2010; Chan et al. 2010). Systemic delivery of drugs for CVD treatments can be exploited due to the basic molecular and physiological processes leading to the development of plaque and the endothelium defects, two components common to all major CVDs. Detection of dysfunctional endothelium along early lesions, for example, may permit timely therapy to reduce leukocyte infiltration within artery walls (Muro et al. 2004). Furthermore, as disease targets within the plaque are characterized, the design of customized treatment strategies for different disease stages could enable patient-specific clinical management.

Molecular Targets of Cardiovascular Diseases

The unique ability of various nanocarriers to be modified on the surface with targeting moieties that recognize specific cardiovascular markers makes them particularly advantageous as potential treatment options in CVDs. The identification of molecular markers in atherosclerotic plaque biology has allowed the development of not only site-specific targeting but also stage-specific targeting of nanocarriers in the atherosclerotic process. Typically, a plaque that is bound to rupture and cause a variety of acute coronary syndromes has certain features. The precursor lesion to such a plaque rupture has been postulated to be the thin-cap fibroatheroma. The precursor lesion has been characterized by a necrotic, macrophage-rich core with an overlying fibrous cap of less than 65 mm (Virmani et al. 2006; Blankstein and Ferencik 2010). Biorecognition moieties attached to the surfaces of nanoparticles, such as peptides, antibodies, or any other receptor ligands, allow for potential targeting to the intended site of treatment delivery. In some cases of CVDs, these targets would be at the site of plaque formation or more remote organs. In other cases, the targets could be in the blood circulation. Strategies for interfacing with key cellular and molecular participants throughout atherosclerotic plaque initiation and progression are needed to enable the development of tools and to facilitate early therapeutic interventions. Table 2.4 shows a list of important molecular targets found during the course of plaque development, which has been investigated in the process of targeting using nanoparticle drug delivery systems.

Early Stage of Atherosclerosis: Endothelial Cell Targets

Early atherosclerotic lesions feature inflammatory activation from the endothelial monolayer. Secretion of various inflammatory molecules, such as cell adhesion molecules (CAMs), promotes the permeation of leukocytes into the vasculature. The overexpression of such molecules at the lesion site offers an opportunity for targeting by therapeutic agents at a very early stage in plaque development. Selectins, CAMs that participate in early leukocyte-endothelial interactions during the inflammatory response of plaque development (Burger and Wagner 2003), have been an effective molecular target for certain nanoparticles. Selectins are stored intracellularly and then translocated to the cell surface as part of the early immune response. Consequently, most selectins (P-selectins) are not expressed in normal arterial endothelium, but become highly expressed in the beginning stages of an artherosclerotic vasculature region. In the early stages of atherosclerosis, 80-nm iron oxide (IO) nanoparticles with an attached P-selectin antibody effectively targeted cells activated *in vivo* (Valat et al. 2010). PLGA [poly(lactic-co-glycolic) acid] nanoparticles with an attached cyclic peptide ligand have also effectively targeted intracellular cell adhesion molecule 1 (ICAM-1) upregulated in human umbilical cord vascular endothelial cells (HUVECs) *in vitro* (Zhang et al. 2008b). The targeted PLGA nanoparticles of around 200 nm observed a significantly higher affinity (two to three times more) for HUVECs than the nontargeted nanoparticles, which were nearly 250 nm in diameter. CAMs expressed at elevated levels

TABLE 2.4

Common Molecular Targets of Drug Delivery Systems

Target	Description	Normal Expression	Atherosclerotic Expression
Endothelial cell	Antibody targeting of cell adhesion molecules, particularly selectins	P-selectin: found only intracellularly; not expressed on cell membrane	P-selectin: translocated to outer plasma membrane surface, making it visible
Macrophage	Presence of high-density lipoprotein (HDL) on surface of arterial macrophages, which become overexpressed in atherosclerosis	Macrophages: X	Macrophages: 4X–10X
Cell apoptosis	High affinity of plasma protein annexin A5 for phosphatidylserine, an intracellular compound that is released prior to apoptosis	Phosphatidylserine: not expressed	Phosphatidylserine: released just prior to apoptosis
Angiogenesis	Attachment of antibody to target a_vb_3 integrin, expressed in the beginning stages of angiogenesis	—	—
Thrombosis	Activated platelets, integrins, and exposed fibrin targeting by antibodies, peptides	Platelets: X	Platelets:10X–20X

Note: X designates the concentration of baseline biological activity (varies from individual to individual).

on the endothelium lining plaques not only play significant roles in leukocyte migration into the subendothelial space but also are endocytosed as part of surface protein recycling. This process has been exploited to internalize CAM-targeted nanocarriers bearing therapeutic agents into endothelial cells (Muro and Muzykantov 2005). These approaches may enable detection and treatment of endothelial dysfunction prior to extensive leukocyte infiltration.

All Stages of Atherosclerosis: Macrophage Targets

Throughout the process of atherosclerotic development, macrophage accumulation in the subendothelial space can be observed, and increased macrophage density is associated with lesion progression and rupture. Consequently, macrophage activity can be an effective potential clinical target for plaque at any stage of development.

One potential molecular target for macrophage upregulation is the presence of high-density lipoproteins (HDLs). HDLs are produced either by the liver and small intestine or on the surface of lipid-enriched macrophages to clear cholesterol from the subendothelial space of arterial walls and are thus of significant therapeutic interest (Toth 2010). Several nanocarrier systems loaded with therapeutic agents have been engineered to mimic the properties of HDLs and their functions *in vivo* (Zhang et al. 2010; Toth 2010). Potential applications of nanomedicine-based treatment systems relevant to the macrophage may include imaging of macrophage density for lesion progression or delivery of relevant therapies within the macrophage to reduce inflammation. It is expected that a large majority of the nanoparticles will accumulate in the liver, and the success of this approach will depend on the ability to deliver a therapeutic drug to the macrophages in the diseased tissue.

Late Stage of Atherosclerosis: Cell Apoptosis Targets

Apoptosis in the vasculature is generally detrimental to vascular integrity and often is a precursor to plaque rupture and subsequent thrombosis. As such, anti-apoptotic therapy may reduce the initiation, progression, or clinical consequences of atherosclerosis (Stoneman and Bennett 2004). As atherosclerosis progresses, lesions exhibit increasingly higher disseminated death due to continual cholesterol deposition and inflammation (Libby 2003). This pathological occurrence can be exploited for targeting of CVDs at stage-specific points. One of the most prominent characteristics of apoptosis is the externalization of phosphatidylserine (PS), a prominent plasma cell membrane phospholipid that is normally sequestered in the inner leaflet of the cell membrane but is translocated to the outer surface in apoptotic cells, primarily foam cells of atherosclerotic plaque (Laufer et al. 2008). Plasma protein annexin A5 has a strong affinity for PS and consequently is able to recognize apoptotic cells by specific molecular interaction with PS. Through the coupling of annexin A5 to various therapeutic agents, potential late-stage atherosclerotic treatment can become feasible.

Targeting of annexin A5 nanoparticles to apoptotic cells has been demonstrated to aid in computed tomographic (CT) and magnetic resonance imaging (MRI) of atherosclerotic lesions *in vivo* using mice models (Smith et al. 2007). Apoptosis of cells, such as macrophages and SMCs, within the plaque has often been associated with vulnerability of plaque rupture; thus nanomedicine-guided targeting of apoptotic regions may have important clinical applications.

Late Stage of Atherosclerosis: Angiogenesis Targets

In advanced CVDs, the aberrant growth of a neovasculature within lesions is believed to promote plaque instability subsequent to hemorrhage and further influx of macrophages within the subendothelial space. Several nanocarrier delivery systems can be loaded with anti-angiogenic drugs and coupled with targeting ligands for plaque-specific inhibition of blood vessel growth. Many approaches have exploited the presence of the a_vb_3 integrin, which is expressed during early angiogenesis but absent on healthy, intact endothelium (Caruthers et al. 2009).

In one such approach, perfluorocarbon nanoparticles bearing the angiostatic reagent fumagillin were coupled with an a_vb_3 integrin-targeted peptidomimetic antibody to target adventitial neovessels *in vivo* using hyperlipidemic rabbits (Winter et al. 2008). The treatment exhibited a sustained anti-angiogenic effect when combined with a concurrent statin therapy as the fumagillin nanoparticles reduced the neovascular signal by 50% to 75% at 1 week and maintained this effect for 3 weeks regardless of diet and drug dose. Perfluorocarbon nanoparticles are versatile candidates for multimodal imaging and therapy of atherosclerotic lesions because of their ability to conjugate ligands and encapsulate physicochemically diverse imaging agents and drugs.

Late Stage of Atherosclerosis: Thrombosis Targets

Rupture of an atherosclerotic plaque exposes collagen and several other plaque components to the bloodstream. This rupture initiates hemostasis in the blood vessel and leads to activation of procoagulant and prothrombotic stimuli, as well as the formation of a thrombus at the site of rupture. Components of thrombi, such as platelets and fibrin, are useful targets for nanoscale platforms for imaging and treatment because they can be elevated by as much as 20 times in injured vasculature in relation to uninjured vasculature (Gighliotti et al. 1998).

A common mechanism used to exploit the upregulation of fibrin in plaque is the use of the clot-binding cyclic peptide, cysteine-arginine-glutamic acid-lysine-alanin (CREKA). In one experiment conducted by researchers at the University of California–San Diego, CREKA-targeted micelles were used to deliver imaging dyes and the thrombin inhibitor hirulog into atherosclerotic plaques in the ApoE-null mouse model *in vivo* (Peters et al. 2009). In addition, platelet-targeted liposomes bearing a glycoprotein IIIb integrin-binding peptide have been shown both *in vitro* and *in vivo* to bind onto platelets and can potentially be engineered to carry therapeutic agents (Srinivasan et al. 2009).

Nanocarrier Drug Delivery Systems for Treatment of CVDs

As discussed in the following sections, many different drug delivery systems have been formulated for treatment of CVDs at different disease stages. The types of nanoparticles used, as well as any targeting surface moiety, can be specifically tailored to seek molecular targets described in the previous section. While many different systems have been described, this section focuses on significant results.

Copolymeric Nanoparticles

Such nanosystems are made from copolymers generally consisting of polyethylene glycol (PEG) conjugated to some other synthetic polymer. The combination of different synthetic polymers at specific ratios allows specific tailoring of material properties. For instance, the conjugation of low molecular weight drugs to synthetic polymers or nanocarriers has been previously shown to increase the circulation time of the agents from minutes to several hours (Zhang et al. 2008a). Moreover, they tend to favor drug delivery to tissues with abnormal vessel architecture (via the enhanced permeability and retention [EPR] effect), such as atherosclerotic plaques.

An important ability of polymeric nanoparticles, in particular those with a PEG outer corona, is their enhanced ability to avoid recognition by the reticuloendothelial system, thereby greatly extending their circulation time (Antoniades et al. 2010). In such systems, the hydrophilic PEG creates an outer surface hydration layer, reducing protein interactions with the nanocarrier, opsonization, and uptake by macrophages. Consequently, the carrier is able to avoid a host immune response and retain increased circulation time. In addition, certain formulations of polymers, in particular those that incorporate PLGA, are able to be degraded and processed easily by the body. These nanocarriers are engineered to be immunocompatible and easily biodegradable (Venkataraman et al. 2005).

Potential treatments of atherosclerosis using synthetic polymeric nanocarriers have been demonstrated utilizing a multitude of engineered formulations with specific targeting ligands. As discussed in the section on potential endothelial targets, PLGA nanoparticles with a cyclic peptide ligand effectively targeted ICAM-1, a surface receptor that is dramatically upregulated on the vascular endothelium in response to the increased production of proinflammatory cytokines (Yang et al. 1999). Yang and coworkers investigated the potential of biocompatible, biodegradable PLGA nanoparticles as a drug delivery system for the passive targeting of vascular SMCs. SMC proliferation is a primary factor involved in accumulation of cells within the intima of blood vessels in atherosclerosis. Formulation of 14-kDa PLGA 50:50 (between 5 and 9 μm) and 17-kDa PLGA 75:25 (between 3 and 6 mm) nanoparticles occurred. A 5% heparin solution was loaded into each of the PLGA formulations and then incubated *in vitro* with cultured human SMCs. A thymidine assay showed 50% reduction in cell proliferation in the cells of the PLGA microsphere formulations when compared to a control of free nonencapsulated heparin (no significant difference in proliferation between PLGA formulations, although release profiles were noticeably dissimilar). Although the *in vitro* results were promising, it is difficult to assess this system due to the lack of *in vivo* data. It is also expected that large particles such as microparticles will have a very short circulation time.

In a novel approach mimicking the method of action of lipoproteins, PEG micelles were functionalized with tyrosine residues, an aromatic lipophilic amino acid. The residues directed the micelle, with average particle diameter of 12 nm, into the lipid-rich areas of atherosclerotic plaque in a population of apolipoprotein mice used as a model of atherosclerosis. PEG micelles modified with 15% tyrosine residues yielded a significant enhancement of the abdominal aortic wall at 6 and 24 hours post-injection and had a half-life 10 times longer compared to the unmodified micelles (Beilvert et al. 2009). These results suggest that modified micelles could be an efficient drug carrier for the treatment of atherosclerosis, but there is a lack of efficacy data *in vivo*.

A particularly significant characteristic of polymeric nanocarriers is their exceptional ability to be easily functionalized or hybridized to obtain a desired behavior. Chan and coworkers demonstrated this with their design of 60-nm hybrid nanoparticles consisting of a polymeric core, a lipid interface, and a PEG outer corona. In addition, peptide ligands with a high affinity for collagen IV, a rich component of vascular basement membranes, were bound onto the outer corona for targeting of SMC proliferation. In this study, paclitaxel conjugates were loaded into the polymer core, which allowed a more delayed drug release profile. The conjugated paclitaxel is released by diffusion when the ester bond of the polyactide core is hydrolyzed. This characteristic, along with the targeting mechanism, allows for unique spatiotemporal control, which was confirmed using both *in vitro* and *in vivo* studies. When administered intra-arterially or intravenously, the targeted nanocarriers showed a greater *in vivo* vascular retention at sites of injured vasculature in the rat models compared to nontargeted carriers. *In vitro*, drug release profiles noted controlled drug release over approximately 10–12 days (Chan et al. 2009), but there is a lack of *in vivo* efficacy data to determine the optimum dose and schedule.

Proteins provide a multitude of desirable properties that can be tailored specifically for the targeted application. A synthetic polymer nanoparticle, for example, conjugated with a native immunocompatible protein will confer the particle longer circulation time and a lower immunological response. In addition, protein conjugation methods are well known and widely established (Siu 2010). However, it is difficult to control the shape and size of the protein conjugates since antibody-enzyme conjugates may consist of one molecule of antibody and drug linked together or several copies of molecules forming clusters. Regardless, protein conjugates are becoming increasingly popular, such as the fusion protein EGFP-EGF1 (enhanced green fluorescent protein-epidermal growth factor 1) PEG-PLA nanoparticles and various bovine serum albumin conjugates. Protein immunoconjugates provide an appealing drug delivery system since they are fully biocompatible, and the degradation products are expelled via natural metabolic pathways (Zhang et al. 2008).

Maximov and coworkers used synthetic biodegradable PLA nanoparticles conjugated with an apolipoprotein B100 (apoB100) antibody to adsorb low-density lipoprotein (LDL) for subsequent delivery to the liver for lysosomal digestion, an important associate to the atherosclerotic process (Maximov et al. 2010). Conjugation occurred through the use of a novel biocompatible photocross-linker, Sulfo-HSAB, which was able to bind the apoB100 antibody to the PLA nanoparticle. A 500-mg/dL suspension of LDL in phosphate-buffered saline (PBS) buffer containing 2% bovine serum albumin was titrated by the nanoparticle-antibody suspension to show that LDL can be adsorbed by antibody-coated nanoparticles in suspension. Titrations were repeated five times to produce a final product of nanoparticle-antibody-LDL complexes with a characteristic size of around 200 nm. The nanoparticle-antibody-LDL suspensions at a concentration of about 400 mg/mL were placed in culture plates containing the mice macrophage cell line RAW 267, which serves as a model for liver Kupffer cells. Cell viability assays suggested lack of cytotoxicity of the complexes as cell lines treated with nanoparticle-antibody-LDL complexes displayed only about 10% less viability after a 12-hour incubation. Fluorescent imaging of the treated cells demonstrated a significant decrease of the fluorescence intensity from labeled complexes over a 24-hour period, indicative of their ingestion and uptake by the macrophage cell line.

Liposome Nanoparticles

Liposomes are a unique material whose use is dated earlier than other nanoscale techniques since liposomes are derivatives of natural biological materials (Schwendener 2008). A liposome is a tiny spherical vesicle consisting of an aqueous core enclosed by a bilayer phospholipid structure. Liposomes are biphasic, a feature that provides them the ability to act as carriers for both hydrophilic and hydrophobic drugs (Mufamadi 2011). In addition, they have good biocompatibility and low-toxicity profiles. However, major drawbacks for liposomes as a carrier for therapeutically active agents do exist. The primary concerns are their inability to achieve sustained drug delivery over a prolonged period of time and limited loading capacity. The binding of hydrophilic biocompatible groups such as PEG to the surfaces of liposomes has been shown to extend circulation time.

One particularly innovative clinical strategy involving liposomal drug carriers was developed by Golomb and colleagues. In this method, bisphosphonates (BPs), a class of drugs used widely in bone-related disorders such as osteoporosis, are encapsulated within a liposomal carrier. Encapsulation of a BP within a particulate delivery system, such as liposomes, deviates these bone-seeking molecules to circulating monocytes and macrophages to induce their apoptosis (van Rooijen et al. 2003; Danenberg et al 2002; Epstein et al. 2007). Since accumulation of macrophages is one of the primary inflammatory initiators of SMC proliferation, partial depletion of them in circulation could potentially help prevent restenosis following coronary interventions such as stent or balloon angioplasty. Golomb and his group showed that the anti-inflammatory effect resulting from monocyte and macrophage depletion by liposomal BPs reduced neointimal hyperplasia and restenosis in animal models (Danenberg et al. 2002; Epstein et al. 2007).

A study compared the bioactivity of liposomal BPs, establishing the relationships between formulation parameters of size, charge, and drug type on internalization and cytokine activation *in vitro* and *in vivo* (Epstein-Barash et al. 2010). In this study, positive and negative charged liposomes encapsulating two different bisphosphonates, alendronate and clodronate, were tested in multiple human and animal lines *in vitro* and in rat and rabbit models *in vivo*. The best formulation observed, in terms of high potency with minimal toxicity, was a negatively charged liposomal formulation of alendronate with a size of 85 nm. The phase I clinical trial showed they were safe; therefore a single intravenous injection of liposomal BPs for prevention of ISR is now under phase II clinical trials in Israel (http://clinicaltrials.gov/ct2/show/NCT00739466). This approach demonstrated that ISR could be due to a systemic rather than local inflammatory response.

In a different approach, Efergan and colleagues (2010) demonstrated the use of phosphatidylcholine liposomes encapsulated with simvastatin, a hypolipidemic drug used to control elevated cholesterol through the inhibition of macrophage/monocyte activity (Tuomisto et al. 2008). Rat models were given a single intravenous injection of 165-nm phosphatidylcholine liposomes loaded with 3 μM simvastatin at the time of angioplasty. Flow cytometry performed on blood specimens determined a nearly 20% decrease in blood monocyte activity in liposomal simvastatin treatment in comparison to the untreated group. *In vitro* studies on RAW264.7, J774 rat macrophage cell and THP-1 human macrophage cells (human acute monocytic leukemia cell line) found that the liposomal simvastatin was one and a half to two times more effective than free drug at suppressing monocyte/macrophage proliferation (Efergan et al. 2010).

Activation of nuclear factor kβ (NF-κβ) leads to the expression of key mediators of inflammatory and immune responses, as well as ICAMs (Collins et al. 1995). Cyclopentenone prostaglandins (CP-PGs) have demonstrated significant anti-inflammatory properties by inhibiting NF-κβ (Homem de Bittencourt et al. 2007). Bittencourt and colleagues developed LipoCardium, a negatively charged, endothelium-directed liposome with adjoined CP-PG and anti-VCAM-1 antibodies, to be used as a delivery system to inhibit NF-κβ. LipoCardium established significant anti-inflammatory properties both *in vitro* and *in vivo*.

Magnetic Nanoparticles

Although the majority of current research in paramagnetic nanoparticles is aimed at their potential use in imaging and diagnostics, a few systems under investigation have therapeutic purposes. Iron oxide (IO) nanoparticles, for instance, have unique properties that generate significant susceptibility effects, resulting in strong contrast at very low concentrations for magnetic resonance imaging (MRI). IO nanoparticles have a long blood retention time, biodegradability, low toxicity, and a large surface area to provide for a large number of functional groups (Ping et al. 2008). These characteristics make IO a primary material for many biomedical applications.

While most therapeutic approaches have involved the systemic administration of cytotoxic drugs, focal therapies, such as those that are light activated, allow control of the localization of the therapeutic effect (McCarthey et al. 2010). One study utilized dextran-coated cross-linked iron oxide (CLIO) nanoparticles modified with near-infrared fluorophores and light-activated therapeutic moieties, which allow for the optical determination of agent localization and phototoxic activation at spectrally distinct wavelengths. The CLIO nanoparticles modified with AlexaFluor 750 fluorophores and CLIO nanoparticles modified with tetra(hydroxyphenyl)chlorin (THPC) were combined in suspension and investigated *in vitro* using RAW 264.7 murine macrophages. As compared to the commonly used chlorin e6, CLIO-THPC was almost 60 times more phototoxic on a chlorin-per-chlorin basis and 1,900-fold more toxic on a molecular level. The *in vivo* localization of the nanoagent to atherosclerotic lesions was then examined in apolipoprotein E-deficient mice. Fluorescent imaging and histological samples of the treated mice illustrated a substantially more successful therapeutic outcome than in the nontreated mice. Thus the modified CLIO nanocarriers were proven to be readily taken up by phagocytic macrophages and demonstrated superior phototoxicity compared to conventional chlorin agents for imaging and therapy. This system is only toxic when activated by the appropriate wavelength of light, thereby minimizing off-target effects. The resulting agent is readily taken up by murine macrophages *in vitro* and is highly phototoxic.

An interesting attempt to reload stents and thereby prevent long-term migration and proliferation of SMCs inside the lumen of coronary stents after stent implantation has been attempted by Johnson and coworkers. This has been demonstrated with biodegradable, superparamagnetic nanoparticles guided by high-gradient magnetic fields to redosing stents with paclitaxel. These nanoparticles had an approximate composition of 30% (w/w) magnetite and 12% (w/w) paclitaxel and were formulated from polylactide and poly(lactide-co-glycolide) polymers employing an emulsification-solvent evaporation methodology. Cell viability assays indicated magnetic nanoparticle dose-dependent cell growth inhibition over an 8-day time span for paclitaxel-loaded formulations. A cell growth arrest of nearly 80% and 100% of cultured vascular SMCs and endothelial cells, respectively, was demonstrated. This was in stark contrast to unloaded drug formulations, which showed negligible differences from the nontreated cells (Johnson et al. 2010).

Chorny and colleagues indicated the need for adjustment of the drug dose and release kinetics to the disease status of the treated vessel and attempted to address this problem with magnetic nanoparticles in a rat carotid model. Magnetic targeting was conducted using a uniform field-induced magnetization effect. Chorny and coworkers showed that magnetic treatment of cultured arterial SMCs with paclitaxel-loaded magnetic nanoparticles caused significant cell growth inhibition, an effect not seen in nonmagnetic conditions. It was also shown that arterial tissue levels of stent-targeted magnetic nanoparticles remained 4- to 10-fold higher in magnetically treated animals versus control over 5 days after delivery. Furthermore, a significant inhibition of ISR with a relatively low dose of magnetic nanoparticle-encapsulated paclitaxel of 7.5 mg of paclitaxel per stent was demonstrated (Chorny et al. 2010).

Conclusions

Numerous new technologies are emerging to provide better therapeutic tools for patients, including local and systemic drug delivery systems. The potential of fully degradable DESs to replace metallic stents has not been shown yet. Efforts to improve current technologies are focused on (a) development of polymer coatings of metallic stents to improve biocompatibility, release drug over a long period of time, and improve endothelial cells proliferation; and (b) development of new designs and synthesis of new materials with enhanced properties. On the other hand, DEB technologies have been described to overcome some of the limitations of DESs, but DEBs are still in early developmental and clinical stages. Typically, these interventional procedures are suitable for later stages of CVD. Overall, the local drug delivery systems have been shown to be promising for some cardiovascular applications in preclinical and clinical studies, but there is a lack of long-term clinical data. The systemic delivery of cardiovascular drugs using nanoparticles that are able to accumulate into the diseased tissue is more recent and has been shown only as proof of concept, and there is a lack of efficacy data using appropriate animal models. This approach has already been successful for oncology, with a number of nontargeted nanoparticle drug delivery systems approved by the FDA and clinical trials of the first targeted nanocarrier. The systemic approach could provide preventive therapy because of the possibility to deliver therapeutics at different stages of CVD, especially at early stages to control plaque formation before it is too late. However, one nanoparticle formulation is currently in a phase II clinical trial to reduce ISR, which occurs at the later stage of disease.

Acknowledgments

Professor Subbu would like to thank the National Research Foundation of Singapore through the Competitive Research Program. Dr. Frank Alexis would like to thank the National Institutes of Health for funding. Kevin Keith would like to thank the Kathryn Sullivan Fellowship and the Honors Research Grant for funding.

References

Alexis F, Pridgen EM, Langer R, Farokhzad OC. 2010. Nanoparticle technologies for cancer therapy: In: Monika Schafer-Korting, ed., *Handbook of Experimental Pharmacology*. Heidelberg: Springer.

Antoniades C., Psarros C., and Tousoulis D. 2010. Nanoparticles: a promising therapeutic approach in atherosclerosis. *Current Drug Delivery* 7:303–11.

Arterial Remodeling Technologies home page. Retrieved April 20, 2011, from http://www.art-stent.com.

Axel D.I., Kunert W., Goggelmann C., et al. 1997. Paclitaxel inhibits arterial smooth muscle cell proliferation and migration *in vitro* and *in vivo* using local drug delivery. *Circulation* 96:636–45.

Beilvert A., Cormode D.P., Chaubet F., et al. 2009. Tyrosine polyethylene glycol (PEG)-micelle magnetic resonance contrast agent for the detection of lipid rich areas in atherosclerotic plaque. *Magnetic Resonance in Medicine* 62:1195–201.

Blankstein R., and Ferencik M. 2010. The vulnerable plaque: can it be detected with cardiac CT? *Atherosclerosis* 211:386–89.

Bolderman R.W., Bruin P., Hermans J.J., Boerakker M.J., Dias A.A., van der Veen F.H., et al. 2010. Atrium-targeted drug delivery through an amiodarone-eluting bilayered patch. *Journal of Thoracic and Cardiovascular Surg*ery 140:904–10.

Burger P., and Wagner D. 2003. Platelet P-selectin facilitates atherosclerotic lesion development. *Blood* 101:2661–66.

Burgess P., Hutt P.B., Farokhzad O.C., Langer R., Minick S., and Zale S. 2010. On firm ground: IP protection of therapeutic nanoparticles. *Nature Biotechnology* 28:1267.

Caruthers S.D., Tillmann C., Winter P.M., Wickline S.A., and Lanza, G. M. 2009. Anti-angiogenic perfluorocarbon nanoparticles for diagnosis and treatment of atherosclerosis. *Wiley Interdisciplinary Reviews: Nanomedicine and Nanobiotechnology* 1:311–23.

Chan J.M., Valencia P.M., Zhang L., Langer R., and Farokhzad O.C. 2010. Polymeric nanoparticles for drug delivery. *Methods in Molecular Biology* 624:163–75.

Chan J.M., Zhang L., Tong R., et al. 2009. Spatiotemporal controlled delivery of nanoparticles to injured vasculature. *Proceedings of the National Academy of Sciences of the United States of America* 107:2213–18.

Chorny M., Fishbein I., Yellen B.B., et al. 2010. Targeting stents with local delivery of paclitaxel-loaded magnetic nanoparticles using uniform fields. *Proceedings of the National Academy of Sciences of the United States of America* 107:8346–51.

Chorny M., Mishaly D., Leibowitz A., Domb A.J., and Golomb G. 2006. Site-specific delivery of dexamethasone from biodegradable implants reduces formation of pericardial adhesions in rabbits. *Journal of Biomedical Material Research A* 78:276–82.

Collins T., Read M.A., and Neish A.S. 1995. Transcriptional regulation of endothelial cell adhesion molecules: NF-B and cytokine-inducible enhancers. *FASEB Journal* 9:899–909.

Cremers B., Speck U., Kaufels N., et al. 2009. Drug-eluting balloon: very short-term exposure and overlapping. *Thrombosis and Haemostasis* 101:201–6.

Danenberg H.D., Fishbein I., Gao J., et al. 2002. Macrophage depletion by clodronate-containing liposomes reduces neointimal formation after balloon injury in rats and rabbits. *Circulation* 106:599–605.

De Labriolle A., Pakala R., et al. 2009. Paclitaxel-eluting balloon: from bench to bed. *Catheterization and Cardiovascular Interventions* 73:643–52.

Dior. 2011. April 20, 2011, from http://www.eurocor.de/products/dior/product_information.

Efergan E., David M., Epstein H., et al. 2010. Liposomal simvastatin attenuates neo-intimal hyperplasia in rats. *American Association of Pharmaceutical Scientists Journal* 12:181–87.

Epstein H., Berger V., Levi I., et al. 2007. Nanosuspensions of alendronate with gallium or gadolinium attenuate neointimal hyperplasia in rats. *Journal of Controlled Release* 117:322–32.

Epstein-Barash H., Gutman D., Markovsky E., et al. 2010. Physicochemical parameters affecting liposomal bisphosphonates bioactivity for restenosis therapy: internalization, cell inhibition, activation of cytokines and complement, and mechanism of cell death. *Journal of Controlled Release* 146:182–95.

Garg S., and Serruys P.W. 2010. Coronary stents current status. *Journal of the American College of Cardiology* 50:S1–42.

Gighliotti G., Waissbluth A., Speidel C., Abenshein D., and Eisenberg P. 1998. Prolonged activation of prothrombin on the vascular wall after arterial injury. *Arteriosclerosis, Thrombosis, and Vascular Biology* 18:250–57.

Gossl M., Rosol M., Malyar N.M., et al. 2003. Functional anatomy and hemodynamic characteristics of Vasa vasorum in the walls of porcine coronary arteries. *The Anatomical Record. Part A, Discoveries in Molecular, Cellular, and Evolutionary Biology* 272:526–37.

Guagliumi G., Sirbu V., et al. 2010a. Strut coverage and vessel wall response to a new-generation paclitaxel-eluting stent with an ultrathin biodegradable abluminal polymer: Optical Coherence Tomography Drug-Eluting Stent Investigation (OCTDESI). *Circulation—Cardiovascular Interventions* 3:367–375.

Guagliumi G., Sirbu V., et al. 2010b. Strut coverage and vessel wall response to zotarolimus-eluting and bare-metal stents implanted in patients with ST-segment elevation myocardial infarction: the OCTAMI (Optical Coherence Tomography in Acute Myocardial Infarction) Study. *JACC Cardiovascular Interventions* 3:680–87.

Habara S., Mitsudo K., Kadota K., et al. 2011. Effectiveness of paclitaxel-eluting balloon catheter in patients with sirolimus-eluting stent restenosis. *JACC Cardiovascular Interventions* 4:149–54.

Holman T.J., Weber J., and Shewe S. Reinforced and drug-eluting balloon catheters and methods for making same. United States Patent 7,491,188 B2, February 17, 2009.

Homem de Bittencourt P.I., Jr., Lagranha D.J., Maslinkiewicz A., et al. 2007. LipoCardium: endothelium-directed cyclopentenone prostaglandin-based liposome formulation that completely reverses atherosclerotic lesions. *Atherosclerosis* 193:245–58.

Igaki-Tamai stent. Searched April 28, 2011, from http://www.kyoto-mp.co.jp/news/081001_en.html.
Jabara R., Chronos N., et al. 2008. Novel bioabsorbable salicylate-based polymer as a drug-eluting stent coating. *Catheterization and Cardiovascular Interventions* 72:186–94.
Jabara R., Pendyala L., et al. 2009. Novel fully bioabsorbable salicylate-based sirolimus eluting stent. *Eurointervention* F58–64.
Jayagopal A., Linton M., and Fazio S. 2010. Insights into atherosclerosis using nanotechnology. *Current Atheroscerosis Reports* 12:209–15.
Johnson B., Toland B., Chokshi R., et al. 2010. Magnetically responsive paclitaxel-loaded biodegradable nanoparticles for treatment of vascular disease: preparation, characterization and *in vitro* evaluation of anti-proliferative potential. *Current Drug Delivery* 7:263–73.
Joner M., Nakazawa G., et al. 2008. Endothelial cell recovery between comparator polymer-based drug-eluting stents. *Journal of the American College of Cardiology* 52:333–42.
Karlberg J.P.E. 2008. Trends in disease focus of drug development. *Nature Reviews Drug Discovery* 7: 639–40.
Laufer E.M., Reutelingsperger C.P., Narula J., and Hofstra, L. 2008. Annexin A5: an imaging biomarker of cardiovascular risk. *Basic Research in Cardiology* 103:95–104.
Learning lessons from Pfizer's $800 million failure. 2011. *Nature Reviews Drug Discovery* 10:163–64.
Lemos P.A., Serruys P.W., et al. 2004. Unrestricted utilization of sirolimus-eluting stents compared with conventional bare stent implantation in the "real world"—The Rapamycin-Eluting Stent Evaluated at Rotterdam Cardiology Hospital (RESEARCH) Registry. *Circulation* 109: 190–95.
Libby P. 2003. Inflammation: a common pathway in cardiovascular diseases. *Dialogues in Cardiovascular Medicine*. 8:59–73.
Liebman S.M., Langer J.C., Marshall J.S., and Collins S.M. 1993. Role of mast cells in peritoneal adhesion formation. *American Journal of Surgery* 165:127–30.
Matsumoto D., Shinke T., et al. 2009. Stent degradation of novel fully bioabsorbable salicylate-based sirolimus-eluting stent evaluated by OCT in pig coronary artery. *American Journal of Cardiology* 104:167D–167D.
Maximov V., Reukov V., Barry J., Cochrane C., and Vertegel A. 2010. Protein–nanoparticle conjugates as potential therapeutic agents for the treatment of hyperlipidemia. *Nanotechnology* 21:265103.
McCarthey J., Korngold E., Weissleder R., and Jafour F. 2010. A light-activated theranostic nanoagent for targeted macrophage ablation in inflammatory atherosclerosis. *Small* 6:2041–49.
Mcfadden E.P., Stabile E., et al. 2004. Late thrombosis in drug-eluting coronary stents after discontinuation of antiplatelet therapy. *The Lancet* 364 (9444):1519–21.
Mori T., Kinoshita Y., Watanabe A., Yamaguchi T., Hosokawa K., and Honjo H. 2006. Retention of paclitaxel on cancer cells for 1 week in-vivo and in-vitro. *Cancer Chemotherapy and Pharmacology* 58:665–72.
Mufamadi M. 2011. A review on composite liposomal technologies for specialized drug delivery. *Journal of Drug Delivery* 2011:939851.
Muro S., Koval M., and Muzykantov V. 2004. Endothelial endocytic pathways: gates for vascular drug delivery. *Current Vascular Pharmacology* 2:281–99.

Muro S., and Muzykantov V.R. 2005. Targeting of antioxidant and anti-thrombotic drugs to endothelial cell adhesion molecules. *Current Pharmaceutical Design* 11:2383–401.

Nakamura T., Brott B.C., Brants I., et al. 2011. Vasomotor function after paclitaxel-coated balloon post-dilation in porcine coronary stent model. *JACC Cardiovascular Interventions* 4:247–55.

Onuma Y., Ormiston J., and Serruys P.W. 2011. Bioresorbable scaffold technologies. *Circulation Journal* 75:509–20.

Opar A. 2007. Where now for new drugs for atherosclerosis? *Nature Reviews Drug Discovery* 6:334–35.

Ormiston J.A., Serruys P.W., et al. 2008. A bioabsorbable everolimus-eluting coronary stent system for patients with single de-novo coronary artery lesions (ABSORB): a prospective open-label trial. *Lancet* 371:899–907.

Peters D., Kastantin M., Kotamraju et al. 2009. Targeting atherosclerosis by using modular, multifunctional micelles. *Proceedings of the National Academy of Sciences Biology* 106:24.

Ping X., Qian X., Mao H., and Wang A. 2008. Targeted magnetic iron oxide nanoparticles for tumor imaging and therapy. *International Journal of Nanomedicine* 3:311–21.

Pinto Slottow T.L., Waksman R. 2007. Overview of the 2006 Food and Drug Administration Circulatory System Devices Panel Meeting on drug-eluting stent thrombosis. *Catheter Cardiovascular Intervention* 69:1064–1074.

Plump, A. 2010. Accelerating the pulse of cardiovascular R&D. *Nature Reviews Drug Discovery* 9:823–24.

Roger V.L., Go A.S., Lloyd-Jones D.M., et al. 2011. American Heart Association Statistics Committee and Stroke Statistics Subcommittee. Heart disease and stroke statistics—2011 update: a report from the American Heart Association. *Circulation* 123(4):e18–e209.

Scheller B., Hehrlein C., Bocksch W., et al. 2006. Treatment of coronary in-stent restenosis with a paclitaxel coated balloon catheter. *New England Journal of Medicine* 355:2113–24.

Scheller B., Hehrlein C., et al. 2008. Two year follow-up after treatment of coronary in-stent restenosis with a paclitaxel-coated balloon catheter. *Clinical Research in Cardiology* 97:773–81.

Scheller B., Speck U., et al. 2003. Contrast media as carriers for local drug delivery. *European Heart Journal* 24:1462–67.

Scheller B., Speck U., Abramjuk C., et al. 2004. Paclitaxel balloon coating, a novel method for prevention and therapy of restenosis. *Circulation* 110:810–14.

Schwendener R.A. 2008. Liposomes in biology and medicine. *Advances in Experimental Medicine and Biology* 620(117):128.

Serruys P.W., Ormiston J.A., et al. 2009. A bioabsorbable everolimus-eluting coronary stent system (ABSORB): 2-year outcomes and results from multiple imaging methods. *Lancet* 373:897–910.

Siu D. 2010. A new way of targeting to treat coronary artery disease. *Journal of Cardiovascular Medicine* 11(1):1–6.

Smith B., Heverhagen J., and Knopp M. 2007. Localization to atherosclerotic plaque and biodistribution of biochemically derivatized superparamagnetic iron oxide nanoparticles (SPIONs) contrast particles for magnetic resonance imaging (MRI). *Biomedical Microdevices* 9:719–27.

Soga Y., Takai S., Koyama T., et al. 2004. Attenuation of adhesion formation after cardiac surgery with a chymase inhibitor in a hamster model. *Journal of Thoracic and Cardiovascular Surgery* 127:72–78.

Srinivasan R., Marchant R.E., and Gupta A.S. 2009. *In vitro* and *in vivo* platelet targeting by cyclic RGD-modified liposomes. *Journal of Biomedical Material Research* 93:1004–15.

Stack R.S., Califf R.M., et al. 1988. Interventional cardiac-catheterization at Duke Medical Center. *American Journal of Cardiology* 62(10):F3–F24.

Stoneman V., and Bennett M. 2004. Role of apoptosis in atherosclerosis and its therapeutic implications. *Clinical Science* 107:343–54.

Tamai H., Igaki K., et al. 2000. Initial and 6-month results of biodegradable poly-l-lactic acid coronary stents in humans. *Circulation* 102:399–404.

Toth P. 2010. Pharmacomodulation of high-density lipoprotein metabolism as a therapeutic intervention for atherosclerotic disease. *Current Cardiology Reports* 12:481–87.

Tsuji T., Tamai H., et al. 2001. Biodegradable polymeric stents. *Current Interventional Cardiology Reports* 3:10–17.

Tuomisto T.T., Lumivuori H., Kansanen E., et al. 2008. Simvastatin has an anti-inflammatory effect on macrophages via upregulation of an atheroprotective transcription factor, kruppel-like factor 2. *Cardiovascular Research* 78:175–84.

U.S. Food and Drug Administration, Circulatory System Devices Panel. Meeting minutes, December 8, 2006, Washington, DC. Accessed September 28, 2010, from http://www.fda.gov/ohrms/dockets/ac/06/transcripts/2006–4253t2.rtf. 2010

Valat M., Deramchia K., and Mornet S. 2010. MRI of inducible P-selectin expression in human activated platelets involved in the early stages of atherosclerosis. *NMR in Biomedicine* doi: 10.1002/nbm.1606 [Epub ahead of print].

van Rooijen N., van Kesteren-Hendrikx E. 2003. In vivo depletion of macrophages by liposome-mediated "suicide." *Methods Enzymology* 373:3–16.

Venkatraman S.S., Jie P., Min F., et al. 2005. Micelle-like nanoparticles of PLA-PEG-PLA triblock copolymers as chemotherapeutic carrier. *International Journal of Pharmaceutics* 298:219–32.

Venkatraman S.S., Ma L.L., Natarajan J.V., and Chattopadhyay S. 2010. Polymer- and liposome-based nanoparticles in targeted drug delivery. *Frontiers in Bioscience* 2:801–14.

Venkatraman S., and Boey F. 2007. Release profiles in drug-eluting stents: issues and uncertainties. *Journal of Controlled Release* 120:149–60.

Virmani R., Burke A.P., Farb A., Kolodgie F.D. 2006. Pathology of the vulnerable plaque. *Journal of the American College of Cardiology* 47:C13–18.

Waksman R., Pakala R. 2009. Drug-eluting balloon: the comeback kid? *Circulation. Cardiovascular Interventions* 2:352–58.

Winter P.M., Caruthers S., Zhang H., et al. 2008. Antiangiogenic synergism of integrin-targeted fumagillin nanoparticles and atorvastatin in atherosclerosis. *JACC: Cardiovascular Imaging* 1(5):624–34.

Yang Z., Birkenhauer P., Julmy F., et al. 1999. Sustained release of heparin from polymeric particles for inhibition of human vascular smooth muscle cell proliferation. *Journal of Controlled Release*, 60:269–77.

Yao Y.L., Ishihara T., Takai S., Miyazaki M., and Mita S. 2000. Association between the expression of mast cell chymase and intraperitoneal adhesion formation in mice. *Journal of Surgical Research* 92:40–44.

Zhang L., Chan J.M., Gu F.X., et al. 2008a. Self-assembled lipid-polymer hybrid nanoparticles: a robust drug delivery platform. *ACS Nano* 2:1696–1702.

Zhang L., Gu F.X., Chan J.M., et al. 2008b. Nanoparticles in medicine: therapeutic applications and developments. *Clinical Pharmacology and Therapeutics* 83:761–69.

Zhang N., Chittasupho C., Duangrat C., Siahaan T., and Berkland C. 2008. PLGA nanoparticle peptide conjugate effectively targets intercellular cell-adhesion molecule-1. *Bioconjugate Chemistry* 19:145–52.

Zhang W., Xiao G., and Hui B. 2010. Nanostructured lipid carriers constituted from high-density lipoprotein components for delivery of a lipophilic cardiovascular drug. *International Journal of Pharmaceutics* 391:313–21.

3

Polymeric Biomaterials for Vascular Tissue Engineering

George Fercana and Dan Simionescu

CONTENTS

Current Options and Clinical Need for Replacements

The total need for vascular grafts has been estimated to be more than 1.4 million in the United States alone (Niklason and Langer 1997). This need can be divided into three categories, in order of decreasing diameter (Table 3.1). The large- and medium-caliber synthetic grafts (>6-mm diameter) are used in the thoracic and abdominal cavities with good long-term outcomes. Common applications include replacement of the aorta, carotid artery, arch vessels, and iliac and femoral arteries. However, synthetic grafts of smaller diameter do not share the same outcomes and fail relatively early due to occlusion. Since tissue engineering holds great potential for development of viable grafts, this chapter delves into research and development of small-diameter vascular grafts using natural polymers.

Almost 200,000 small-caliber grafts (<6 mm) are used every year for vascular access, to relieve peripheral lower limb ischemia, or for coronary artery bypass graft (CABG); autologous veins or arteries are the "gold standard" for replacement of small-caliber arteries, but in 30–40% of patients these are not

TABLE 3.1

Overview of Sizes and Preferential Choices for Vascular Grafts

	Vascular Regions				
Vascular Substitute Choice	**Large-Caliber Arteries (≥ 8 mm)**	**Medium-Caliber Arteries (6–8 mm)**	**Small-Caliber Arteries (≤6 mm)**	**Venous Reconstructions**	**Hemodialysis Arteriovenous Access**
	Aorta, arch vessels, iliac and common femoral arteries	Carotid, subclavian, common femoral, visceral, and above-the-knee arteries	Coronary, below-the-knee, tibial, and peroneal arteries	Superior and inferior vena cava, iliofemoral veins, portal vein, visceral veins	Upper > lower extremity
First choice	Prosthesis (Dacron, ePTFE)	Prosthesis or autograft (equal)	Arterial or venous autograft	Saphenous spiral vein graft, deep venous autograft	Native material
Second choice	Allograft, deep venous autograft	Prosthesis or autograft	Composite graft, vein interposition, prosthesis (ePTFE, Dacron), allograft, biosynthetic	Allografts, ePTFE, Dacron, biografts	ePTTE, PU, xenografts, biografts. TEBV (clinical trial)

Source: Chlupac, J., Filova, E., and Bacakova, L. 2009. Blood vessel replacement: 50 years of development and tissue engineering paradigms in vascular surgery. *Physiological Research* 58(Supplement 2):S119–39. With permission.

available due to prior harvesting or preexisting conditions. In these last cases, synthetic grafts are used, but they provide poor outcomes as 50% of these will occlude within 5 years (Veith et al. 1986), potentially leading to amputation.

In the search for small-caliber vascular substitutes, a range of materials and methodologies has been evaluated (Bezuidenhout and Zilla 2004), but most exhibited poor midterm performance. These included (a) synthetic grafts such as expanded polytetrafluoroethylene (ePTFE), polyethylene-terephthalate (PET), polyurethanes, polyglycolic (PG), and polylactide polyglycolide (PL) (Zdrahala 1996) and (b) bioprosthetic grafts (homologous, heterologous), each with different conformations that are better suited for particular applications (Table 3.2 and Table 3.3). Most synthetic polymers exhibit good biostability, compliance, and hemocompatibility but are prone to infections and dilation and variable healing patterns and endothelialization potential. Taken together, as multiple bypasses are sometimes required and availability of autologous arteries or veins is limited, there is clearly a significant unmet clinical need for small-caliber vascular grafts.

Tissue engineering using appropriate tubular scaffolds seeded with autologous living stem cells holds promise to solve this need by providing living tissue substitutes capable of integration, remodeling, and long-term patency. Mechanical conditioning of cell-seeded grafts before implantation is required for cell differentiation and adaptation to dynamic conditions. Notably, a tissue-engineered graft scaffold is required to be capable of immediately re-establishing blood flow; thus mechanical properties, including burst pressure and compliance, need to be engineered *in vitro* before implantation.

Necessary Properties for the Ideal Vascular Graft

In the realm of biomedical polymeric engineering, a large breadth of materials has been investigated for vascular replacement applications to achieve necessary properties intrinsic to the ideal vascular replacement (Barrett and Yousaf 2010). The properly functioning vascular graft needs to accommodate physiological properties such as adequate burst pressure, the capacity to recoil, and radial compliance.

Burst pressure is an intrinsic property of tubular materials and is tested by cannulating both ends of the graft and connecting a piezoelectric digital pressure transducer at one end and a peristaltic pump (or syringe pump) at the opposite end. The system is filled with saline, and pressure is slowly increased. Burst pressure is recorded when a sharp drop in internal graft pressure occurs. At times, it is useful to document the pattern of tissue failure by photography, as this may provide clues to the presence of weaker components in the graft structure. Native arteries exhibit a burst pressure of 1,500–2,200 mmHg,

TABLE 3.2

Brief Overview of Characteristics and History of Biological Vascular Grafts, where IND Denotes Internodal Distance

	Synthetic Vascular Grafts					
	PET (Dacron, Terylen)		**ePTFE (Teflon, Gore-Tex)**		**Polyurethane**	
	Woven	**Knitted**	**Low Porosity (<30 μm IND)**	**High Porosity (>45 μm IND)**	**Fibrillar**	**Foamy**
Advantages	Better stability, lower permeability and less bleeding	Greater porosity, tissue ingrowth and radial distensibility	Biostability, no dilation over time	Biostability, better cell ingrowth	Compliance, good hemo- and biocompatibility, less thrombogenicity	
Disadvantages	Reduced compliance and tissue incorporation, low porosity,fraying at edges, infection risk	Dilation over time, infection risk	Stitch bleeding, limited incorporation, infection risk, perigraft seroma formation	Late neointimal desquamation in 90 μm IND, infection risk	Biodegradation in first generation, infection risk, carcinogenic?	
Healing	Inner fibrinous capsule, outer collagenous capsule, scarce endothelial islands	Fibrin luminal coverage, very sporadic endothelium, trans-anastomotic endothelialization in animals	Luminal fibrin and platelet carpet, connective tissue capsule with foreign body giant cells, no transmural tissue ingrowth	Macrophages and polymorphonuclear invasion, capillary sprouting, fibroblast migration, certain angiogenesis, thicker neointima, endothelialization in animals	Thin inner fibrin layer, outside foreign body cells, limited ingrowth	Better ingrowth with bigger pores
First use	Ku et al. 1957		Norton and Eiseman 1975		Boertos and Pierce 1967	
Review, for example	Xue and Greisler 2003		Nishabe et al. 2004		Tiwari et al 2002	

Source: From Chlupac, J., E. Filova, and L. Bacakova, 2009. *Blood vessel replacement: 50 years of development and tissue engineering paradigms in vascular surgery*. Physiological Research 58(2): S119–S139.

TABLE 3.3

Brief Overview of Properties of Biological and Synthetic Scaffolds

	Biological Scaffolds	Synthetic Scaffolds
Advantages	Naturally occurring, nontoxic Favorable for cell binding Generally biocompatible	Precise control over material properties Easily available and cheap Easy to process Little or no batch-to-batch variation
Disadvantages	May degrade rapidly Weak mechanical property unless cross-linked Inconsistency between different batches Chance of disease transmission	Toxic residual monomers or catalysts and degradation by-products may illicit inflammation Poor cellular interaction

Source: Patel, A., et al. 2006. Elastin biosynthesis: the missing link in tissue-engineered blood vessels. *Cardiovascular Research* 71:40–49. With permission.

which in theory is redundant by a safety factor of about 100. Currently, it is not known what the most tolerable safety factor for an engineered graft should be, but scientists aim at reaching at least 300–500 mmHg.

Physiological compliance is defined as the increase in graft diameter as pressure increases from 80 to 120 mmHg. Compliance measurement is performed as follows: Grafts are cannulated with one end connected to a piezoelectric digital pressure transducer and the other adapted to a saline reservoir. The reservoir is raised until the transducer reads 80 mmHg hydrostatic pressure, and digital images are taken for external diameter measurement. Then, the pressure is increased to 120 mmHg, and the diameter is measured again (Figure 3.1). Typically, a native artery exhibits 10–15% compliance. This is an important parameter to engineer because of known effects of compliance mismatch on graft performance.

In addition to the aforementioned qualities, vascular grafts will require adequate performance regarding implant biocompatibility, such as resistance to calcification, thrombosis, and infection (Sarkar et al. 2007), which are typically modulated using alterations to the material's surface or bulk chemistry via known anticoagulants, such as variations of heparin (Murugesan et al. 2008; Rabenstein 2002), or treating the material to resist calcification (Simpson et al. 2007; Simionescu 2004; Isenburg et al. 2005).

Once satisfactory material properties have been established for the proposed vascular graft, the material must also prove to be noncytotoxic and porous and allow retention of shear resistant endothelial cells (ECs) in the intima, vascular smooth muscle cells (VSMCs) in the media, and fibroblasts (FBs) in the adventitia, the three tunics native to blood vessels (Figure 3.2). Pending infiltration of these cell types, the material must permit degradation and matrix remodeling by the host's own cells to produce a patient-tailored, autologous replacement according to the recent paradigm of regenerative medicine (Chlupac et al. 2009).

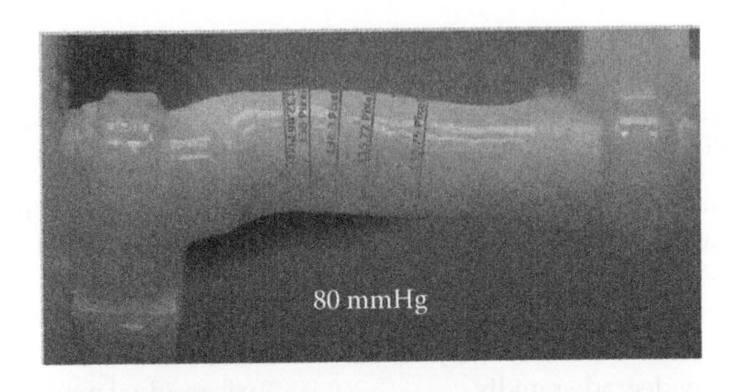

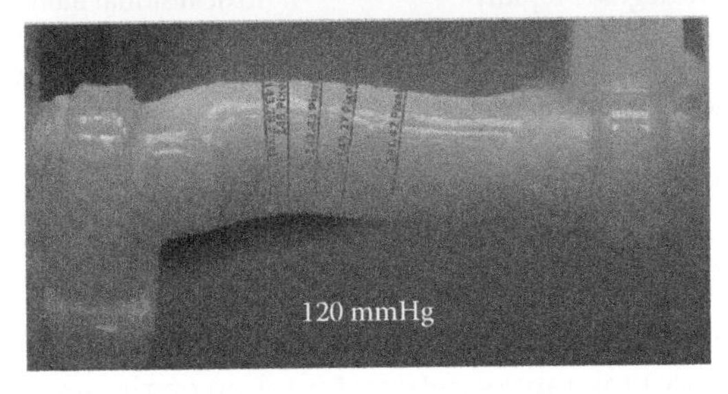

FIGURE 3.1
Setup for measurement of vascular graft compliance. The graft is mounted using barbed adapters and subjected to physiological pressures; digital pictures are taken for diameter measurements.

Small-Diameter Prosthetic Grafts: Research Fueling Implant Improvement

The available amount of polymeric options for any surgical procedure is quite large, but over the years ePTFE has remained the material of choice for small-diameter vascular replacement due to its decreased inflammatory and thrombogenic activity in comparison to other implant graft materials. Research on vascular replacements began with Voorhees and colleagues on the introduction of woven Vinyon N as a vascular replacement material (Voorhees et al. 1952). This research sparked studies of other polymeric materials; however, the work of Creech and colleagues established PET (Dacron) and ePTFE as the most resistant to degradation when compared to the other tested materials, including nylon, Orlon, and Ivalon (Creech et al. 1957). Since this discovery, much work has been done on improving ePTFE for vascular replacement. Although ePTFE retains properties that decrease thrombogenicity and inflammation to improve overall implant biocompatibility, the material will still fall prey to the body's innate defense mechanisms of platelet adhesion, protein adsorption, and other processes intrinsic to the coagulation cascade, starting at the blood-biomaterial interface. Problem areas for all polymeric vascular grafts are the interfaces between the (a) material and

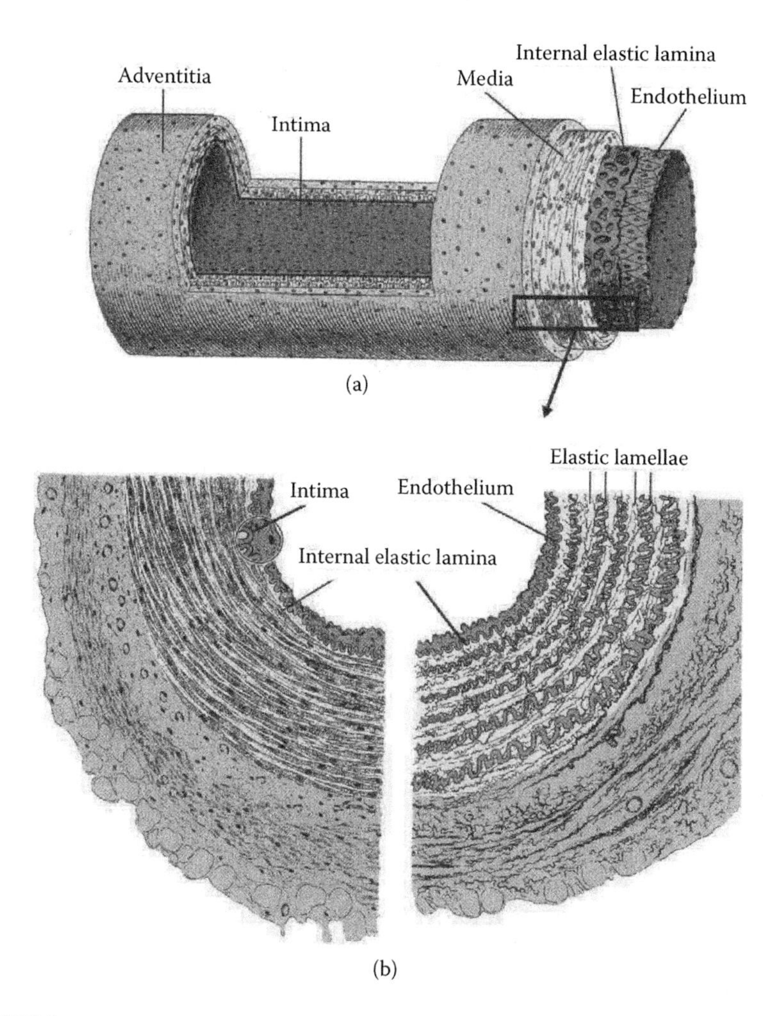

FIGURE 3.2
(a) Representation of the three tunics native to a blood vessel. Intima, ECs; media, VSMCs; adventitia, FBs. (From Junqueira, L.C., and J. Cameiro, eds. 2005. *Basic Histology: Text and Atlas.* 11th ed. New York: McGraw Hill, pp. 206–7.) (b) Structural differences between muscular arteries (left) and elastic arteries (right); note differences in elastin content dependent on artery type. (From Junqueira, L.C., and J. Cameiro, eds. 2005. *Basic Histology: Text and Atlas.* 11th ed. New York: McGraw Hill, pp. 206–7.)

blood, (b) tissue and blood, and (c) sites of anastomosis, keeping in mind the "intimal" and "adventitial" regions of the material will both be exposed to the body's defense mechanisms. Improving the biocompatibility of ePTFE and other polymeric vascular replacements includes research into promoting endothelialization of the intimal surface of the implant material and decreasing VSMC proliferation while retaining quiescent phenotype in the tissue immediately adjacent to the implant graft (Nishibe et al. 2007). Several groups have chosen a different route of improvement and dedicated their efforts to surface modification with known anticoagulants commonly utilized in the medical field in hopes of decreasing long-term thrombogenicity of synthetic implant materials (Murugesan et al. 2008; Rabenstein 2002).

The Allure of Natural Biopolymers

When deciding on the optimum material for a vascular graft, one should keep in mind the aforementioned "ideal" properties for such a scaffold. The two main categories of available scaffolds are biological and synthetic (Table 3.4). Biological scaffolds are naturally occurring biocompatible molecules to which cells readily bind and onto which cells proliferate; however, biological scaffolds generally have insufficient mechanical properties and have a tendency to degenerate rapidly after implantation. These properties can be better controlled using chemical or physical methods of cross-linking or stabilization, which reduce biodegradability and enhance tensile strength. Synthetic scaffolds share the major advantages that material properties can be tailored to the target tissue or organ, are easy to process, and are consistent between batches. Some polymers exhibit poor cellular interactions and may also leach residual monomers, catalysts, and degradation by-products that may be toxic or elicit inflammation.

Choosing the appropriate source of scaffolds depends greatly on desired properties of the target tissue. If the implant needs to function mechanically immediately after implantation (e.g., heart valve, artery, knee replacement), a strong scaffold is needed that allows few changes in mechanical properties with time as this will impair functionality. For skin and wound dressing regeneration, it is beneficial that the scaffold degrades completely and allows rapid regeneration; thus a rapidly degradable biological scaffold may be optimal. If the targeted tissue is metabolically active (liver, pancreas), one may choose a strong, porous biocompatible scaffold that degrades slowly.

What often leads researchers to use biopolymers such as collagen- or elastin-based proteins are the unique properties of said biopolymers, which often already provide ideal characteristics due to their natural origins. For example, elastin provides elasticity to tissues to achieve necessary compliance and cyclic fatigue strength and has been shown to function as a completely nonthrombogenic surface (Wise et al. 2009; Waterhouse et al. 2011). Collagen-based scaffolds, conversely, provide rigidity that will not only impart mechanical strength and the potential for rapid degradation and remodeling, but also contribute to thrombus formation due to the material's known high thrombogenicity.

One example of successful biological polymers currently in use would be bioprosthetic heart valves, which essentially are highly cross-linked,

TABLE 3.4
Brief Overview of Characteristics and History of Biological Vascular Grafts

	Biological Vascular Grafts			
	Autografts		Allografts (Homografts)	Xenografts (Heterografts)
	Arterial	Venous	Arterial	Venous
Advantages	Closest approximation, less diameter mismatch, internal mammary artery anatomically nearby, excellent function	Durable and versatile, good results, infection resistance, relative availability	Off-the-shelf availability, better resistance to infection, transplant-recipient patients	
Disadvantages	Availability, vasospasm (radial artery), donor site morbidity	Availability, harvest injury, vein graft disease	Antigenicity, graft deterioration, early occlusions, chronic rejection, intake of drugs, infection risk	
Healing	Intimal thickening, myointimal hyperplasia (radial artery)	Endothelial desquamation, vein dilation, wall thickening, arterialization, reendothelialization	Endothelial denudation, immune response, fibrotization	
First use	Jaboulay and Briau 1896	Goyannes 1906	Gross et al. 1948	Linton 1955
Review, for example	Nezic et al. 2006	Cooper et al. 1996	Fahner et al. 2006	Dardik et al. 2002 Schmidt and Baier 2000

Source: Chlupac, J., Filova, E., and Bacakova, L. 2009. Blood vessel replacement: 50 years of development and tissue engineering paradigms in vascular surgery. *Physiological Research* 58(2):S119–39. With permission.

nondegradable animal tissue scaffolds. These biomaterials perform very well mechanically and do not require anticoagulant or immunosuppressive therapies but fall prey to degeneration and calcification (Simionescu 2004; Bracher et al. 2001).

With the combination of necessary mechanical properties and coveted *in vivo* biocompatibility, biopolymers are often the "natural" choice for researchers. Interestingly, researchers observe that neither purified collagen- nor elastin-based vascular replacements retain sufficient mechanical properties when used separately for functional vascular replacements in arterial positions (Patel et al. 2006). This has prompted investigators to attempt to upregulate elastin biosynthesis to supplement three-dimensional scaffolds in hopes of improving scaffold mechanical and biocompatibility properties, as well as capitalizing on elastin's recently discovered bioactivity and nonthrombogenicity (Patel et al. 2006; Daamen et al. 2007; Waterhouse et al. 2011).

Current Biopolymer Options: Collagen

The extracellular matrix (ECM) protein collagen exists in the body in numerous forms, including fine fibers, intricate fibrils, delicate bundles, or strong flat sheets. Collagen has a rapid turnover and is deposited rapidly into *in vivo* implants in the form of either a fibrous capsule surrounding the implant, indicating a host response that can lead to implant rejection, or a neocollagen formation within the matrix of the implant. Such neocollagen formation often indicates a positive implant remodeling. As the most abundant protein in the body (Isenburg, B.C. et al. 2006), collagen is readily available and has been experimented with thoroughly in the literature for the purpose of engineering vascular grafts; an example of such is discussed next.

One current methodology for using this ECM protein includes electrospinning (Figure 3.3), a process in which the fibers are spun with varying voltages, distances between the plate and needle, and solvents to dissolve the fiber for the process. Readers are directed to a thorough review of electrospinning technology and the potential applications of the methodology by Prabhakaran and coworkers (2011). With experimentation into hydrogel-based substrates generally producing inadequate mechanical properties for the vascular constructs as discussed by Patel and colleagues (Patel et al. 2006), researchers began to investigate mechanical conditioning on hydrogels in hopes of elucidating keys to increased mechanical strength for hydrogel-based vascular constructs. It was later suggested by L'Heureux and coworkers (1993) that mechanical forces should be applied to collagen gels to induce alignment of collagen fibrils and seeded smooth muscle cells in circumferential fashion, as seen in natural vessels (Barocas et al. 1998; Grassl et al. 2003). When this methodology was first applied in attempts to produce

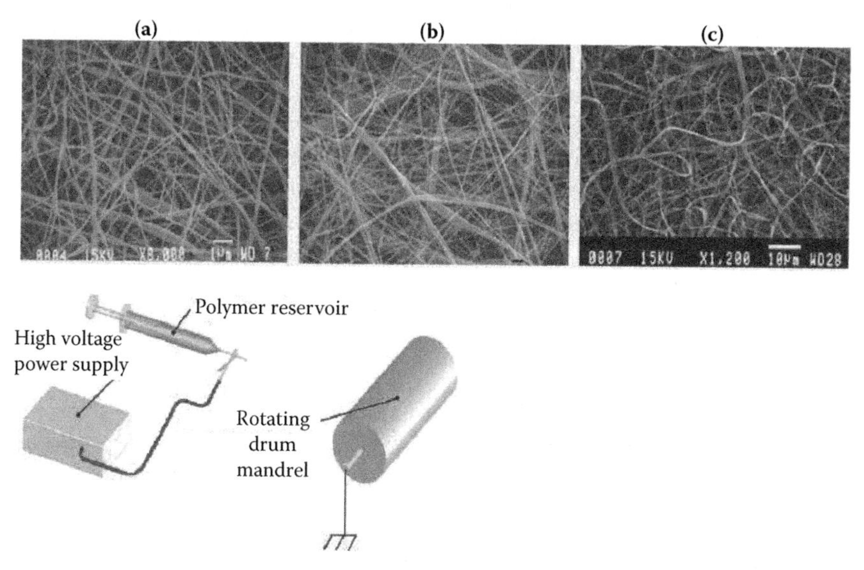

FIGURE 3.3
Scanning electron micrographs of (a) electrospun type I collagen (×8,000, scale bar 1.0 mm); (b) electrospun type III collagen (×4,300, scale bar 1.0 mm); and (c) electrospun collagen type IV collagen (×1,200, scale bar 10 mm). (Figure 3.3a from Boland, E.D., et al. 2004. Electrospinning collagen and elastin: preliminary vascular tissue engineering. *Frontiers in Bioscience: A Journal and Virtual Library* 9:1422–32. With permission. Figures 3.3b and 3.3c reprinted from Barnes, C.P., et al. 2007. Nanofiber technology: Designing the next generation of tissue engineering scaffolds. *Advanced Drug Delivery Reviews* 59:1413–33, copyright 2007. With permission.) (Bottom) Schematic representation of simple electrospinning setup using a grounded rotating drum as a collection mandrel. (Reprinted from Sell, S.A., et al. 2009. Electrospinning of collagen/biopolymers for regenerative medicine and cardiovascular tissue engineering. *Advanced Drug Delivery Reviews* 61:1007–19. With permission.)

a hollow, cylindrical artery using a mandrel-based approach by Hirai and Matsuda (1996), mechanical strength was not sufficient for implantation into arterial positions. Follow-up experimentation utilized glycation mechanisms in addition to lysyl oxidase-based cross-linking of fibers; however, again, mechanical strength of the collagen-based gels proved to be insufficient (Girton et al. 2000; Elbjeirami et al. 2003). These findings suggest that vascular grafts based on collagen require supplementation with smooth muscle cells that maintain matrix homeostasis, elastin to improve resilience, and finally an endothelial cell layer to prevent thrombogenicity (Patel et al. 2006).

Current Biopolymer Options: Elastin

Elastin is a very hydrophobic, "rubbery," highly cross-linked insoluble protein endowed with one of the slowest turnover rates in the human body. Due to this property, once elastin is degraded or significantly altered (as in aortic aneurysms, Marfan's syndrome, medial arterial elastocalcinosis), elastin is not replenished by resident cells. Elastin provides properties tantamount to a functional tissue-engineered vessel and is widely known for the resilience it imparts to biological tissues (Wise et al. 2009). For a tissue engineered vascular graft to be remodeled by the host with acceptable mechanical properties, said construct should induce elastin biosynthesis during remodeling *in vivo* or perhaps somehow graft tropoelastin to existing matrix fibers to endow the implant with increased elasticity and resilience. However, currently there have been no large successes in elastin biosynthesis or tropoelastin grafting for tissue engineered constructs.

An example of previous efforts conducted in the field to incite elastin biosynthesis utilized combinations of fibrin and collagen. Other growth factors and conditions involving smooth muscle cells known to produce the coveted elastin were utilized in these experiments, but no elastin was produced by the efforts of said groups (Weinberg and Bell 1986; L'Heureux et al. 1993; Hirai and Matsuda 1996; Long and Tranquillo 2003). Research into differences between fibrin- and collagen-based hydrogel scaffolds conducted by Long and Tranquillo did, however, elucidate that when murine neonatal smooth muscle cells are seeded into both collagen and fibrin gels, the fibrin gels produce significantly more elastin than those made of collagen, indicating that perhaps fibrin is a much more favorable substrate for elastin biosynthesis (Long and Tranquillo 2003). Investigating the effects of another hydrogel substrate on elastin biosynthesis, work done by Ramamurthi's group compared performance of neonatal rat smooth muscle cells in both hyaluronan gels and monolayer conditions on tissue culture polystyrene. The results showed that elastin was indeed produced and in the fenestrated form native to the internal elastic lamina and concentric lamellae inside the media of blood vessels (Ramamurthi and Vesely 2005). The research from these groups suggested that elastin biosynthesis is upregulated when used in specific 3D substrates, but the key ingredients necessary to repeatedly and dependably produce elastin are not fully understood.

Tissue Decellularization: The Alternative to Polymeric Fabrication

The act of gathering specific biologically inspired polymers and integrating them methodically and precisely into a mechanically stable structure via hydrogels, mandrels, or other commonly utilized substrates is a technique favored by many research groups. This particular methodology can easily be included in the category of a "bottom-up" fabrication approach in which a biologically viable scaffold is essentially "created from scratch." This process retains advantages due to the seemingly unlimited variability afforded by such a technique, in which the researcher specifically selects the desired components and implements them into a scaffold.

However, investigators in the field are also adopting a more "top-down" approach for scaffold fabrication. For this process, donor tissue of either xenogenic or human origin is meticulously treated to remove the undesired antigens, soluble proteins, and cellular remnants. This step, referred to as *decellularization*, is essential because of the possibility of immune rejection on implantation. A second prerequisite is to ensure that the ECM composition and 3D integrity are fully retained after decellularization. This in turn will determine mechanical properties of the scaffolds. This process is also similarly advantageous in that researchers can fine-tune their approach to retain specific ECM compositions and porosities while further augmenting their process by choosing a different donor tissue as deemed necessary. An example of such would be the choice of either a muscular or elastic artery for decellularization and scaffold treatment: Each artery type will provide different mechanical properties and porosity, which is discussed more thoroughly in this chapter.

With the advent of decellularization for production of tissue-engineered scaffolds came numerous questions regarding the extent of decellularization needed to retain necessary mechanical properties (Gilbert et al. 2006). However, the question of the extent of decellularization with respect to leftover nucleic acids and the consequences of such a presence in a scaffold has been explored thoroughly since then (Crapo et al. 2011). With this newfound understanding, researchers often are combining several known decellularization methods, such as detergents, acids/bases, alcohols, and biologic agents such as nucleases and proteases. Crapo and coworkers clarified that the choice of the optimum decellularization medium is often determined by four components: (a) cell density, (b) total cell content, (c) lipid content, and (d) thickness (Crapo et al. 2011). Readers are directed to this excellent review for further details regarding current clinical options and mechanisms utilized to deliver the necessary treatment agents to the tissue as well as a general overview of possible sterilization options for biological scaffolds, and their consequences of use, before implantation and use.

Following successful decellularization of a scaffold, the researcher must then characterize the scaffold with respect to mechanical properties, biological properties, and host cell ingrowth potential as well as porosity of the scaffold as described previously (see the section "Necessary Properties for the Ideal Vascular Graft") (Sarkar et al. 2007). Pending *in vitro* properties, the scaffold is then ready for the initial *in vivo* biocompatibility test for scaffolds, subcutaneous implantation in a small animal model, to assess the potential for inflammation and calcification on functional implantation. A functional implantation utilizes a large-animal model and necessitates the implantation of the fully prepared scaffold in the position it was originally intended; evaluation for mechanical and biocompatible properties follows. For example, a tissue-engineered aortic valve would be implanted in the position of the aortic valve within a large animal. Pending successful large-animal studies, the potential for clinical trials arises in which the scaffold is implanted in human patients; efficacy is then again evaluated. The Food and Drug Administration (FDA) investigation begins, with positive results holding promise for finally bringing the device to market.

Application of Decellularization in Vascular Tissue Engineering

Before the Holy Grail of getting a tissue-engineered scaffold to market, extensive research is necessary (Figure 3.4). Research from our group focuses on decellularization mechanisms of scaffold preparation and is applied to vascular grafts, heart valves, myocardium, and the nucleus pulposus found in intervertebral discs (Chuang et al. 2009; Sierad et al. 2010; Tedder et al. 2011; Mercuri et al. 2011; Isenburg et al. 2005; Simionescu et al. 2011), all of which make use of natural polymers. For vascular scaffolds in particular, this route of scaffold production has the advantage of retaining mature elastin, a highly cross-linked protein no longer turned over past neonatal development (Patel et al. 2006), inside the scaffold; the benefits of such have been described previously. However, Isenburg and colleagues clearly demonstrated that simply retaining elastin inside a scaffold is not sufficient for producing a biologically viable scaffold (Isenburg et al. 2004) because of its natural tendency to hastily degrade *in vivo* (Chuang et al. 2009) as a result of matrix-degrading proteases.

To circumvent this issue, our approach is to stabilize scaffolds with compounds that bind to matrix components and decrease their degradation *in vivo* but not completely annihilate them. Our group utilizes naturally derived phenolic tannins to achieve this partial and reversible fixation, thereby remaining in the realm of "natural" components for vascular tissue engineering.

Penta-galloyl-glucose (PGG) is a polyphenol (Tedder et al. 2009) naturally derived from tannic acid (Figure 3.5) that shows particularly high affinity for proline-rich proteins (Charlton et al. 1996) such as collagen and elastin (Luck et al. 1994), to which it binds strongly via hydrophobic and hydrogen bonds. Our group has reported the use of PGG to stabilize cardiovascular collagen scaffolds (Tedder et al. 2009) in addition to vascular elastin scaffolds (Chuang et al. 2009). Furthermore, we have showed that treatment with PGG diminishes vascular calcification (Chuang et al 2009). PGG is a

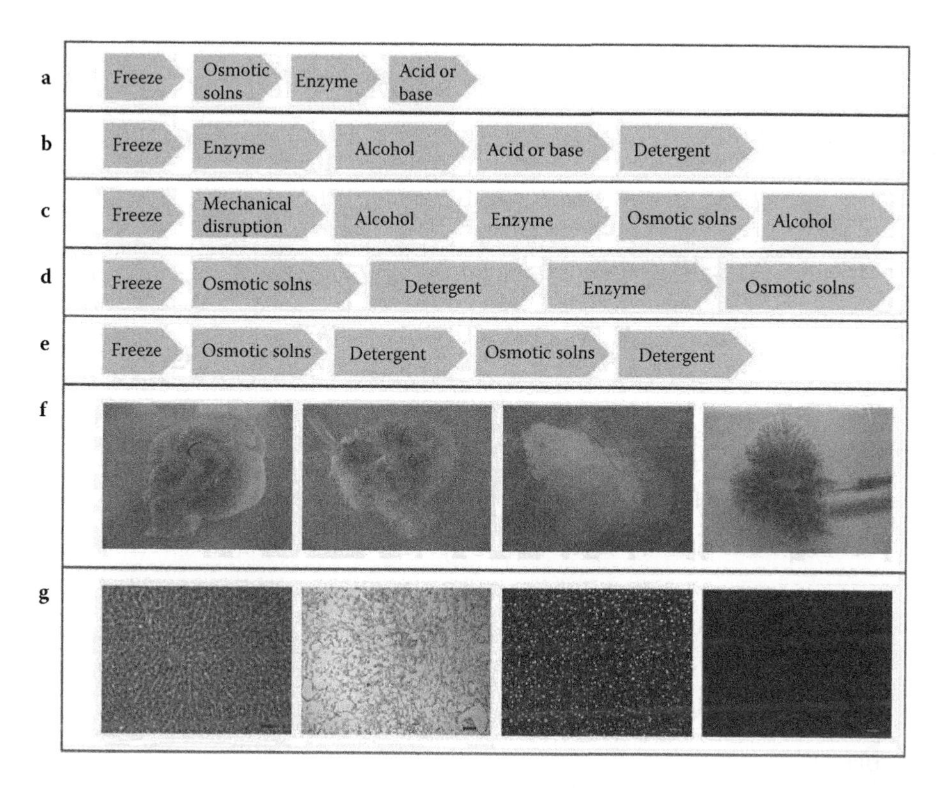

FIGURE 3.4 (see color figure)
Example decellularization protocols for (a) thin laminates such as pericardium; (b) thicker laminates such as dermis; (c) fatty, amorphous tissues such as adipose; (d) composite tissues or whole simple organs such as trachea; and (e) whole vital organs such as liver. Arrow lengths represent relative exposure times for each processing step. Rinse steps for agent removal and sterilization methods are not shown to simplify comparison. (f) Representative images of the gross appearance of intact rat liver subjected to decellularization (left to right): before, during, and after decellularization; decellularized liver perfused with blue dye. (g) Representative photomicrographs showing no nuclear staining after whole-organ decellularization (left to right): native rat liver hematoxylin and eosin (H&E); decellularized liver ECM H&E; native rat liver DAPI (4′,6-diamidino-2-phenylindole); liver ECM DAPI. Scale bars are 50 mm. (From Crapo, P.M., Gilbert, T.W., and Badylak, S.F. 2011. An overview of tissue and whole organ decellularization processes. *Biomaterials* 32:3233–43. With permission.)

strong antioxidant (Piao et al. 2008; Choi et al. 2002), inhibits many proteases, reduces inflammation and antigenicity (Haslam 1989), and is not cytotoxic (Isenburg J.C. et al. 2007; Isenburg B.C. et al. 2006) and thus can be used safely in tissue-engineering applications. In addition to the properties that fixation with PGG grants a tissue, the created bonds degrade over time to bestow robust mechanical strength initially on implantation and gradually allow for implant remodeling *in vivo* (Tedder et al. 2009), a desired biological property of all tissue-engineered constructs.

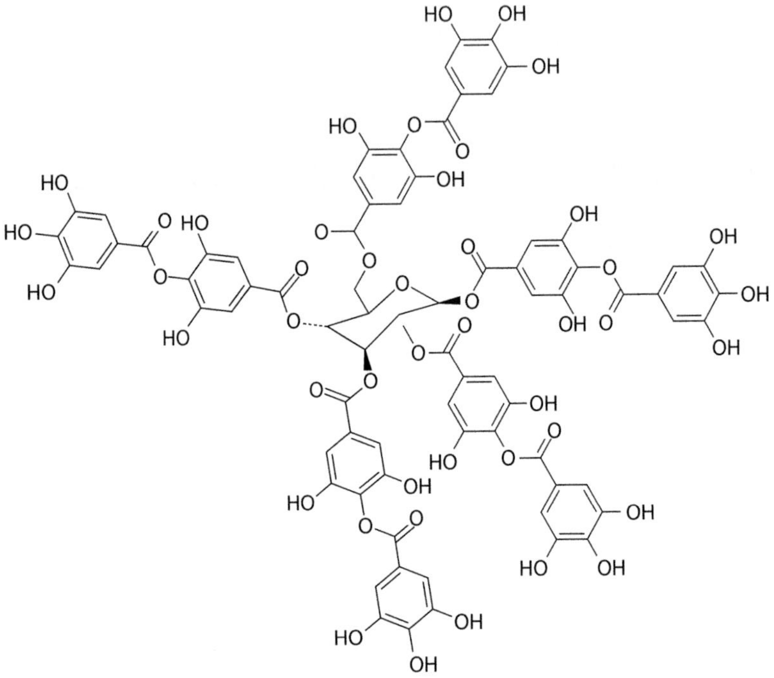

FIGURE 3.5
Structure of tannic acid. A central glucose molecule is esterified with gallic acid at all five hydroxyl moieties, resulting in a penta-galloyl glucose core. This may be further derivatized by gallic acid residues, yielding a deca-galloyl-glucose, as necessary. (Isenburg, J.C., Simionescu, D.T. and Vyavahare, N.R.. 2004. Elastin stabilization in cardiovascular implants: improved resistance to enzymatic degradation by treatment with tannic acid. *Biomaterials* 25:3293–302. With permission.)

The Future of Bioengineering: Clinically Translational Research

Most researchers in the field are familiar with the briefly discussed and highly difficult process of bringing a medical device or implant to clinical trials. Such successful individuals have accomplished the task of producing clinically viable implants. However, few researchers are able to consolidate their science into a small device easily usable by clinicians, nurses, and other medical faculty in a hospital setting without any supervision by the inventor of said technology. With the majority of "translational" literature surrounding the often-discussed topic of stem cell treatments (Banjeree et al. 2011), the potential for improvement in this area is recognized. Furthermore, fully automated machines remove the issue of batch-to-batch reproducibility that is innate to anything that has to be done by hand with human supervision.

By incorporating a researcher's science into a theoretical device capable of creating patient-tailored implants at the push of a button, one has created a translational device, a device that successfully bridges the gap between lab bench and patient bedside. Although a lofty goal for all researchers, this is arguably the future of regenerative medicine, one in which implanted devices will be unique to each patient and not require meticulous sizing in operating rooms, as is currently done with the majority of cardiovascular implantation procedures. Time will tell if such dreams are valid and whether we have the resources to bring science to the patient, our prime target as bioengineers.

References

Banerjee, C. 2011. Stem cells therapies in basic science and translational medicine: current status and treatment monitoring strategies. *Current Pharmaceutical Biotechnology* 12:469–87.

Barnes, C.P., et al. 2007. Nanofiber technology: designing the next generation of tissue engineering scaffolds. *Advanced Drug Delivery Reviews* 59:1413–33.

Barocas, V.H., Girton, T.S., and Tranquillo, R.T. 1998. Engineered alignment in media equivalents: magnetic prealignment and mandrel compaction. *Journal of Biomechanical Engineering* 120:660–66.

Barrett, D.G., and Yousaf, M.N. 2010. Thermosets synthesized by thermal polyesterification for tissue engineering applications. *Soft Matter* 6:5026–36.

Bezuidenhout, D., and Zilla, P. 2004. Vascular grafts. In *Encyclopaedia of Biomaterials and Biomedical Engineering*. G.L. Bowlin and G.E. Wnek, Eds., Informa Healthcare, NY.

Boland, E.D., et al. 2004. Electrospinning collagen and elastin: preliminary vascular tissue engineering. *Frontiers in Bioscience: A Journal and Virtual Library* 9:1422–32.

Bracher, M., et al. 2001. Matrix metalloproteinases and tissue valve degeneration. *Journal of Long-Term Effects of Medical Implants* 11:221–30.

Charlton, A.J., et al. 1996. Tannin interactions with a full-length human salivary proline-rich protein display a stronger affinity than with single proline-rich repeats. *FEBS Letters* 382(3):289–92.

Chlupac, J., Filova, E., and Bacakova, L. 2009. Blood vessel replacement: 50 years of development and tissue engineering paradigms in vascular surgery. *Physiological Research* 58(Supplement 2):S119–39.

Choi, B.M., et al. 2002. 1,2,3,4,6-Penta-O-galloyl-beta-D-glucose protects rat neuronal cells (Neuro 2A) from hydrogen peroxide-mediated cell death via the induction of heme oxygenase-1. *Neuroscience Letters* 328:185–89.

Chuang, T.H., et al. 2009. Polyphenol-stabilized tubular elastin scaffolds for tissue engineered vascular grafts. *Tissue Engineering Part A* 5:2837–51.

Crapo, P.M., Gilbert, T.W., and Badylak, S.F. 2011. An overview of tissue and whole organ decellularization processes. *Biomaterials* 32:3233–43.

Creech, O.J., et al. 1957. Vascular prostheses; report of the Committee for the Study of Vascular Prostheses of the Society for Vascular Surgery. *Surgery* 41:62–80.

Daamen, W.F., et al. 2007. Elastin as a biomaterial for tissue engineering. *Biomaterials* 28:4378–98.

Elbjeirami, W.M., et al. 2003. Enhancing mechanical properties of tissue-engineered constructs via lysyl oxidase crosslinking activity. *Journal of Biomedical Materials Research Part A* 66:513–21.

Gilbert, T.W., Sellaro, T.L., and Badylak, S.F. 2006. Decellularization of tissues and organs. *Biomaterials* 27:3675–83.

Girton, T.S., et al. 2000. Mechanisms of stiffening and strengthening in media-equivalents fabricated using glycation. *Journal of Biomechanical Engineering* 122:216–23.

Grassl, E.D., Oegema, T.R., and Tranquillo, R.T. 2003. A fibrin-based arterial media equivalent. *Journal of Biomedical Materials Research Part A* 66:550–61.

Haslam, E. 1989. Plant polyphenols; vegetable tannins revisited. In *Chemistry and Pharmacology of Natural Products,* ed. J. Phillipson. Cambridge, UK: Cambridge University Press, pp. 167–195.

Hirai, J., and Matsuda, T. 1995. Self-organized, tubular hybrid vascular tissue composed of vascular cells and collagen for low-pressure-loaded venous system. *Cell Transplantation* 4:597–608.

Hirai, J., and Matsuda, T. 1996. Venous reconstruction using hybrid vascular tissue composed of vascular cells and collagen: tissue regeneration process. *Cell Transplantation* 5(1):93–105.

Isenberg, B.C., Williams, C., and Tranquillo, R.T. 2006. Small-diameter artificial arteries engineered *in vitro*. *Circulation Research* 98(1):25–35.

Isenburg, J.C., Simionescu, D.T., and Vyavahare, N.R. 2004. Elastin stabilization in cardiovascular implants: improved resistance to enzymatic degradation by treatment with tannic acid. *Biomaterials* 25:3293–3302.

Isenburg, J., Simionescu, D.T., and Vyavahare, N.R. 2005. Tannic acid treatment enhances biostability and reduces calcification of glutaraldehyde fixed aortic wall. *Biomaterials* 26:1237–45.

Isenburg, J.C., et al. 2006. Structural requirements for stabilization of vascular elastin by polyphenolic tannins. *Biomaterials* 27:3645–51.

Isenburg, J.C., et al. 2007. Elastin stabilization for treatment of abdominal aortic aneurysms. *Circulation* 115:1729–37.

Jaboulay M., Briau E. 1896. Recherches expérimentelles sur la suture et la greffe artérielles. *Lyon Méd* 81:97–99.

Junqueira, L.C., and J. Cameiro, eds. 2005. *Basic Histology: Text and Atlas.* 11th ed. New York: McGraw Hill, pp. 206–7.

L'Heureux, N., et al. 1993. *In vitro* construction of a human blood vessel from cultured vascular cells: a morphologic study. *Journal of Vascular Surgery* 17:499–509.

Long, J.L., and Tranquillo, R.T. 2003. Elastic fiber production in cardiovascular tissue-equivalents. *Matrix Biology: Journal of the International Society for Matrix Biology* 22:339–50.

Luck, G., et al. 1994. Polyphenols, astringency and proline-rich proteins. *Phytochemistry* 37:357–71.

Mercuri, J.J., Gill, S.S., and Simionescu, D.T. 2011. Novel tissue-derived biomimetic scaffold for regenerating the human nucleus pulposus. *Journal of Biomedical Materials Research Part A* 96:422–35.

Murugesan, S., Xie, J., and Linhardt, R.J. 2008. Immobilization of heparin: approaches and applications. *Current Topics in Medicinal Chemistry* 8:80–100.

Niklason, L.E., and Langer, R.S. 1997. Advances in tissue engineering of blood vessels and other tissues. *Transplant Immunology* 5:303–6.

Nishibe, T., et al. 2007. Optimal prosthetic graft design for small diameter vascular grafts. *Vascular* 15:356–60.

Patel, A., et al. 2006. Elastin biosynthesis: the missing link in tissue-engineered blood vessels. *Cardiovascular Research* 71:40–49.

Piao, X., et al. 2008. Antioxidative activity of geranium (*Pelargonium inquinans* Ait) and its active component, 1,2,3,4,6-penta-O-galloyl-beta-D-glucose. *Phytotherapy Research* 22:534–38.

Prabhakaran, M.P., Ghasemi-Mobarakeh, L., and Ramakrishna, S. 2011. Electrospun composite nanofibers for tissue regeneration. *Journal of Nanoscience and Nanotechnology* 11:3039–57.

Rabenstein, D.L. 2002. Heparin and heparan sulfate: structure and function. *Natural Product Reports* 19:312–31.

Ramamurthi, A., and Vesely, I. 2005. Evaluation of the matrix-synthesis potential of crosslinked hyaluronan gels for tissue engineering of aortic heart valves. *Biomaterials* 26:999–1010.

Sarkar, S., et al. 2007. Achieving the ideal properties for vascular bypass grafts using a tissue engineered approach: a review. *Medical and Biological Engineering and Computing* 45:327–36.

Sell, S.A., et al. 2009. Electrospinning of collagen/biopolymers for regenerative medicine and cardiovascular tissue engineering. *Advanced Drug Delivery Reviews* 61:1007–19.

Sierad, L.N., et al. 2010. Design and testing of a pulsatile conditioning system for dynamic endothelialization of polyphenol-stabilized tissue engineered heart valves. *Cardiovascular Engineering and Technology* 1:138–53.

Simionescu, A., et al. 2011. Lectin and antibody-based histochemical techniques for cardiovascular tissue engineering. *Journal of Histotechnology* 34:20–29.

Simionescu, D.T. 2004. Prevention of calcification in bioprosthetic heart valves: challenges and perspectives. *Expert Opinions in Biological Therapy* 4:1971–85.

Simpson, C.L., et al. 2007. Toward cell therapy for vascular calcification: osteoclast-mediated demineralization of calcified elastin. *Cardiovascular Pathology* 16:29–37.

Tedder, M.E., et al. 2009. Stabilized collagen scaffolds for heart valve tissue engineering. *Tissue Engineering Part A* 15:1257–68.

Tedder, M.E., et al. 2011. Assembly and testing of stem cell-seeded layered collagen constructs for heart valve tissue engineering. *Tissue Engineering Part A* 17:25–36.

Veith, F.J., et al. 1986. Six-year prospective multicenter randomized comparison of autologous saphenous vein and expanded polytetrafluoroethylene grafts in infrainguinal arterial reconstructions. *Journal of Vascular Surgery* 3:104–14.

Voorhees, A.B., Jr., Jaretzki, A., 3rd, and Blakemore, A.H. 1952. The use of tubes constructed from vinyon "N" cloth in bridging arterial defects. *Annals of Surgery* 135:332–36.

Waterhouse, A., et al. 2011. Elastin as a nonthrombogenic biomaterial. *Tissue Engineering Part B* 17:93–99.

Weinberg, C.B., and Bell, E. 1986. A blood vessel model constructed from collagen and cultured vascular cells. *Science* 231:397–400.

Wise, S.G., Mithieux, S.M., and Weiss, A.S. 2009. Engineered tropoelastin and elastin-based biomaterials. *Advances in Protein Chemistry and Structural Biology* 78:1–24.

Zdrahala, R.J. 1996. Small caliber vascular grafts. Part II: Polyurethanes revisited. *Journal of Biomaterials Applications* 11:37–61.

4

Polymeric Materials for Vascular Grafts

Shawn J. Peniston and Georgios T. Hilas

CONTENTS

Introduction

Background and Clinical Relevance

The search for a patent vascular graft has attracted much attention from researchers and physicians due to the significant number of mortalities in the Western world each year from vascular disease. Vascular bypass grafting for coronary artery and peripheral vascular disease (atherosclerosis) account for the majority of bypass procedures; in addition, the repair of thoracic and abdominal aneurysms is also a prominent use of vascular grafts. Several procedures are now available for physicians to treat vascular disease.

The development of minimally invasive endovascular procedures such as percutaneous angioplasty, atherectomy, stenting, and laser angioplasty can open occluded vessels. However, these procedures require access using the catheter technique and are not effective if access is physically impossible or extensive occlusion has developed. Consequently, an open bypass surgical procedure using an autologous or prosthetic vascular graft is the only clinical alternative. As a result, 600,000 coronary and peripheral bypass procedures (Ravi, Qu, and Chaikof 2009) are performed each year in the United States, most commonly with the saphenous vein or internal mammary artery. However, 30% of patients (Veith, Moss, Sprayregen, and Montefusco 1979) have inadequate or insufficient tissue. These patients require the use of a substitute vascular conduit.

Prosthetic vascular grafts comprised of polyethylene terephthalate (PET) and polytetrafluoroethylene (PTFE) are the primary clinical options. These grafts are biocompatible in the sense that they are stable in the biologic environment and nontoxic, but they are not blood compatible and do not possess the viscoelastic or biomechanical properties of the native artery. The success of using prosthetic vascular grafts has been acceptable for large (12- to 38-mm) arteries, marginal for medium (6- to 12-mm) arteries, and not viable for small arteries (<6 mm). In the case of coronary arteries, the replacement size is less than 6 mm. In part, the lack of a suitable synthetic option accounts for the high fatality rates from coronary artery disease, highlighting the clinical necessity of a vascular graft with improved patency. The development of a patent vascular graft for use in all bypass procedures has enormous commercial and humanitarian benefits. To this end, research has focused on improving vascular grafts by developing more compliant and blood-compatible biomaterials. In addition, the potential of regenerating vascular tissue has received significant attention in the last decade due the advancement of tissue engineering.

Biology of the Artery

To better grasp the challenges of duplicating the function of the artery, it is important to understand the basic biology of vascular tissue. The vascular wall functions as a dynamic, closed-loop system rather than an inactive conduit for blood. It is composed primarily of endothelial cells (ECs), smooth muscle cells (SMCs), fibroblasts, collagen, elastin, and glycosaminoglycans (GAGs). The vascular cells and the unique three-dimensional matrix of structural proteins have a high degree of interaction to function and remodel.

The vascular wall is commonly segmented into three layers based primarily on function: the intima, media, and adventitia (Figure 4.1). The intima is the blood contact surface and consists of a single layer of polygonal ECs. The vascular endothelium is responsible for several functions:

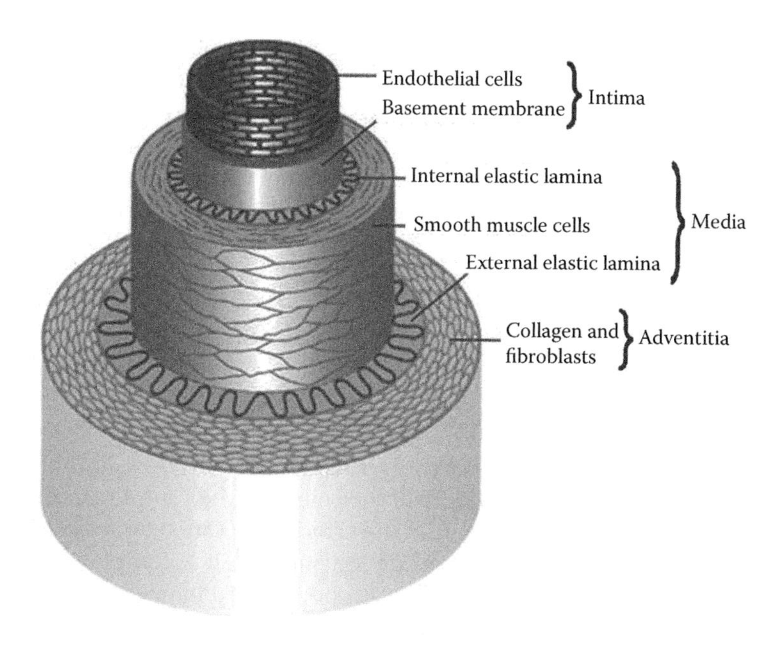

FIGURE 4.1
The anatomy of an artery depicted in layers. (From Sarkar S., Schmitz-Rixen T., Hamilton G., Seifilian A. 2007. Achieving the ideal properties for vascular bypass graft using tissue engineering approach: A review. *Med Biol Eng Comput* 45:327–36. With permission.)

hemostasis, regulation of vascular tone, synthesis of cytokines and growth factors, angiogenesis, selective transmission of inflammatory cells (diapedesis), and provision of a barrier function between blood and all other tissues. Under homeostatic conditions, ECs provide continuous chemical and physical signals to circulating blood components to prevent thrombosis and coagulation. Thrombosis formation occurs when platelets encounter a foreign material (collagen or synthetic polymer), resulting in the adhesion and release of adenosine diphosphate (ADP) and thromboxane. The release of ADP signals other platelets, and thromboxane promotes additional platelet aggregation. Furthermore, degranulated platelets initiate the formation of thrombin, which then converts blood-soluble fibrinogen into insoluble fibrin fibers resulting in coagulation. As such, ECs play a unique and critical role in maintaining the balance between being able to react quickly to a site of injury yet prevent potentially life-threatening blood-clotting episodes.

The endothelium is anchored to the media by a tie layer of connective tissue called the basement membrane, which is made up of type IV collagen, laminin, and fibronectin proteins. The internal- and external-elastic lamina are pronounced layers of elastic connective tissue that give arteries their unique balance of compliance, elastic recoil, and strength. The media is comprised of radial aligned sheets of elastin, cross-linked elastic connective tissue fibers, similar to the internal and external lamina, but less pronounced and separated by layers of SMCs. The media is largely responsible for the biomechanics of the artery, generating the contractile forces and participating in the elastic recoil within the arterial wall. The adventitia is constructed of axially aligned type I collagen fibers that provide radial resistance to arterial blood pressure and prevent excessive dilation. Overall, the artery wall is a complex composite structure with layers that each have specific functions yet interact to transport blood to tissue efficiently.

Vascular Graft Functional Requirements

The development of a patent vascular graft has proven to be exceptionally difficult. In part, the specialized nature of the cells and the complex structure of the extracellular matrix (ECM) within the arterial wall are responsible for this challenge. Consequently, vascular grafts must replicate a complex myriad of chemical signals and possess anisotropic, nonlinear biomechanical properties to function with a high degree of biocompatibility. Table 4.1 provides a summary of loosely categorized requirements for a vascular graft, with an understanding that there is significant interaction and overlap between categories. The degree of biocompatibility increases as the vascular graft design incorporates more of the requirements. In addition, for clinical acceptance the design of vascular grafts must consider the regulatory pathway, meet user needs within the surgical suite, and be commercially cost effective.

Clinically Relevant Vascular Grafts

Materials

Polyethylene Terephthalate

Polyethylene terephthalate (PET) is a synthetic polymer, commonly known under the trade name Dacron, that has been a viable vascular graft material for medium and large arterial replacements. PET is a heterochain linear aromatic polymer ($-C_{10}H_8O_4-$) with the characteristic feature of two ester linkages on either side of an aromatic ring in the backbone of the polymer chain. Consequently, the polymer is slightly polar, more hydrophilic, and more hygroscopic than homochain hydrocarbon polymers. The ester groups create chemically liable sites that are susceptible to hydrolysis. However, local hydrophobic moieties and high crystallinity slow this reaction considerably. The strong dipole-dipole-type van der Waals-London forces between adjacent carbonyl groups contribute to its high-strength characteristics.

TABLE 4.1

Vascular Graft Biocompatibility Requirements

Physical and Structural
Assortment of calibers and lengths to accommodate the patient population
Adequate porosity for tissue ingrowth and angiogenesis without significant blood loss
Confluent and intact intimal surface
Stratified vascular wall structure
Material
Low inflammatory response
Nonimmunogenic
Noncarcinogenic
Nonthrombogenic
Chemical stability in the biologic environment (permanent scaffolds)
Predictable degradation of absorbable scaffold materials
No leachable low molecular weight fractions (monomer, oligomer, impurities)
Resistance to infection for aseptic implantation
Biomechanical
Kink resistant
Elastic recoil
Mechanical strength to resist luminal burst pressure and axial stress
Viscoelasticity to accommodate efficient pulsatile blood flow
Compliance (radial and axial)
Tear resistance to secure sutures
Creep resistance
Fatigue resistance
Mechanical stability of the intimal surface to resist wall shear stress
Biochemical and Cellular Signaling
Ability to be repopulated and remodeled by the host cells
Active regulation of vascular tone
Development and maintenance of cell phenotype (biomechanical influence as well)
Continuous production of chemical factors to maintain thromboresistance
Selective permeability to inflammatory cells (diapedesis)

PET grafts are produced from multifilament yarn, which is woven or knitted into a fabric tube. Grafts produced using a woven structure show minimal fluid permeability and are mechanically stiff. In contrast, knitted grafts are more flexible and have increased porosity, leading to a higher degree of tissue ingrowth (Zilla, Bezuidenhout, and Human 2007). However, these properties are lost shortly after implantation due to tissue integration (Ravi, Qu, and Chaikof 2009). In addition, PET grafts are often crimped longitudinally or have external coils added to provide additional compression and kink resistance (Kannan, Salacinski, Butler, Hamilton, and Seifalian 2005). Although PET has been used as a vascular graft material since the 1970s, it does induce protein absorption, thrombosis, and leukocyte activation and migration. After 18 months in the *in vivo* environment, a pseudointema containing an inner layer of fibrin, an intermediate layer of foreign body giant cells, and an outer connective tissue layer develop to form a relatively thick, compact layer over the graft surface, with the greatest thickness at the proximal and distal ends and less in the midgraft region (Kannan, Salacinski, Butler, Hamilton, and Seifalian 2005; Greisler 2003). When PET is used for an aortal or thoracic arterial conduit, the relatively large diameter and high blood flow are forgiving to occlusions. In addition to blood compatibility issues, knitted PET grafts have shown a tendency to dilate with time (Kannan, Salacinski, Butler, Hamilton, and Seifalian 2005). This may be attributed to the susceptibility of PET to hydrolysis, possibly accelerated by enzymatic and oxidative attack by macrophages or foreign body giant cells, which are present after the first week of implantation and remain for the life of the implant (Smith, Oliver, and Williams 1987). However, due to their construction, PET grafts are more compliant than other commercially available materials. PET grafts used for aortic bypass have 5-year patency rates of 93%, and peripheral grafts have a 3-year patency rate of less than 45% (Xue and Greisler 2003). For these reasons, currently PET grafts are the preferred material for the replacement of large arteries.

Expanded Polytetrafluoroethylene

Polytetrafluoroethylene (PTFE) is a linear homochain polymer constructed of a carbon backbone saturated with fluorine atoms ($-CF_2-$). The characteristic feature of PTFE is its inert nature due to the extreme stability of the carbon-fluorine bond. Although highly crystalline, the intermolecular attraction between PTFE molecules is very small, which results in bulk properties that are inferior to other engineered polymers. The extreme perfection of the crystalline lattice of PTFE results in a melting point that is very close to its degradation temperature. As a result, PTFE does not possess a meaningful melt processing window. Accordingly, PTFE is manufactured by stretching and sintering a solid melt-extruded tube. This process gives rise to the "expanded" precursor designation (ePTFE). The result is a microporous node-fibril structure in which solid nodes connect through fine fibrils with an average internodal distance of 30 mm for a standard graft (Xue and Greisler 2003). The formation of micropores does increase graft compliance and create a porous substrate for the attachment of a pseudointema. However, standard ePTFE grafts are still two or three times stiffer than the natural artery. In an attempt to improve compliance, thin-walled ePTFE grafts have been developed that have an elastic stiffness 1.6 times that of the coronary artery (Jorgensen and Paaske 1998).

Small-diameter vascular grafts in low-flow conditions, such as below the knee, are prone to short-term occlusion from acute thrombosis. Although the blood compatibility of ePTFE is considered poor, its electronegative luminal surface lessens the onset of platelet adhesion and produces a thinner pseudointema. As a consequence, ePTFE has gained popularity in peripheral bypass applications for which occlusion results from thrombosis (Venkataraman, Boey, and Luciana 2008). However, in a multicenter, prospective, randomized trial investigating the use of a PET or ePTFE graft for femoropopliteal bypass surgery, there was no difference in patency rate after 3 years (Post et al. 2001). It was observed that PET performed slightly better than ePTFE in above-knee applications and worse in below-knee applications, but with no statistical difference. Roll and coworkers conducted a systemic evaluation and meta-analysis of randomized controlled trials comparing PET and ePTFE for peripheral bypass procedures and showed no evidence of an advantage of one synthetic material over the other (Roll et al. 2008). The preference of ePTFE grafts over PET for femoropopliteal bypass surgery is relatively unjustified since no significant difference in patency rates exists between the two materials (Lau and Cheng 2001). Overall, like PET grafts, the compliance mismatch and the lack of a functional endothelium account for ePTFE grafts having poor patency.

Polyurethanes

Polyurethanes are copolymers composed of alternating hard and soft segments, with the hard segments comprised of urethane linkages and the soft segments typically composed of ether or ester moieties. By varying the ratios of hard and soft segments, polyurethanes can be tailored to be elastic and compliant. They have been researched for years as a desirable biomaterial for vascular grafts because of their excellent compliance, fatigue resistance in flexure, tensile strength, high ultimate elongation, and relatively good blood compatibility. Unfortunately, the traditional polymer containing ester or ether soft segment linkages has *in vivo* stability issues with hydrolysis and oxidation, respectively. Consequently, the development of more hydrolytically and oxidatively stable variants that employ a polycarbonate polyol as the polymer soft segment has been investigated.

The first human trials have been initiated in Europe for a poly(carbonate) urethane-based prosthesis (Cardiopass, CardioTech International). In past studies on the predicate device to Cardiopass called MyoLink, the *in vivo* biostability of the poly(carbonate) urethane was challenged by exposing the polymer to *in vitro* solutions of hydrolytic, oxidative, peroxidative, and biological media. The findings showed excellent hydrolytic stability, especially when compared to conventional poly(ether) urethane controls (Salacinski, Odlyha, Hamilton, and Seifalian 2002; Salacinski, Tai, et al. 2002). In addition, a long-term biocompatibility study was completed *in vivo* on canine models that resulted in acceptable mechanical biostability at 3 years (Seifalian et al. 2002). The compliant nature of the MyoLink graft is due to a microporous, single-layer structure comprised of an inner and outer skin with a spongy, elastic middle section. When a bolus of blood enters the graft, the

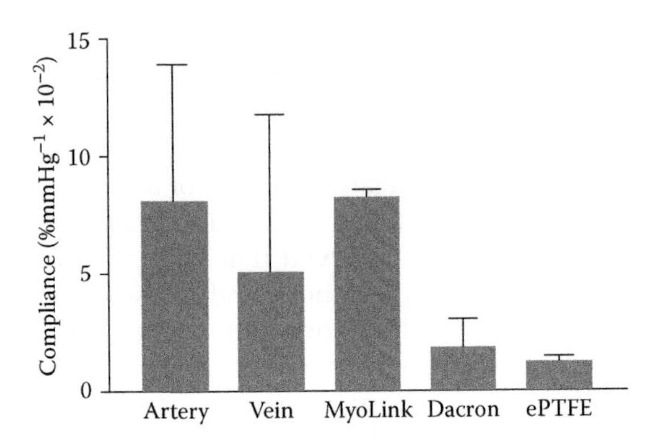

FIGURE 4.2
A comparison of the compliance values for several vascular graft materials and natural tissue. (From Tiwari A., Salacinski H., Seifalian A.M., Hamilton G. 2002. New prostheses for use in bypass grafts with special emphasis on polyurethanes. *Cardiovasc Surg* 10:191–97. With permission.)

inner diameter expands in an elastic manner, while the outside diameter remains relatively unchanged. This design provides radial compliance and conserves the energy of the pulsatile flow of blood through the prosthesis, which maintains a relatively constant wall shear stress (WSS). In addition, the compliant wall produces minimal bleeding from suture holes because the elastic nature of the poly(carbonate) urethane collapses together around the suture after the needle is pulled through the wall. Figure 4.2 compares the compliance of an artery, vein, PET, and ePTFE to MyoLink.

Other poly(carbonate) urethane-based vascular grafts have been developed that showed promising patency rates in rabbits (Ishii et al. 2007, 2008). This system possessed a microporous luminal lining of absorbable collagen and hyaluron that could incorporate heparin and sirolimus for time-controlled release. Heparin functions as an anticoagulant, while sirolimus reduces the proliferation of SMCs in a similar manner to its use in drug-eluting coronary stents. However, of primary concern is the development of an endothelium on the graft intimal surface. The use of sirolimus in drug-eluting coronary stents proved relatively unsafe as the drug prevented endothelialization of the stent surfaces, leading to thrombus formation and an increased risk for myocardial infarction (Luscher et al. 2007). In addition, a potential issue with a drug-eluting graft is that the drug will be exhausted prior to the required period of efficacy.

Poly(dimethyl siloxane) (PDMS) is another attractive soft segment for vascular grafts. PDMS-based polyurethanes show excellent biostability due to their hydrolytically and oxidatively stable siloxane groups (Martin et al. 2000; Simmons, Padsalgikar, Ferris, and Poole-Warren 2008). In addition, siloxanes produce chemically inert biomaterials, and thrombogenicity testing has revealed good blood compatibility (Tepe et al. 2006). A preliminary *in vivo* study in a sheep model was conducted to determine the blood and tissue compatibility of a novel compliant small-diameter vascular graft

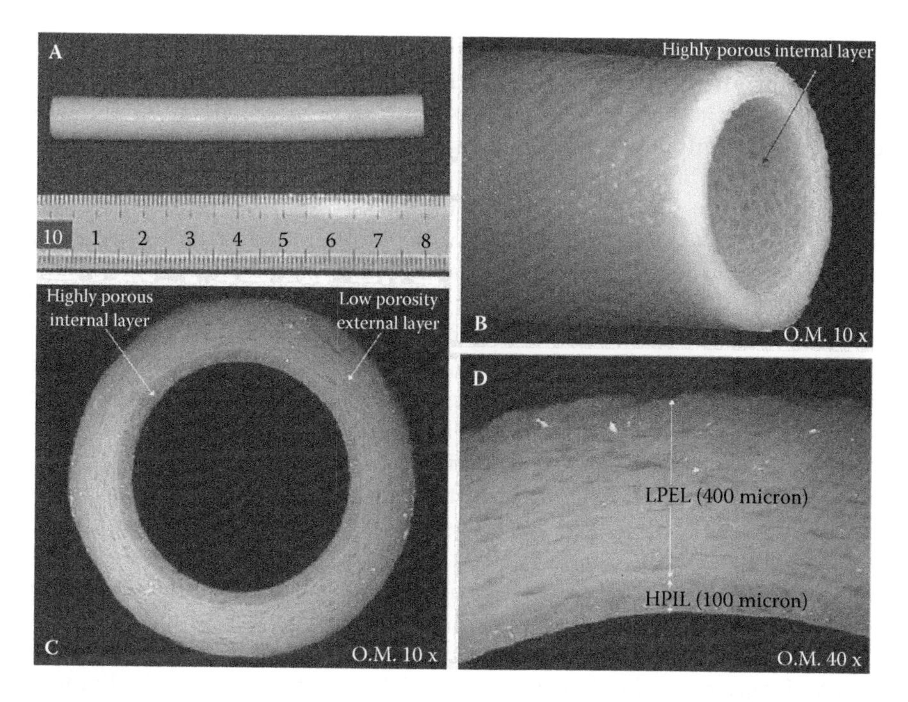

FIGURE 4.3
Representative poly(ether)urethane-PDMS semi-interpenetrating polymeric network used in a sheep model: (A) longitudinal view of graft, (B) tilted view of graft, (C) cross-sectional view of graft showing the sponge-like appearance of the graft wall (original magnification ×10), (D) higher magnification of the graft wall (original magnification ×40).

constructed from a poly(ether)urethane-PDMS semi-interpenetrating polymeric network (Figure 4.3) (Soldani et al. 2009). The graft had a highly porous inner layer and low-porosity external layer constructed using a spray phase-inversion technique. At 6 months, 50% of the ePTFE control grafts were occluded, while all of the PDMS-based grafts were still patent, with neointima formation and no signs of calcification. At 24 months, all PDMS-based grafts were patent, and the luminal surfaces were covered with a neointima. These results indicate that a PDMS-based polyurethane as a vascular graft material may be feasible for use in small-diameter graft applications.

Limitations and Insufficiencies of Current Vascular Grafts

Mechanical Compatibility

The importance of matching the compliance of vascular grafts to the native artery was first established in a canine model using autologous tissue

(Abbott, Megerman, Hasson, L'Italien, and Warnock 1987). Compliance matching or mismatching using carotid artery (1:1) and femoral artery (2:5) autografts resulted in 85% or 37% patency at 90 days postimplantation, respectively. Compliance mismatch is a significant challenge to long-term patency because it causes intimal hyperplasia (IH), which leads to graft occlusion. IH is a condition of tissue ingrowth into the luminal space that causes occlusion of the lumen due to the proliferation of SMCs from the media to the intima. Compliance mismatch between synthetic grafts and natural arteries causes hemodynamic disturbances at the anastomosis that can lead to turbulent flow and changes in WSS (Sarkar, Sales, Hamilton, and Seifalian 2007). Evidence suggested that both high and low shear stress can stimulate IH (Fei, Thomas, and Rittgers 1994). This response is complex, and the mechanisms and interactions are not completely understood; however, IH formation within the *in vivo* period of 2 to 24 months has been reported to be the primary cause of bypass graft failure (Sarkar, Salacinski, Hamilton, and Seifalian 2006). Furthermore, it has been demonstrated that a linear correlation between graft compliance and percentage patency exists (Figure 4.4) (Salacinski et al. 2001). IH can also be induced from size mismatch (Weston, Rhee, and Tarbell 1996). Divergent geometry can reduce WSS and may induce flow separation and turbulence, whereas convergent geometry will increase WSS and may cause EC injury and platelet activation. However, diameter mismatch has been reported to be less of a factor than compliance mismatch in the formation of IH (Perktold et al. 2002).

ePTFE and PET vascular grafts are incompliant, isotropic, biomechanically inactive, homogeneous conduits compared to the native artery, which is an elastic, anisotropic, dynamic, three-dimensional composite structure. As such, current vascular grafts lack the ability to provide mechanical transduction to developing neotissue that controls cell phenotype and ECM production. The viscoelasticity of the arterial wall is an important factor in

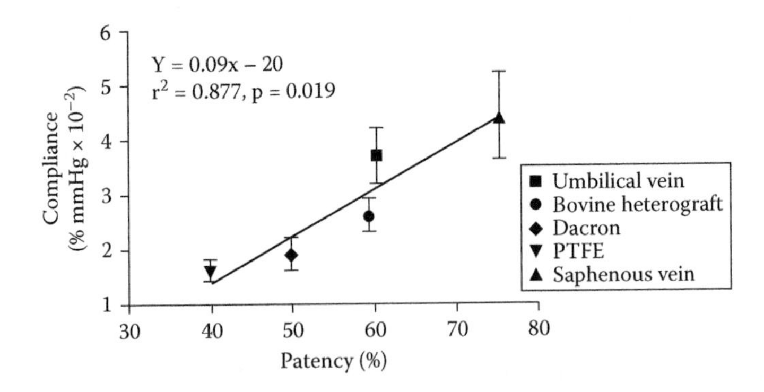

FIGURE 4.4
Data reported for the compliance of various biological and prosthetic grafts versus percentage patency. (From Salacinski H.J., Goldner S., Giudiceandrea A., et al. 2001. The mechanical behavior of vascular grafts: a review. *J Biomater Appl* 15:241–78. With permission.)

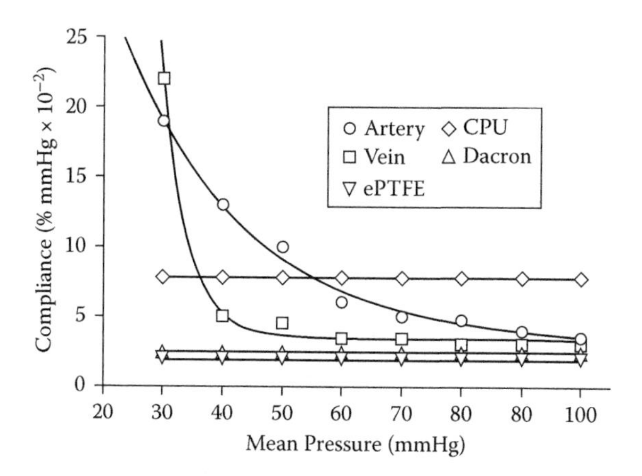

FIGURE 4.5 (see color figure)
Modulation of compliance as a function of mean pressure for different vascular conduits. (From Sarkar S., Salacinski H.J., Hamilton G., Seifalian A.M. 2006. The mechanical properties of infrainguinal vascular bypass grafts: their role in influencing patency. *Eur J Vasc Endovasc Surg* 31:627–36. With permission.)

preserving hemodynamic energy within pulsatile blood flow and maintaining WSS. In part, the success of autologous vein grafts results from their ability to respond dynamically to arterial pressure pulse waves in a manner similar to the native artery (Baird and Abbott 1976). Figure 4.5 shows the modulation of compliance as a function of changes in mean pressure for different vascular conduits. ECs perceive changes in WSS and via physical and chemical pathways transmit signals to the vessel wall that change vessel diameter, tone, SMC proliferation, lumen thrombogenicity, and ECM organization (Isenberg, Williams, and Tranquillo 2006). Synthetic vascular grafts are relatively incompliant and do not reproduce these dynamic characteristics (Tai, Salacinski, Edwards, Hamilton, and Seifalian 2000). An artery can increase its compliance in response to a decrease in blood pressure (shock or trauma) to preserve pulsatile energy (Salacinski et al. 2001).

Porosity and Surface Characteristics

Porosity, characterized by pore size and percentage pore area, is a major determining factor for tissue ingrowth at the suture lines and to facilitate the development of a luminal lining (Matsuda 2004). However, the porosity must be balanced between the competing requirements of tissue integration and minimal blood leakage through the graft wall *in situ*. Preclotting with either the patient's blood or using cross-linked coatings of proteins, such as albumin or gelatin, is used to prevent blood leakage through the graft at the time of implantation. In general, woven PET vascular grafts have smaller pores, while knitted grafts produce looping fibers (velour technique) that result in larger pores and facilitate greater tissue ingrowth (Bowald, Busch, and Eriksson 1979). For ePTFE grafts, animal models have indicated that internodal distance is a determining factor for tissue integration (Nagae, Tsuchida, Peng, Furukawa, and Wilson 1995). The ideal range of pore sizes has been suggested to be between 10 and 45 mm to facilitate significant fibrovascular tissue infiltration (He and Matsuda 2002). However, long-term human explants of ePTFE grafts have revealed that the luminal surface is not well covered with tissue. Rather, thin and irregular layers of fibrin are generally found interspersed with areas of exposed ePTFE (Guidon et al. 1993). In addition, infiltration occurred mainly at the proximal and distal ends of the explanted vascular grafts and increased with the duration of implantation. The surface charge of the luminal surface can be a determining factor for the amount and type of cell adhesion and retention under flow conditions. As a result, more electronegative surfaces, such as that of ePTFE, tend to incur lower levels of thrombosis (Akers, Du, and Kempczinski 1993) and cell attachment. In addition, the hydrophobicity of ePTFE and PET grafts is a factor in cell proliferation and healing characteristics, with surfaces that are more hydrophilic producing greater proliferation (Wildevuur et al. 1987). As such, graft microporosity and surface characteristics influence graft integration, cell proliferation, and the formation of a neointimal layer.

Blood Compatibility

The long-term success of implants is heavily influenced by cell-biomaterial interactions, even more so for vascular grafts as they are in constant contact with platelets, various proteins, complement, and leukocytes. The lack of blood compatibility of PET and ePTFE vascular grafts leads to poor patency when used in medium-diameter applications such as in peripheral vascular surgery, for which 5-year primary patency rates for ePTFE grafts have been reported to be as low as 39% (Klinkert, Post, Breslau, and van Bockel 2004). Therefore in an attempt to create a more blood-compatible surface and increase patency rates, a large amount of research has been focused on the development of thromboresistant coatings and surfaces. Research in this field has been concentrated in two areas: (a) coating the surface of vascular grafts with blood-compatible molecules or polymers and (b) coating the surface with biomaterials that release antithrombogenic molecules. Each approach attempts to simulate a subset of the properties provided by a functional endothelium. In addition, a confluent, functional EC layer is considered the most ideal "coating" for making synthetic vascular grafts blood compatible. However, protein coatings currently used to seal vascular grafts have not shown evidence of endothelium formation (Francois, Chakfe, Durand, and Laroche 2009).

The coating of vascular grafts with native proteins to reduce thrombogenicity has been examined since the 1980s with varied success. One such protein, albumin, has been extensively studied after it was discovered that it had the ability to reduce thrombosis. Although *in vitro* studies and *in vivo* animal models have shown promising results, in humans the albumin coating is absorbed into the blood in about 2 months (Xue and Greisler 2003). Coated PET grafts have shown patency rates similar to standard uncoated grafts (Kudo, Nishibe, Miyazaki, Flores, and Yasuda 2002; al-Khaffaf and Charlesworth 1996). Consequently, clinical outcomes for albumin have been largely disappointing; therefore, other protein systems have been investigated. The structural protein elastin and other elastic tissue components, namely fibrilin and fibulin, have also been explored as a thrombosis-resistant coating. These proteins are interesting as coatings in vascular applications because they (a) show a reduction in platelet adhesion, (b) have the ability to inhibit the proliferation of SMCs (IH), and (c) facilitate the attachment of ECs (Ito, Ishimaru, and Wilson 1998; Williamson, Shuttleworth, Canfield, Black, and Kielty 2007). This approach provides a pathway for establishing an endothelium on the surface of a synthetic vascular graft.

Ideally an intact endothelium will prevent thrombosis through a number of physical and chemical mechanisms, resist protein and procoagulant deposition, and secrete prostacyclin and nitric oxide (NO), which inhibit platelet adherence and SMC proliferation (Parikh and Edelman 2000). For the natural function of the endothelium and SMCs, the regulation of the cell phenotype must be controlled. *In vivo* EC growth, differentiation, barrier function, migration, and survival are regulated in a complex manner by the surrounding ECM, cell-cell contacts, growth factors, and mechanical cues (McGuigan and Sefton 2007). In particular, hemodynamic forces on ECs stimulate mechanosensor mechanisms and produce junctions, cytoskeleton, and integrin reorganization that alter ECM organization, EC morphology, and EC gene expression. In addition, hemodynamic forces affect the expression and secretion of proteins that control vascular tone, fibrinolysis, surface adhesion, and coagulation promoters and inhibitors. Although research involving the coating of proteins that have the ability to promote endothelialization is promising, sufficient testing is yet to be conducted to show its efficacy in a clinical situation.

Another approach used to create thromboresistant surfaces is the immobilization of anticoagulants on the surface of a synthetic vascular conduit. One such anticoagulant, heparin, has been widely used and shown to be effective *in vitro*, but clinical trials have yielded mixed results (Heyligers et al. 2006). In a randomized multicenter study, patency rates were higher for heparin-bonded PET grafts compared to standard ePTFE at 3 years, but at 5 years the difference was not statistically significant (Devine and McCollum 2004).

In spite of these results, research with heparin as a vascular graft coating is ongoing, with special emphasis placed on the immobilization of heparin to increase efficacy. One such technique, known as end-point immobilization, involves (a) depolymerization of the reducing end of the linear heparin chain to yield an aldehyde group, which is then (b) conjugated to a primary amine on the vascular graft surface. *In vitro* studies of graft materials using this method of heparin attachment have shown effective inhibition of initial contact activation enzymes by an antithrombin-mediated mechanism (Elgue, Blomback, Olsson, and Riesenfeld 1993; Sanchez, Elgue, Riesenfeld, and Olsson 1998). This led to the development of a heparin-coated PTFE vascular graft in which heparin is bound via end-point immobilization (Propaten Graft, W. L. Gore & Associates). Currently, only 1-year patency rates have been reported, but the data indicate that heparin-bound grafts are more patent than standard ePTFE grafts in femoropopliteal bypass surgery (Lindholt et al. 2011). Although initial results appear promising, 5-year patency rates are needed to determine the long-term efficacy of this prosthesis.

NO is a bioactive molecule released from the endothelium that prevents platelet activation. Interestingly, this molecule can be released by polymers that contain diazeniumdiolate groups ([N(O)NO]$^-$), which on decomposition in physiological fluids spontaneously generate NO (Vanin et al. 1990). A number of approaches for preparing NO-releasing polymers have been studied and include (a) the physical blending of the [N(O)NO]$^-$ complex into a bulk polymer, (b) the incorporation of a group (nucleophile) containing [N(O)NO]$^-$ as a side chain into the polymer, and (c) the incorporation of [N(O)NO]$^-$ into the polymer backbone (Figure 4.6).

A polymer coating composed of a cross-linked poly(ethylenimine) where [N(O)NO]$^-$ was directly attached to the polymer chain was studied in a baboon animal model to examine thrombus formation and show feasibility of such a coating in vascular applications (Smith et al. 1996). In this particular study, the polymer containing [N(O)NO]$^-$ was coated onto a ePTFE graft, which was then exposed to flowing blood via an artery-to-vein shunt for 1 hour; results showed substantially less thrombus formation in the graft coated with [N(O)NO]$^-$.

Although promising, one of the major limitations of NO-generating coatings is the eventual exhaustion of NO donors. The maximum reported NO release period is 2 months (Ho-wook, Taite, and West 2005). Due to this limitation, research has focused on the development of sustainable release mechanisms

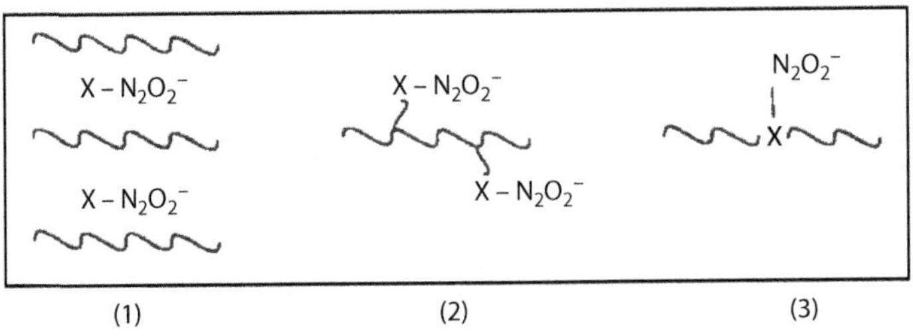

FIGURE 4.6
Generalized polymer types for the addition of [N(O)NO]$^-$: X = nucleophile residue, $N_2O_2^-$ = NO releasing unit, ~ = polymer backbone. (From Smith D.J., Chakravarthy D., Pulfer S., et al. 1996. Nitric oxide-releasing polymers containing the [N(O)NO]$^-$ group. *J Med Chem* 39:1148–56.) (1) the physical blending of the [N(O)NO]$^-$ complex into a bulk polymer, (2) the incorporation of a group (nucleophile) containing [N(O)NO]$^-$ as a side chain into the polymer, (3) the incorporation of [N(O)NO]$^-$ into the polymer backbone.

based on the catalytic generation of NO from endogenous nitrite via polymeric films doped with lipophilic Cu(II) complexes (Oh and Meyerhoff 2004). Using this process, NO has the ability to be generated at therapeutic levels for extended periods far beyond the previous 2-month maximum.

Immune and Inflammatory Response

Along the vascular wall, blood contacts an endothelium, which interacts with a high concentration of leukocytes and complement. For synthetic vascular conduits, the blood-biomaterial interface is under constant surveillance by both the inflammatory and immune systems. As such, the introduction of a foreign surface to blood triggers a series of events, including protein adsorption, complement and leukocyte adhesion, and the acute activation of platelets and coagulation. This intense immune and inflammatory response to synthetic vascular grafts contributes to their poor blood biocompatibility and subsequent complications.

It is well established that polymers of biologic origin activate a strong immune response mediated by the classical pathway of the complement system. As a consequence of the collagen, albumin, gelatin, or other biologic coating used to seal the intimal surface, the immune response is activated by the perceived antigen. Several studies have recognized the humoral and cell-mediated immune response to coated PET vascular grafts (Schlosser et al. 2002, 2005; Wilhelm et al. 2007). On the other hand, the "nonself" surface of polymeric biomaterials often results in spontaneous low-rate complement activation via the alternative pathway. To date, blood compatibility issues have focused on minimizing coagulation and platelet adhesion or activation through systemic drug therapy. Considering that blood clot formation is a special case of inflammation, the direct, local control of thrombosis and coagulation may be possible. However, this requires a more complete understanding of the role of leukocytes in blood-biomaterial interaction.

This subject has been reviewed by Gobert and Sefton with emphasis on complement activation as a prelude to thrombosis and the role of leukocytes in coagulation (Gorbet and Sefton 2004). To demonstrate, Hong and coworkers showed that without leukocytes the formation of thrombin was negligible when blood was exposed to a biomaterial (Hong, Nilsson Ekdahl, Reynolds, Larsson, and Nilsson 1999). Following exposure to polyvinyl chloride, levels of thrombin were negligible in plasma and platelet-rich plasma, but significant in whole blood (i.e., presence of leukocytes). Therefore leukocyte activation and cytokine production were a prerequisite for coagulation.

Monocytes and macrophages play a pivotal role in synthetic vascular graft complications. Unfortunately, ePTFE and PET elicit a chronic inflammatory response that starts with early leukocyte adhesion and can ultimately assist in late graft failure (Parikh and Edelman 2000). For example, macrophages have been implicated in the chemical signal that stimulates SMC proliferation resulting in IH (Simon, Xu, Ortlepp, Rogers, and Rao 1997). In addition, it has also been suggested that the potent cytokines secreted by chronically active macrophages are inhibitors to angiogenesis, which significantly reduces neovascularization (Salzmann, Kleinert, Berman, and Williams 1999). Constructed from permanent biomaterials, current vascular grafts produce chronic inflammatory responses from the seemingly unlimited local supply of leukocytes within blood. In a subcutaneous rat study investigating the macrophage response to PET and ePTFE, it was shown that PET produced a more intense initial inflammatory response than ePTFE. This may be the result of the more inert surface of ePTFE, which reduces early leukocyte adhesion. However, ePTFE produced a delayed proliferating cell response, with 4% at 3 weeks and 21% at 5 weeks, compared to PET, with 23% at 3 weeks and 8% at 5 weeks (Hagerty, Salzmann, Kleinert, and Williams 2000). These results underlined the importance of minimizing the long-term inflammatory response, which impedes healing and the population of native vascular cells within vascular grafts. In addition, a better understanding of the role of leukocytes in vascular graft complications may hold the key to improving patency.

Tissue-Engineered Vascular Grafts

Scaffolds for the Next Generation

Due to the poor patency of current vascular grafts, motivation to create the ideal prosthesis has stimulated and challenged current tissue-engineering practices. Tissue engineering a patent vascular graft remains an enormous task as the list of prerequisites is long and requires a multidisciplinary approach with input from bioengineers, clinicians, and researchers. The three basic elements that are required to accomplish this task are a structural scaffold, vascular cells, and a nurturing environment (Kakisis, Liapis, Breuer, and Sumpio 2005). The implementation of these elements is wide and varied due to the many choices for scaffold materials, cell types and sources, and the choice of an *in vitro* or *in vivo* nurturing environment. The vast number of choices provides flexibility but adds to the complexity of finding the ideal solution that meets all, or most, of the prerequisites. To make matters even more difficult, the device design must have clinical acceptance, and the approach must not require excessive preparation time or effort.

Synthetic Absorbable Scaffolds

Synthetic polymers can be engineered to have a range of different mechanical and chemical properties, manufactured easily and consistently, and processed using a variety of methods into various forms (e.g., films, nanofibers, yarns). As a result, polymers, and their copolymers, represent a class of materials that provide extensive design flexibility and are cost effective. Hydrolytically degrading and bioabsorbable polymers for use as tissue-engineered vascular graft scaffolds possess the ability to modulate temporal degradation and strength retention, support cell ECM production and proliferation, and absorb to be replaced by functional remodeling vascular tissue. In the long term, this approach leaves the implant site absent of any foreign material. However, early attempts to produce fully absorbable vascular grafts from polyglycolide (PG) did not perform well due to aneurysm formation (Xue and Greisler 2003). This can be attributed to the relatively fast loss of mechanical integrity of PG, which preceded the development of sufficient tissue strength. To overcome this issue, partially absorbable scaffolds have been developed that combine a fast-degrading absorbable polymer supported by a nondegradable polymer (Yu and Chu 1993; Yu, Ho, and Chu 1994; Izhar et al. 2001). However, research has focused mainly on the use of compliant, fully absorbable scaffolds based mostly on linear, aliphatic copolyesters with the major molecular component being polylactide (PL) or polycaprolactone (PCL). These polymeric systems provide significantly longer strength retention.

Crapo and Wang investigated two fully absorbable scaffolds with the hypothesis that elastomeric scaffolds under dynamic conditions would develop strong and compliant arterial constructs. To this end, scaffolds composed of either rigid poly(lactide-co-glycolide) (PLGA) or elastomeric poly(glycerol sebacate) (PGS) were seeded with baboon SMCs and *in vitro* cultured under dynamic mechanical stimulation for 10 days (Crapo and Wang 2010). Their results found that initial scaffold compliance was a determining factor in tissue development and postconditioning mechanical properties. Furthermore, the elastic PGS graft produced significant amounts of elastin within days, while the stiff PLGA graft produced no appreciable elastin.

Other attempts to fabricate elastic scaffolds that can withstand mechanically dynamic conditions have been developed using poly(glycolide-co-caprolactone) (Lee et al. 2003) and poly(lactide-co-caprolactone) (PLCL) (Inoguchi et al. 2006). In the former, scaffolds were produced by solvent casting and NaCl leaching to create a compliant, porous tube. Mechanical testing showed that radial strains up to 120% provided 98% recovery, and failure occurred at 250% elongation, indicating excellent compliance and viscoelasticity. Cyclic loading at an applied strain of 10% and a frequency of 1 Hz for 2 days produced less than 5% permanent deformation. To develop a mechanically active small-diameter graft, scaffolds of PLCL were prepared using the electrospinning technique to produce fabrics of different wall thickness (50 to 340 mm) (Inoguchi et al. 2006). Thinner-walled vessels were shown to pulsate synchronously, approaching the native artery, to dynamic pulsatile flow conditions.

The use of electrospinning is another novel solution to construct a fully absorbable vascular prosthesis that is complaint. This technology offers the benefit of being able to incorporate synthetic and biologic polymers simultaneously and control composition, structure, and mechanical properties (Stitzel et al. 2006; Tillman et al. 2009). Scaffold preparation using collagen type I, elastin, and poly(D,L lactide-co-glycolide) (PDLGA) was electrospun onto a tubular mandrel to a thickness of 1 mm and a length of 12 cm (Stitzel et al. 2006). *In vitro* mechanical testing produced burst pressures of 1,425 mmHg, nearly 12 times systolic pressure, with 40% strain at failure. Tissue compatibility results showed a confluent monolayer of ECs on the inner surface after 4 days and SMCs on the outer surface after 3 days. This approach has advantages in the clinical setting as different geometries, compositions, and tailored mechanical properties can be produced reliably.

Another proposed construction utilizing the mechanical stability of PLGA was a hybrid scaffold using porous freeze-dried marine collagen as a cell interface with a fibrous PLGA elecrospun structural scaffold (Jeong et al. 2007). Following EC and SMC seeding, an *in vitro* pulsatile perfusion system was utilized to provide radial distension. Results indicated that expressions of smooth muscle (SM) α-actin, SM myosin heavy chain, EC von Willebrand factor, and NO were observed. As such, normal cell phenotype activity was preserved.

The ideal tissue-engineered scaffold may incorporate both synthetic and naturally derived tissues to take advantage of the mechanical stability and cell attachment and signaling characteristics, respectively. An improved understanding of cell phenotype regulation and cell responses to chemical and mechanical stimulation will be a key factor in the development of a patent tissue-engineered vascular graft.

PCL is a slow-degrading polyester that is not as widely used as its other absorbable counterparts (PL, PG); however, it offers several advantages for use in vascular graft tissue engineering (Woodruff and Hutmacher 2010). For example, PCL provides much longer strength retention to facilitate tissue maturation for elderly patients or those with comorbidities. This greater strength retention may be required for such a high-risk device, for which failure may result in mortality. In addition, due to fewer ester groups, the degradation products are released over a longer period of time, which reduces the likelihood of local pH changes to an acidic environment, as is known to occur with PL and PG.

The use of a PL/PCL-based scaffold seeded with autologous bone marrow-derived mononuclear cells (BMMCs) has shown excellent patency in a pediatric clinical study of patients born with a single-ventricle defect, a life-threatening condition (Hibino, McGillicuddy et al. 2011; Naito et al. 2011; Matsumura, Hibino, Ikada, Kurosawa, and Shin'oka 2003; Shin'oka et al. 2005). Twenty-five grafts were implanted, and there was no graft-related mortality, evidence of aneurysm formation, graft rupture, infection, or ectopic calcification. Within the first 7 years, the only graft-related complication was stenosis, affecting approximately 16% of the grafts (Naito et al. 2011). To better understand the underlying mechanisms, canine (Watanabe et al. 2001), lamb (Brennan et al. 2008), and mice (Goyal et al. 2006; Lopez-Soler et al. 2007; Roh et al. 2008, 2011) studies were initiated by researchers using a miniaturized model of that used in the clinical trial. Results indicated that BMMCs had an indirect rather than direct impact on the regeneration of vascular tissue. Rather than BMMCs incorporating into the graft, they instead stimulated monocyte activity, which triggered an inflammatory response, leading to the recruitment of ECs and SMCs from adjacent normal vessels (Hibino, Villalona et al. 2011). In a short time, the seeded cells were gone, and the host cells were incorporated. This investigation has shown that the innate repair mechanisms can be used to create new tissues with seeded cells as only precursors to initiate the response.

Overall, tissue-engineered vascular grafts based on absorbable synthetic copolymers have shown feasibility to produce a viable temporary scaffold that will accommodate vascular cells and maintain structural integrity during cell proliferation and ECM development under hemodynamic conditions; however, the engineered scaffold that will meet all prerequisites is still unclear. In addition, the logistics of acquiring cells, the long culturing periods, and the limited or variable cell proliferation capacity are all potential clinical limitations (Ravi, Qu, and Chaikof 2009).

Polymers of Natural Origin

The use of biologic materials derived from proteins and polysaccharides has many advantages. For example, biopolymers have the potential to preserve or re-create structural characteristics and mechanical function, the ability to be naturally remodeled, and the ability to provide chemical signals and intrinsic sites for cell attachment and growth. Polymers of natural origin exhibit the ability to augment the healing and remodeling process and are not subject to some of the insufficiencies of synthetic absorbable polymers, which include the release of acidic by-products and marked inflammatory responses (Turner, Kielty, Walker, and Canfield 2004). However, like PG, biopolymers have a strength retention profile that is inadequate for many load-bearing applications. Although several methods of incorporating natural materials into scaffolds have been investigated, one primary approach is using decellularized ECM biomaterials.

Decellularized tissues attempt to mimic arterial physiology by decellularizing a donor tissue, typically using a series of physical, chemical, and enzymatic approaches to isolate the ECM and remove all of the highly immunogenic cellular matter. Chemical methods vary greatly and include alkaline/acidic treatments, nonionic and ionic detergents, zwitterionic detergents, hypotonic and hypertonic treatments, tri(n-butyl) phosphate (TBP), and various chelating agents to achieve decellularization (Gilbert et al. 2006). Once decellularized, the ECM graft can then be repopulated with cardiovascular cells using either an *in vitro* seeding or *in vivo* infiltration method to approximate a biomimetic structure. In addition, *in vitro* seeding approaches often involve the use of some type of vessel bioreactor, which functions to mimic the physiological vessel environment, including the cyclic strain and shear stresses seen in the body, with the end goal of having a fully functional vessel at the time of surgery (Sorrentino and Haller 2011). ECM scaffolds can be derived from human and several animal sources; they are composed of various structural and functional proteins, ranging from collagen, to elastin, to a number of growth factors, and to proteoglycans, making them ideal for use as graft scaffold materials (Piterina et al. 2009; Badylak, Freytes, and Gilbert 2009). The primary sources of decellularized scaffolds that have been studied include human umbilical arteries and veins, ureters (porcine, bovine, or canine), and carotid arteries (porcine and canine).

Gui and colleagues showed successful decellularization of a human umbilical artery with maintenance of graft mechanical strength using a CHAPS (3-[(3-cholamidopropyl)-dimethylammonio]-1-propane sulfonate)/sodium dodecyl sulfate buffer treatment followed by incubation in EC growth media (Gui, Muto, Chan, Breuer, and Niklason 2009). *In vivo* testing using an abdominal aorta rat model revealed retained function for up to 8 weeks. In another study, decellularized canine ureters showed only 20% patency at 1 week when implanted in a canine carotid artery without cell seeding, while the EC-seeded versions showed 100% patency at 24 weeks (Narita et al. 2008). Cell seeding prior to implantation appears to be a key factor in determining the success of a decellularized, protein-based vascular graft material.

Although the use of decellularized tissues as scaffolds seems attractive, there are a number of hurdles that have yet to be overcome. One of the largest of these is stabilization of the decellularized ECM. On implantation, unmodified natural polymers will degrade due to chemical and enzymatic degradation, seriously decreasing the life of the prosthesis (Schmidt and Baier 2000). In addition, graft calcification and immunological recognition can occur, possibly due to the presence of residual cellular components. A recent examination of a decellularized bovine ureter graft indicated that graft failure with aneurysmal dilation and thrombus formation may be due to an acute and chronic inflammatory response caused by residual cellular components not removed during the decellularization process (Spark, Yeluri, Derham, Wong, and Leitch 2008).

For these reasons, and the need for sterilization, naturally derived biomaterials typically require chemical pretreatment with cross-linking reagents such as glutaraldehyde. However, this leaves the scaffold susceptible to cytotoxic effects on repopulated cells. Increased cross-linking produces a structure more resistant to degradation, but at the cost of mechanical compliance. Other cross-linking agents, such as polyepoxy compounds, showed reduced levels of calcification, decreased antithrombogenicity, and increased flexibility, resulting in improved patency compared to vascular grafts treated with other chemicals (Schmidt and Baier 2000).

Another noted challenge associated with decellularized vessels is incomplete repopulation, generally caused by the inability of seeded cells to penetrate the densely packed collagen-elastin network. In an attempt to solve this issue, Kurane and colleagues preferentially removed the collagen of decellularized porcine carotid artery grafts to increase their porosity in addition to loading the grafts with basic fibroblast growth factor (Kurane, Simionescu, and Vyavahare 2007). Cell infiltration was analyzed from the histological evaluation of subdermal implanted tubular constructs. Overall, improved cellular infiltration was noted.

Another investigated avenue for attaining a tissue-engineering scaffold is using biological proteins or polysaccharides as raw materials for constructing vascular grafts. This concept of reconstituting a vascular graft from natural materials was first introduced by Weinburger and Bell over 20 years ago with the formation of a tubular type I collagen gel that was seeded or loaded with various cell types that are contained in natural vascular tissues (Weinburger and Bell 1986). Although the general idea remains the same, techniques and material types have since evolved to employ the use of various materials, such as elastin, fibrin, collagen, silk, and hyaluronan. While many of these constructs have excellent cell compatibility, they generally lack the mechanical properties (strength, compliance, and elasticity) required for vascular applications. To address this issue, Wise and colleagues developed a composite graft material using elastin and PCL through the use of an electrospinning technique (Wise et al. 2011). The resulting grafts had mechanical properties similar to human internal mammary arteries, with excellent EC attachment/proliferation and blood compatibility.

Fibroin has also shown promise as a vascular graft material. Fibroin is the core protein component of silk that remains after the removal of sericin, the gum-like protein surrounding silk fibers (Altman et al. 2003). Enomoto and coworkers constructed small-caliber (1.5-mm diameter) vascular grafts by weaving silk fibroin thread and implanted them in an abdominal aorta rat model (Enomoto et al. 2010). They showed a significant increase in patency rates (85.1% vs. 30%) at 1 year compared to ePTFE controls. In addition, ECs and SMCs successfully migrated into the scaffolds, with a significant increase in SMC migration between 1 and 3 months (Enomoto et al. 2010).

Hyaluronan, or estrified hyaluronic acid, is another versatile tissue-engineering tool due to its many desirable characteristics. From a standpoint of physical properties, it is a GAG with variable molecular weight, a negative charge that attracts water, and controllable cross-linking properties, making load-bearing hydrogels possible (Leach and Schmidt 2005). The *in vivo* biological advantages include tissue organization, wound healing, angiogenesis, cell adhesion, regulation of inflammation, and nonimmunogenicity, and when degraded by hyaluronidases during neotissue formation, the resulting products induce production of ECM (Hoenig, Campbell, Rolfe, and Campbell 2005; Remuzzi et al. 2004). In addition, hydrogels can be produced by photopolymerization of glycidyl methacrylate and hyaluronic acid to comprise bioactive, degradable, hydrated, and pliable materials that can be modified with peptide moieties for protein therapy (Hoenig, Campbell, Rolfe, and Campbell 2005). In vascular graft research, hyaluronan-based materials have been shown to promote endothelial and SMC attachment while displaying hemocompatibility properties (Turner, Kielty, Walker, and Canfield 2004; Remuzzi et al. 2004; Amarnath, Srinivas, and Ramamurthi 2006). Although these results seem promising, like protein-based biomaterials, hyaluronan vascular grafts may have inadequate *in vivo* mechanical stability with time.

Conclusions

Autologous vascular tissue has been used successfully for decades to replace diseased vessels. However, after significant effort by bioengineers and clinicians, synthetic alternatives are not equivalent to autologous vessels. This endeavor has provided an appreciation for blood-biomaterial interactions, the importance of cell integration, and the biomechanical properties required to achieve a highly patent vascular prosthesis. Future advances in the patency of vascular grafts will likely occur as stepwise improvements, rather than a single novel discovery that alleviates all of the complications. In the short term, the next advances will likely come from the use of poly(carbonate) urethane grafts, which have improved blood compatibility and more closely match the compliance of an artery. The development of new materials or coatings that support a functional endothelium will be required to produce the first small-diameter graft for use in coronary bypass procedures and to improve the patency of medium-diameter grafts. While the field of tissue engineering continues to search for a solution to total vascular tissue regeneration, more emphasis on reliably producing an endothelium would have the greatest short-term impact on patient care.

At the current rate of advancements in tissue engineering, it is likely that in the next two decades vascular grafts as we know them today will be obsolete and replaced by cell-based scaffolds. Although the realization of tissue-engineered devices has been slow, the investment in cell-based technologies will eventually result in a highly patent vascular graft. Although the optimal implementation of tissue-engineered conduits remains uncertain, and significant challenges remain ahead, it is likely that polymeric scaffolds will have a role in supporting the application of a cell-based vascular graft technology.

The translation of a tissue-engineered vascular graft from research to clinical use will be challenging. All cellular, mechanical, and physical characteristics of a tissue-engineered vascular graft must be controlled as they relate to the design, manufacturing processes, and equipment used in the construction of the device. Research is beginning to uncover some of the significant variables for achieving success. However, the translation to clinical use requires that the critical design variables are well understood and controlled, with either validation or verification to ensure efficacy for all high-risk design features. The Food and Drug Administration (FDA) requires that all design and manufacturing activities are risk based. In other words, as the risk of a design feature failing causes injury or mortality, the level of control and understanding must increase to mitigate the risk. It is easy to anticipate that tissue-engineered vascular grafts would have a significant number of design risks related to controlling cell phenotype, ECM production and quality, and endothelialization. In addition, the process of producing a tissue-engineered vascular graft must be predictable and reproducible to a high degree of statistical significance. Patient age and comorbidities will mean that cell-seeded grafts will inherently have a high degree of variability. As such, the validation of such a process will be difficult, if not impossible. Therefore verification of each graft produced will be required using an elaborate series of tests that ensure safety and efficacy of the specific graft intended for implantation. With design verification, several issues can arise. How is the failure of a graft to meet predetermined specifications handled? Do you continue with conditioning the implant in a bioreactor or start over? What about the patient? Can the patient wait, or is intervention critical? These are just a few examples of the many challenges ahead as cell-based vascular graft technologies translate from research to the clinical setting.

References

Abbott W.M., Megerman J., Hasson J.E., L'Italien G., Warnock D.F. 1987. Effect of compliance mismatch on vascular graft patency. *J Vasc Surg* 5:376–82.

Akers D.L., Du Y.H., Kempczinski R.F. 1993. The effect of carbon coating and porosity on early patency of expanded polytetrafluoroethylene grafts: an experimental study. *J Vasc Surg* 18:10–15.

al-Khaffaf H., Charlesworth D. 1996. Albumin-coated vascular prostheses: a five-year follow-up. *J Vasc Surg* 23:686–90.

Altman G.H., Diaz F., Jakuba C., et al. 2003. Silk-based biomaterials. *Biomaterials* 24:401–16.

Amarnath L.P., Srinivas A., Ramamurthi A. 2006. *In vitro* hemocompatibility testing of UV-modified hyaluronan hydrogels. *Biomaterials* 27:1416–24.

Badylak S.F., Freytes D.O., Gilbert T.W. 2009. Extracellular matrix as a biological scaffold material: structure and function. *Acta Biomater* 5:1–13.

Baird R.N., Abbott W.M. 1976. Pulsatile blood-flow in arterial grafts. *Lancet* 2(7992):948–50.

Bowald S., Busch C., Eriksson I. 1979. Arterial regeneration following polyglactin 910 suture mesh grafting. *Surgery* 86:722–29.

Brennan M.P., Dardik A., Hibino N., et al. 2008. Tissue-engineered vascular grafts demonstrate evidence of growth and development when implanted in a juvenile animal model. *Ann Surg* 248:370–77.

Crapo P.M., Wang Y. 2010. Physiologic compliance in engineered small-diameter arterial constructs based on an elastomeric substrate. *Biomaterials* 31:1626–35.

Devine C., McCollum C. 2004. Heparin-bonded Dacron or polytetrafluorethylene for femoropopliteal bypass: five-year results of a prospective randomized multicenter clinical trial. *J Vasc Surg* 40:924–31.

Elgue G., Blomback M., Olsson P., Riesenfeld J. 1993. On the mechanism of coagulation inhibition on surfaces with end point immobilized heparin. *Thromb Haemost* 70:289–93.

Enomoto S., Sumi M., Kajimoto K., et al. 2010. Long-term patency of small-diameter vascular graft made from fibroin, a silk-based biodegradable material. *J Vasc Surg* 51:155–64.

Fei D.Y., Thomas J.D., Rittgers S.E. 1994. The effect of angle and flow rate upon hemodynamics in distal vascular graft anastomoses: a numerical model study. *J Biomech Eng* 116:331–36.

Francois S., Chakfe N., Durand B., Laroche G. 2009. A poly(L-lactic acid) nanofibre mesh scaffold for endothelial cells on vascular prostheses. *Acta Biomater* 5:2418–28.

Gilbert T.W., Sellaro T.L., Badylak S.F. 2006. Decellularization of tissues and organs. *Biomaterials* 27:3675–83.

Gorbet M.B., Sefton M.V. 2004. Biomaterial-associated thrombosis: roles of coagulation factors, complement, platelets and leukocytes. *Biomaterials* 25:5681–703.

Goyal A., Wang Y., Su H., et al. 2006. Development of a model system for preliminary evaluation of tissue-engineered vascular conduits. *J Pediatr Surg* 41:787–91.

Gui L., Muto A., Chan S.A., Breuer C.K., Niklason L.E. 2009. Development of decellularized human umbilical arteries as small-diameter vascular grafts. *Tissue Eng Part A* 15:2665–76.

Guidon R., Chafke N., Maurel S., et al. 1993. Expanded polytetrafluoroethylene arterial prosthesis in humans: a histopathological study of 298 surgically excised grafts. *Biomaterials* 14:678–93.

Hagerty R.D., Salzmann D.L., Kleinert L.B., Williams S.K. 2000. Cellular proliferation and macrophage populations associated with implanted expanded polytetrafluoroethylene and polyethyleneterephthalate. *J Biomed Mater Res* 49:489–97.

He H., Matsuda T. 2002. Arterial replacement with compliant hierarchic hybrid vascular graft: biomechanical adaptation and failure. *Tissue Eng* 8:213–24.

Heyligers J.M., Verhagen H.J., Rotmans J.I., et al. 2006. Heparin immobilization reduces thrombogenicity of small-caliber expanded polytetrafluoroethylene grafts. *J Vasc Surg* 43:587–91.

Hibino N., McGillicuddy E., Matsumura G., et al. 2011. Late-term results of tissue-engineered vascular grafts in humans. *J Thorac Cardiovasc Surg* 139:431–36, 436e1–2.

Hibino N., Villalona G., Pietris N., et al. 2011. Tissue-engineered vascular grafts form neovessels that arise from regeneration of the adjacent blood vessel. *FASEB J* 25:2731–39.

Hoenig M.R., Campbell G.R., Rolfe B.E., Campbell J.H. 2005. Tissue-engineered blood vessels: alternative to autologous grafts? *Arterioscler Thromb Vasc Biol* 25:1128–34.

Hong J., Nilsson Ekdahl, K., Reynolds H, Larsson R., Nilsson B. 1999. A new *in vitro* model to study interaction between whole blood and biomaterials. Studies of platelet and coagulation activation and the effect of aspirin. *Biomaterials* 20:603–11.

Ho-wook J., Taite J., West J. 2005. Nitric oxide releasing polyurethanes. *Biomacromolecules* 6:838–844.

Inoguchi H., Kwon I.K., Inoue E., et al. 2006. Mechanical responses of a compliant electrospun poly(L-lactide-co-epsilon-caprolactone) small-diameter vascular graft. *Biomaterials* 27:1470–78.

Isenberg B.C., Williams C., Tranquillo R.T. 2006. Small-diameter artificial arteries engineered *in vitro*. *Circ Res* 98:25–35.

Ishii Y., Kronengold R.T., Virmani R., et al. 2007. Novel bioengineered small caliber vascular graft with excellent one-month patency. *Ann Thorac Surg* 83:517–25.

Ishii Y., Sakamoto S., Kronengold R.T., et al. 2008. A novel bioengineered small-caliber vascular graft incorporating heparin and sirolimus: excellent 6-month patency. *J Thorac Cardiovasc Surg* 135:1237–45; discussion 1245–46.

Ito S., Ishimaru S., Wilson S.E. 1998. Application of coacervated alpha-elastin to arterial prostheses for inhibition of anastomotic intimal hyperplasia. *ASAIO J* 44(5):M501–5.

Izhar U., Schwalb H., Borman J.B., et al. 2001. Novel synthetic selectively degradable vascular prostheses: a preliminary implantation study. *J Surg Res* 95:152–60.

Jeong S.I., Kim S.Y., Cho S.K., et al. 2007. Tissue-engineered vascular grafts composed of marine collagen and PLGA fibers using pulsatile perfusion bioreactors. *Biomaterials* 28:1115–22.

Jorgensen C.S., Paaske W.P. 1998. Physical and mechanical properties of ePTFE stretch vascular grafts determined by time-resolved scanning acoustic microscopy. *Eur J Vasc Endovasc Surg* 15:416–22.

Kakisis J.D., Liapis C.D., Breuer C., Sumpio B.E. 2005. Artificial blood vessel: the Holy Grail of peripheral vascular surgery. *J Vasc Surg* 41:349–54.

Kannan R.Y., Salacinski H.J., Butler P.E., Hamilton G., Seifalian A.M. 2005. Current status of prosthetic bypass grafts: a review. *J Biomed Mater Res B Appl Biomater* 74:570–81.

Klinkert P., Post P.N., Breslau P.J., van Bockel J.H. 2004. Saphenous vein versus PTFE for above-knee femoropopliteal bypass. A review of the literature. *Eur J Vasc Endovasc Surg* 27:357–62.

Kudo F.A., Nishibe T., Miyazaki K., Flores J., Yasuda K. 2002. Albumin-coated knitted Dacron aortic prostheses. Study of postoperative inflammatory reactions. *Int Angiol* 21:214–17.

Kurane A., Simionescu D.T., Vyavahare N.R. 2007. *In vivo* cellular repopulation of tubular elastin scaffolds mediated by basic fibroblast growth factor. *Biomaterials* 28:2830–38.

Lau H., Cheng S.W. 2001. Is the preferential use of ePTFE grafts in femorofemoral bypass justified? *Ann Vasc Surg* 15:383–87.

Leach J.B., Schmidt C.E. 2005. Characterization of protein release from photocross-linkable hyaluronic acid-polyethylene glycol hydrogel tissue engineering scaffolds. *Biomaterials* 26:125–35.

Lee S.H., Kim B.S., Kim S.H., et al. 2003. Elastic biodegradable poly(glycolide-co-caprolactone) scaffold for tissue engineering. *J Biomed Mater Res A* 66:29–37.

Lindholt J.S., Gottschalksen B., Johannesen N., et al. 2011. The Scandinavian Propaten™ Trial—1-year patency of PTFE vascular prostheses with heparin-bonded luminal surfaces compared to ordinary pure PTFE vascular prostheses—a randomised clinical controlled multi-centre trial. *Eur J Vasc Endovasc Surg* 41:668–73.

Lopez-Soler R.I., Brennan M.P., Goyal A., et al. 2007. Development of a mouse model for evaluation of small diameter vascular grafts. *J Surg Res* 139:1–6.

Luscher T.F., Steffel J., Eberli F.R., et al. 2007. Drug-eluting stent and coronary thrombosis: biological mechanisms and clinical implications. *Circulation* 115:1051–58.

Martin D.J., Warren L.A., Gunatillake P.A., et al. 2000. Polydimethylsiloxane/polyether-mixed macrodiol-based polyurethane elastomers: biostability. *Biomaterials* 21:1021–29.

Matsuda T. 2004. Recent progress of vascular graft engineering in Japan. *Artif Organs* 28:64–71.

Matsumura G., Hibino N., Ikada Y., Kurosawa H., Shin'oka T. 2003. Successful application of tissue engineered vascular autografts: clinical experience. *Biomaterials* 24:2303–8.

McGuigan A.P., Sefton M.V. 2007. The influence of biomaterials on endothelial cell thrombogenicity. *Biomaterials* 28:2547–71.

Nagae T., Tsuchida H., Peng S.K., Furukawa K., Wilson S.E. 1995. Composite porosity of expanded polytetrafluoroethylene vascular prosthesis. *Cardiovasc Surg* 3:479–84.

Naito Y., Shinoka T., Duncan D., et al. 2011. Vascular tissue engineering: towards the next generation vascular grafts. *Adv Drug Deliv Rev* 63:312–23.

Narita Y., Kagami H., Matsunuma H., et al. 2008. Decellularized ureter for tissue-engineered small-caliber vascular graft. *J Artif Organs* 11:91–99.

Oh B.K., Meyerhoff M.E. 2004. Catalytic generation of nitric oxide from nitrite at the interface of polymeric films doped with lipophilic CuII-complex: a potential route to the preparation of thromboresistant coatings. *Biomaterials* 25:283–93.

Parikh S.A., Edelman E.R. 2000. Endothelial cell delivery for cardiovascular therapy. *Adv Drug Deliv Rev* 42:139–61.

Perktold K., Leuprecht A., Prosi M., et al. 2002. Fluid dynamics, wall mechanics, and oxygen transfer in peripheral bypass anastomoses. *Ann Biomed Eng* 30:447–60.

Piterina A.V., Cloonan A.J., Meaney C.L., et al. 2009. ECM-based materials in cardiovascular applications: inherent healing potential and augmentation of native regenerative processes. *Int J Mol Sci* 10:4375–417.

Post S., Kraus T., Muller-Reinartz U., et al. 2001. Dacron vs. polytetrafluoroethylene grafts for femoropopliteal bypass: a prospective randomised multicentre trial. *Eur J Vasc Endovasc Surg* 22:226–31.

Ravi S., Qu Z., Chaikof E.L. 2009. Polymeric materials for tissue engineering of arterial substitutes. *Vascular* 17 Suppl 1:S45–54.

Remuzzi A., Mantero S., Colombo M., et al. 2004. Vascular smooth muscle cells on hyaluronic acid: culture and mechanical characterization of an engineered vascular construct. *Tissue Eng* 10:699–710.

Roh J.D., Nelson G.N., Brennan M.P., et al. 2008. Small-diameter biodegradable scaffolds for functional vascular tissue engineering in the mouse model. *Biomaterials* 29:1454–63.

Roh J.D., Sawh-Martinez R., Brennan M.P., et al. 2011. Tissue-engineered vascular grafts transform into mature blood vessels via an inflammation-mediated process of vascular remodeling. *Proc Natl Acad Sci U S A* 107:4669–74.

Roll S., Muller-Nordhorn J., Keil T., et al. 2008. Dacron vs. PTFE as bypass materials in peripheral vascular surgery—systematic review and meta-analysis. *BMC Surg* 8:22.

Salacinski H.J., Goldner S., Giudiceandrea A., et al. 2001. The mechanical behavior of vascular grafts: a review. *J Biomater Appl* 15:241–78.

Salacinski H.J., Odlyha M., Hamilton G., Seifalian A.M. 2002. Thermo-mechanical analysis of a compliant poly(carbonate-urea)urethane after exposure to hydrolytic, oxidative, peroxidative and biological solutions. *Biomaterials* 23:2231–40.

Salacinski H.J., Tai N.R., Carson R.J., et al. 2002. *In vitro* stability of a novel compliant poly(carbonate-urea)urethane to oxidative and hydrolytic stress. *J Biomed Mater Res* 59:207–18.

Salzmann D.L., Kleinert L.B., Berman S.S., Williams S.K. 1999. Inflammation and neovascularization associated with clinically used vascular prosthetic materials. *Cardiovasc Pathol* 8:63–71.

Sanchez J., Elgue G., Riesenfeld J., Olsson P. 1998. Studies of adsorption, activation, and inhibition of factor XII on immobilized heparin. *Thromb Res* 89:41–50.

Sarkar S., Salacinski H.J., Hamilton G., Seifalian A.M. 2006. The mechanical properties of infrainguinal vascular bypass grafts: their role in influencing patency. *Eur J Vasc Endovasc Surg* 31:627–36.

Sarkar S., Sales K.M., Hamilton G., Seifalian A.M. 2007. Addressing thrombogenicity in vascular graft construction. *J Biomed Mater Res B Appl Biomater* 82:100–8.

Sarkar S., Schmitz-Rixen T., Hamilton G., Seifilian A. 2007. Achieving the ideal properties for vascular bypass graft using tissue engineering approach: a review. *Med Biol Eng Comput* 45:327–36.

Schlosser M., Wilhelm L., Urban G., et al. 2002. Immunogenicity of polymeric implants: long-term antibody response against polyester (Dacron) following the implantation of vascular prostheses into LEW.1A rats. *J Biomed Mater Res* 61:450–57.

Schlosser M., Zippel R., Hoene A., et al. 2005. Antibody response to collagen after functional implantation of different polyester vascular prostheses in pigs. *J Biomed Mater Res* A 72:317–25.

Schmidt C.E., Baier J.M. 2000. Acellular vascular tissues: natural biomaterials for tissue repair and tissue engineering. *Biomaterials* 21:2215–31.

Seifalian A., Salacinski H., Tiwari A., et al. 2002. *In vivo* biostability of poly(carbonate-urea)urethane graft. *Biomaterials* 24:2549–57.

Shin'oka T., Matsumura G., Hibino N., et al. 2005. Midterm clinical result of tissue-engineered vascular autografts seeded with autologous bone marrow cells. *J Thorac Cardiovasc Surg* 129:1330–38.

Simmons A., Padsalgikar A.D., Ferris L.M., Poole-Warren L.A. 2008. Biostability and biological performance of a PDMS-based polyurethane for controlled drug release. *Biomaterials* 29:2987–95.

Simon D.I., Xu H., Ortlepp S., Rogers C., Rao N.K. 1997. 7E3 monoclonal antibody directed against the platelet glycoprotein IIb/IIIa cross-reacts with the leukocyte integrin Mac-1 and blocks adhesion to fibrinogen and ICAM-1. *Arterioscler Thromb Vasc Biol* 17:528–35.

Smith D.J., Chakravarthy D., Pulfer S., et al. 1996. Nitric oxide-releasing polymers containing the $[N(O)NO]^-$ group. *J Med Chem* 39:1148–56.

Smith R., Oliver C., Williams D. 1987. The enzymatic degradation of polymers *in vitro*. *J Biomed Mater Res* 21:991–1003.

Soldani G., Losi P., Bernabei M., et al. 2009. Long term performance of small-diameter vascular grafts made of a poly(ether)urethane-polydimethylsiloxane semi-interpenetrating polymeric network. *Biomaterials* 31:2592–2605.

Sorrentino S., Haller H. 2011. Tissue engineering of blood vessels: how to make a graft. *Tissue Eng* 2:263–78.

Spark J.I., Yeluri S., Derham C., Wong Y.T., Leitch D. 2008. Incomplete cellular depopulation may explain the high failure rate of bovine ureteric grafts. *Br J Surg* 95:582–85.

Stitzel J., Liu J., Lee S.J., et al. 2006. Controlled fabrication of a biological vascular substitute. *Biomaterials* 27:1088–94.

Tai N.R., Salacinski H.J., Edwards A., Hamilton G., Seifalian A.M. 2000. Compliance properties of conduits used in vascular reconstruction. *Br J Surg* 87:1516–24.

Tepe G., Schmehl J., Wendel H.P., et al. 2006. Reduced thrombogenicity of nitinol stents—*in vitro* evaluation of different surface modifications and coatings. *Biomaterials* 27:643–50.

Tillman B.W., Yazdani S.K., Lee SJ., et al. 2009. The *in vivo* stability of electrospun polycaprolactone-collagen scaffolds in vascular reconstruction. *Biomaterials* 30:583–88.

Tiwari A., Salacinski H., Seifalian A.M., Hamilton G. 2002. New prostheses for use in bypass grafts with special emphasis on polyurethanes. *Cardiovasc Surg* 10:191–97.

Turner N.J., Kielty C.M., Walker M.G., Canfield A.E. 2004. A novel hyaluronan-based biomaterial (Hyaff-11) as a scaffold for endothelial cells in tissue engineered vascular grafts. *Biomaterials* 25:5955–64.

Vanin A.F., Vedernikov Iu I., Galagan M.E., et al. 1990. [Angeli salt as a producer of nitrogen oxide in animal tissues]. *Biokhimiia* 55:1408–13.

Veith F.J., Moss C.M., Sprayregen S., Montefusco C. 1979. Preoperative saphenous venography in arterial reconstructive surgery of the lower extremity. *Surgery* 85:253–56.

Venkataramen S., Boey F., Luciana L. 2008. Implanted cardiovascular polymers: natural, synthetic, and bio-inspired. *Prog Polym Sci* 33:853–74.

Watanabe M., Shin'oka T., Tohyama S., et al. 2001. Tissue-engineered vascular autograft: inferior vena cava replacement in a dog model. *Tissue Eng* 7:429–39.

Weinburger C.B., Bell, E. A blood vessel model constructed from collagen and cultured vascular cells. *Science* 1986;231:397–400.

Weston M.W., Rhee K., Tarbell J.M. 1996. Compliance and diameter mismatch affect the wall shear rate distribution near an end-to-end anastomosis. *J Biomech* 29:187–98.

Wildevuur C.R., van der Lei B., Schakenraad J.M. 1987. Basic aspects of the regeneration of small-calibre neoarteries in biodegradable vascular grafts in rats. *Biomaterials* 8:418–22.

Wilhelm L., Zippel R., von Woedtke T., et al. 2007. Immune response against polyester implants is influenced by the coating substances. *J Biomed Mater Res A* 83:104–13.

Williamson M.R., Shuttleworth A., Canfield A.E., Black R.A., Kielty C.M. 2007. The role of endothelial cell attachment to elastic fibre molecules in the enhancement of monolayer formation and retention, and the inhibition of smooth muscle cell recruitment. *Biomaterials* 28:5307–18.

Wise S.G., Byrom M.J., Waterhouse A., et al. 2011. A multilayered synthetic human elastin/polycaprolactone hybrid vascular graft with tailored mechanical properties. *Acta Biomater* 7:295–303.

Woodruff M.A., Hutmacher D.W. 2010. The return of a forgotten polymer: polycaprolactone in the 21st century. *Prog Polym Sci* 35:1217–56.

Xue L., Greisler H.P. 2003. Biomaterials in the development and future of vascular grafts. *J Vasc Surg* 37:472–80.
Yu T.J., Chu C.C. 1993. Bicomponent vascular grafts consisting of synthetic absorbable fibers. I. *In vitro* study. *J Biomed Mater Res* 27:1329–39.
Yu T.J., Ho D.M., Chu C.C. 1994. Bicomponent vascular grafts consisting of synthetic absorbable fibers: part II: *in vivo* healing response. *J Invest Surg* 7:195–211.
Zilla P., Bezuidenhout D., Human P. 2007. Prosthetic vascular grafts: wrong models, wrong questions and no healing. *Biomaterials* 28:5009–27.

5

Endovascular Stents

G. Lawrence Thatcher

CONTENTS

Introduction

This chapter presents an introduction to the development of polymeric endovascular stents, with the indications-for-use in peripheral and coronary revascularization. Tsuji and Tamai and coworkers stated, "The success of biodegradable stents depends on not only the biocompatibility of the stent materials but also the ability of the *manufactured* stent itself" [1]. Because the ultimate goal is to have a device that is both clinically and commercially viable, the process of product realization is woven into this discussion with examples drawn from current clinical and preclinical experience. The objective is to present the story of polymeric endovascular stents, in a translational approach, putting the current body of work into context of the development path, and to draw attention to some of the multitude of interactions that can affect device efficacy and viability. What are commonly referred to as "stent-grafts," for the exclusion of aneurysms of the abdominal aorta, will only be mentioned in regard to the potential for a polymeric primary stent platform, leaving fuller discussion of the polymers used for their outer and inner lining constructs to chapters discussing vascular grafts and tissue engineering of blood vessels. Polymer stent platforms may also be considered for the controlled release of active pharmaceutical ingredients (APIs), in addition to their drug eluting coatings, however, details of polymer systems for drug release are to be addressed in a separate chapter. Since about 2006, concern has been raised regarding the increased risk of late and very late stent thrombosis occurring with drug eluting stents (commonly referred to as DES) constructed of a permanent metal platform with various drug release coatings. Therefore this chapter focuses primarily on polymeric fully bioresorbable scaffolding.

Clinical Prelude

The tools and paradigms for the treatment of atherosclerotic vascular disease have undergone both revolutionary and evolutionary changes that have fueled the current desire to develop fully bioresorbable stents [2,3]. Some developments, particularly in the arena of imaging, such as multislice spiral computed tomography (MSCT), quantitative coronary angiography (QCA), intravascular ultrasound (IVUS), and optical coherence tomography (OCT) (Figure 5.1), have not only improved diagnoses and interventional treatment but also dramatically improved our means to evaluate new stent designs and stent materials.

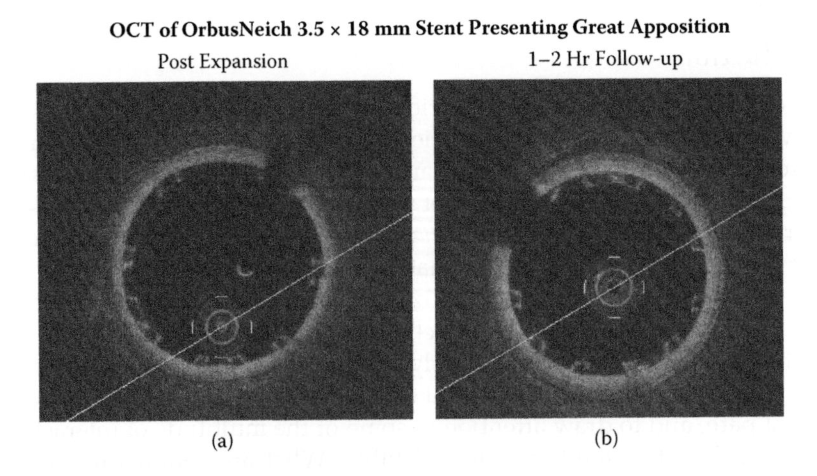

FIGURE 5.1
OCT image of the OrbusNeich stent in a porcine left internal mammary artery: (a) immediately after deployment with great apposition and no thrombus and (b) 1 hour postdeployment with great apposition and no thrombus. The stent struts present as highlighted black boxes against the artery wall. (Courtesy of OrbusNeich, Fort Lauderdale, FL. With permission.)

Labinaz and coworkers [4] summarized Dr. Russell Ross's response-to-injury model to explain the development of atherosclerosis. Ross suggested that when the endothelium was injured, a complex cascade of events and healing responses formed a plaque comprised of various cells, fats or cholesterol, and fibrous tissue. These lesions could progress, possibly calcify, and eventually form a blockage (stenosis) in the artery, leading to reduced blood flow. Reduced blood flow, as well as a plaque rupture forming a clot, can cause a heart attack. This cascade of events has been the focus of significant research, and the response-to-injury model has been refined not only to help us understand responses to interventional therapies but also to target the development of new designs or materials.

In 1977, a decade after the introduction of coronary artery bypass grafting, balloon angioplasty was introduced. With the use of a percutaneous balloon catheter, blockages in arteries could be treated, improving blood supply. Onuma and Serruys characterized this treatment milestone as the first revolution in the field of revascularization [3].

Initial catheters were not easy to steer or navigate to the stenosis. Subsequent numerous technical innovations with guide catheters, guide wires, and angioplasty balloons led to increased use of this procedure. Success over previous treatments was profound but suffered some important limitations. Injury to the artery intimal wall would occur when extensive dilation was needed to remodel plaque, particularly with calcified and eccentric lesions. Sometimes, a tear in the blood vessel lining or a dissection of the plaque could occur, creating an obstructive flap with abrupt thrombus formation, resulting in acute blood vessel blockage. Some cases respond to an immediate repeat procedure, while others may require emergency bypass surgery. Successful balloon angioplasty restored vessel patency and allowed vascular remodeling and late luminal enlargement. Frequently, however, restenosis would occur caused by elastic recoil, neointimal hyperplastic healing response to the vessel trauma, and what is termed constrictive remodeling. A variety of adjunctive therapies was examined as well as alternate treatments such as several atherectomy devices and ablative laser catheters to remove atherosclerotic material from inside the artery.

The treatment of atherosclerotic vascular disease evolved, was driven, to address the less-than-perfect outcome as well as treatment-induced complications of balloon angioplasty. The concept of placing a metal scaffold to support the artery from recoil and to seal plaque or intimal flaps, thus preventing acute stenosis, was introduced by Charles Dotter in 1967. However, it was not until 1986 that the self-expanding Wallstent™ (Schneider Inc.) was first successfully used in human coronary arteries. This was followed by the balloon expandable Gianturco-Roubin (Cook Inc.) and the Palmaz-Schatz (Johnson & Johnson) stainless steel bare metal stents (BMSs). Various stent designs progressively emerged to reduce the intensity of vessel wall injury and subsequent influence on neointimal proliferation, as well as improved crossing profiles, improved stent placement, reduced side branch occlusion, and so on.

Providing a valuable solution to some of the complications of "simple" balloon angioplasty also resulted in some new complications. Neointimal hyperplasia was more significant than with balloon angioplasty alone, occurring now inside the stent, frequently requiring repeat treatment. Two advantageous healing responses, late luminal enlargement and vascular remodeling with vasomotion, were now also physically inhibited by a permanent metal scaffold.

Stents coated with a drug-eluting polymer were developed to mitigate the profound neointimal hyperplasia experienced with BMSs [5,6]. The first of these drug-eluting stents (DESs) became commercially available in about 2002. The polymer coatings are compounded with an antiproliferative or anti-inflammatory active pharmaceutical ingredient that elutes over time, inhibiting tissue ingrowth. The first-generation DES employed nonbiodegradable polymers in the coatings. As early as 2004, Virmani and colleagues [7] warned that there might be a risk of late and very late stent thrombosis in patients after implantation of DESs. Her examination of autopsy specimens revealed struts that remained uncovered with new endothelium, as well as some persistent inflammatory reaction [8]. It was suggested that this might have occurred because the polymer caused the inflammatory response or possible persistent drug release. Additional concerns have also been expressed related to discontinuities, or cracks, in the surface coatings, presenting poststent expansion. This has led to the development of a second-generation DES based on various bioresorbable polymer coatings. Having a clear clinical need has now renewed the drive toward the development of fully bioresorbable stent platforms and prompted excitement that they will not only mitigate these new complications but also allow for restoration of the endothelial structure and function and vessel remodeling. This reinforces what Stack and Clark called for as the "ideal stent design" [2] in 1994 and has since become called "vascular restoration therapy" and the fourth revolution in interventional cardiology by Wykrzykowska, Onuma, and Serruys [9]. In addition, a fully bioresorbable stent platform would allow for the use of newer diagnostic imaging, such as magnetic resonance imaging (MRI) and MSCT, which are becoming the noninvasive imaging of choice, and easier reintervention, avoiding the full metal jacket syndrome.

Polymeric Stent Development Background

In 1988, just 2 years after the first successful use of a metallic self-expanding stent in humans, Stack and Clark at Duke University were making the case for the bioabsorbable stent. They reported on their poly-L-lactide (PLLA), braided-strand construct, self-expanding stent. The results after up to 18 months *in vivo* were judged biocompatible with a low thrombotic response,

TABLE 5.1

Cleveland Clinic/Mayo Clinic Biodegradable Test Polymers

	Polymer Name	Degradation Products	Degradation Rate
PGLA	Poly(D, L-lactide/glycolide): copolymer 85% lactide/15% glycolide	D-Lactic acid L-Lactic acid Hydroxyacetic (glycolide) acid	100% in 60 to 90 days (rat subcutaneous model)
POE	Polyorthoester	Cyclohexanedimethanol 1,6-Hexanediol Pentaerythritol Propionic acid	60% in 46 weeks (in saline, pH 7.4 at 37°C)
PHBV	Poly(hydroxybutyrate/ hydroxyvalerate) copolymer: 22% valerate	Hydroxybutyric acid Hydroxyvaleric acid	0 to 20% in 182 days (rat subcutaneous model)
PCL	Polycaprolactone	Hydroxycaproic acid	52% in 1,491 days (rabbit subcutaneous model)

Source: Adapted from Zidar, J.P., A.M. Lincoff, R.S. Stack. 1994. Biodegradable stents. In *Textbook of Interventional Cardiology*, 2nd ed., ed. E.J. Topol, 787–802. New York: Saunders.

minimal neointimal response, and low inflammatory reaction. They stated that it was a "specialized form of poly-L-lactide" [2] that proved most suitable. This gave an early indication of how important not only polymer selection is to the outcome but also polymer processing and morphology development to achieve the requirements for a stent.

This foundational work was followed by the Cleveland/Mayo Clinic healing response study (a joint effort between the Cleveland Clinic, Mayo Clinic, and Thoraxcenter, Erasmus University), reported in 1992. This study examined the healing response to four bioresorbable polymer films (other than PLLA) solvent cast on a portion of a balloon-expandable tantalum wire coil stent. Table 5.1 shows the biodegradable test polymers in the Cleveland/ Mayo Clinic healing response study. The outcome from this study was less than encouraging for the bioresorbable polymers tested, which presented significant inflammatory responses. This prompted some confusion as some had anticipated that bioabsorbable polymers would be noninflammatory based on both the Duke study results and then-current successes with fracture fixation, wound closure, and drug delivery. Further testing repeating the same protocol but with several biodurable polymers (polyether urethane urea, silicone, and polyethylene terephthalate [PET]) attempted to differentiate between an inflammatory response to the polymer degradation products or the presence of a polymer implant itself. The results showed similar inflammatory responses even though these three biodurable polymers had previously demonstrated good graft or implant experience.

Equally conflicting results with biodurable polymeric stents made from PET were also reported in porcine trials. Murphy and coworkers developed and reported on a self-expanding PET stent [10]. It was reported that at 4 to 6 weeks after implantation, all stent deployment sites were occluded due to neointimal proliferation "with chronic foreign body inflammatory response surrounding the stent filaments and marked neointimal proliferative response in the center of the vessel." van der Giessen and colleagues [11] reported the opposite response, with their PET stent showing patent vessels after 4 weeks with minimal neointimal hyperplasia.

Dennis Jamilokowski shared a favorite axiom of his with participants at the Medical Device and Manufacturing conference on bioresorbable polymers in February 2011: "The devil is in the details." This is evident when confronted with conflicting study outcomes, and we are looking for root causes for better understanding. It is easy to overlook what seem to be "just details" when focusing on the inflammatory response associated with a polymer. We have come to understand, for example, that some implants in these studies were sterilized and others not.

Tamai also showed us that even changing stent construct design had an influence on the inflammatory response [3,12]. The presence of residual solvents from solution casting could foster differing cellular responses and stimulus for intimal proliferation. Even though there was an effort to rule this out in the Mayo study, we have since come to understand better how difficult it is to remove trace solvent as it has been shown that a solvent-cast polyactide acid (PLA) sample had trace chloroform even after several years under high vacuum. More recent work by Vipule Dave with solvent-cast stent blanks resorted to supercritical CO_2 extraction to remove residual solvent sufficiently [13].

Differences in the polymers due to their synthesis can also influence outcome. Residual monomers or solvents from the polymerization alone can induce inflammatory responses. Differences in the chain transfer agents used will change a polymer's end group and could precipitate different reactivity and cellular response. Separate work by Lincoff and coworkers [14] and Tamai and colleagues [12] suggested that high molecular weight PLLA is more quiescent in the artery than lower molecular weight polymer. Various nuances in the methods of manufacture of a stent aside from the polymer itself will also influence the morphology and subsequent properties as well as degradation kinetics.

Such apparently conflicting data led some research teams to examine more closely the healing response to proposed bioresorbable polymers before committing to further costly stent and stent delivery system development. Accordingly, Yoklavich and coworkers [15] reported in 1996 a favorable healing response at 52 weeks follow-up to a novel bioabsorbable stent (Cordis/TESco) (Figure 5.2), injection molded from a hybrid blend of PLLA and a trimethylene carbonate copolymer (TMC), deployed in the iliac artery in both canine and porcine models. This approach used a delivery balloon briefly heated to 70°C, allowing expansion of the stent at above its glass transition temperature T_g, then cooling back to 37°C. Because of questions regarding possible heat damage to the intimal wall, the alternate artery branch was used as a

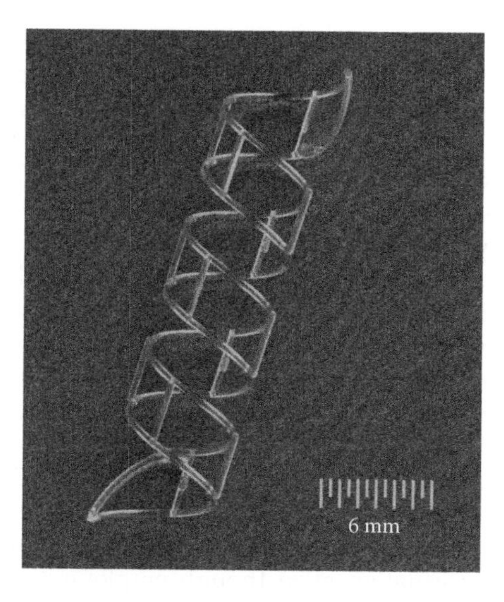

FIGURE 5.2
Cordis-TESco Hybrid PLA/TMC intravascular prototype stent. (Courtesy of TESco Associates Inc., Tyngsborough, MA. With permission.)

control with only the heated balloon. The concept of the novel hybrid polymer was to provide a mechanism that would be friendly to balloon expansion versus a braided, self-expanding construct used previously by Stack and Clark. The hybrid polymer system was developed also to have a quiescent breakdown even to the extent that the TMC moiety prevailed longer than the lactide, so that on loss of physical integrity the breakup would be soft or compliant within the endothelium.

Reports of early either mixed or disappointing results may have hampered general enthusiasm for bioresorbable stents, just as early disappointments with inflammatory response from the first polyglycolic first proximation pins hampered development of other bioresorbable orthopedic devices. The first to market pins suffered even though polyglycolide had been well received as a suture. The new pins made from the same suture material presented a larger bolus than previously experienced, prompting an inflammatory response to the amount of dye as well as the larger amount of polymer degradation product. It was found that even the cutting of the pins during surgery left ends of the pins that caused localized inflammation. These kinds of responses prompt us to look beyond a small sample of material, breaking out of the research mode and into the reality of manufacturing. In particular, they suggest the need to examine how the ends of braid or other filament-type constructs are cut and sealed and if they present a risk of physical inflammatory response.

Stack continued work with Zidar and colleagues to develop a PLLA stent [2] and in 1999 reported placement for 18 months in canine femoral arteries without inflammatory reaction. At about the same time, Tamai and coworkers [12] reported good biocompatibility, also using high molecular weight PLLA in a self-expanding stent. These studies, along with the Yoklavich (Cordis/TESco) stent, successfully used high molecular weight PLLA or a PLLA hybrid polymer to establish quiescent degradation.

Lincoff and colleagues [14], in their work on coated stents, also suggested better compatibility with higher molecular weight PLLA. Both of the Stack and Tamai stents used high molecular weight PLLA filaments draw oriented and crystallized to impart the requisite strength and self- or semi-self-expansion. The Tamai stent, however, introduced a significant change in the stent design and delivery, changing from a braided construct to zigzag form elements. The delivery became semi-self-expanding, requiring balloon expansion with contrast dye heated to 50°C for 13 seconds. The stent would otherwise take considerably longer to self-expand at 37°C. This design change demonstrated less intimal damage by stent implantation (with a concomitant reduction in neointimal proliferation and inflammatory response) and less thrombus formation even though employing a similar polymer. Missing from this snapshot picture are the substantive details in polymer synthesis and processing actually to make the oriented filaments and stent constructs.

These early works seemed focused more on polymer safety, that is, low inflammatory response, than on design efficacy. With the challenges to develop an efficacious bioresorbable stent platform and delivery system seeming formidable, and especially prior to a clear and immediate clinical need, attention appeared directed more toward what appeared to be a less-complicated path of coating current metal platforms developing DESs to resolve BMS problems.

The Design Envelope

When developing polymeric endovascular scaffolding, one needs to reflect on the complex interactions that influence successful development of a safe, efficacious, and cost-beneficial stent system. "This 'process' of product realization involves understanding the *entire* product life cycle" (italics mine) [16], p. 95. This process is just as applicable to endovascular stents as it was proposed for orthopedic implants. It involves developing an understanding not only of the device's clinical task but also all of its life cycle, starting with polymer synthesis and ending, as in the case of a fully bioresorbable polymer stent, with its degradation and final elimination of the polymer degradation products from the body. This life-cycle understanding becomes layered with risk assessment of the ability to reach each objective, including that of commercial viability within various cost or time constraints. James Oberhauser and coworkers [17] presented a review of the clinical portion of the life cycle divided into three phases: revascularization, restoration, and resorption. To these phases, we need to add an understanding of the manufacturing as well as the intervention procedure, or delivery, of the device. So, as we continue the discussion of polymeric endovascular stents, it is as much about the process as it is the polymer itself. Vipul Dave [13] suggested an interaction of polymer materials, stent design, and drug delivery with novel processes, and James Oberhauser [18] reinforced the emphasis on polymer processing to deliver clinical utility, not just simple polymer selection. Robert Cottone [19] proposed the formation of a design envelope to guide the development of bioresorbable stent platforms; an adaption of this is shown in Figure 5.3.

When we explore the four main groups in this design envelope, we can break some of these into subsets more dependent on when or where the requirement presents within the life cycle. Cottone suggested the main requirement groups in an overview detailed in Table 5.2.

It is important to establish how entwined these criteria sets are; when one part of an interdisciplinary development team begins to address one issue, it can dramatically affect other requirements or change the constraint window.

One may think, for example, that the process of polymer selection starts with establishing the biocompatibility of a polymer. However, what really needs to be considered is biocompatibility of the stent system. As mentioned, there is a complex cascade of events that represent the healing response to the implant, starting with insult to the intimal wall and inner elastic lamina of the vessel when the stent is delivered and deployed at the lesion. Thus acute

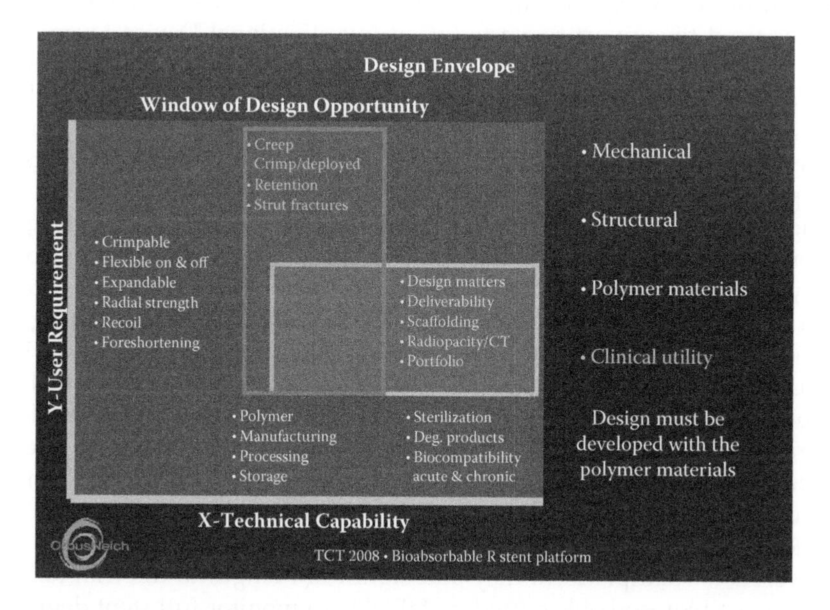

FIGURE 5.3 (see color figure)
Design envelope. (Courtesy of Cottone, R. 2008. Bioabsorbable R stent design concepts. Presentation at the Transcatheter Cardiovascular Therapeutics Conference, Washington, DC, October. With permission.)

TABLE 5.2

Requirement Groups

Mechanical	Structural	Polymer Materials	Clinical Utility
Crimpable	Creep	Polymer	Design matters
Expandable	Crimp deployed	Manufacturing	Deliverability
Radial strength	Retention	Processing	Scaffolding
Recoil	Strut fractures	Storage	Radiopacity
Foreshortening		Sterilization	Enables a full product portfolio
Flexible on and off (delivery catheter)		Degradation products	
		Biocompatibility (both acute and chronic)	

Source: Adapted from Cottone, R.J. 2010. Fully absorbable vascular scaffold with combination CD34 ab cell capture and abluminal sirolimus eluting coating. Presentation at the Transcatheter Cardiovascular Therapeutics, Washington, DC, September 21–25.

biocompatibility is dependent not only on the immediate polymer chemistry but also on many other factors, for example, how the polymer was made; residual contaminants from synthesis; effects of processing on the polymer, on both degradation and contaminants; design of the stent and how it is manufactured and deployed. These interactions become challenges under design control requirements and planning for validation. The team needs to estimate when in the design review process to impose a design lock. This typically occurs when starting long-term preclinical trials in which the data is to be used to support requests for an Investigational Device Exemption (IDE) and the start of human clinical trials. Changes implemented to address manufacturing and performance issues may necessitate additional preclinical trials and the restarting of clinical trials. It follows, then, that early in the process there should be a discussion of the regulatory hurdles or risks as they pertain to the proposed theater of sales and the different and constantly changing regulatory environments. This especially weighs heavy depending on the regulatory theaters considered and the need to demonstrate both safety and efficacy for approval to market. For example, at this date, obtaining a European CE mark requires demonstrating device safety (meeting the essential safety requirement of the EU directive), whereas obtaining U.S. Food and Drug Administration (FDA) approval to market requires establishing both safety and efficacy. In addition, a new device is expected to demonstrate improved efficacy or equivalent efficacy, but at a lower cost, over the current standard of treatment. I learned the cost for a human clinical trial in the United States for a coronary stent is estimated to be between $20 and $30 million for an initial primary indication for use. In addition, a full bioresorbable stent platform may add significant length to the trial follow-up, versus a bioresorbable coated metal DES, to monitor full stent degradation and absorption as well as potential late responses. Joseph Berglund and coworkers [20] referred to the "technical challenges *to develop and commercialize* a successful bioabsorbable stent," (italics mine) (p. F72) underscoring that this is all about commercial product development, not just esoteric research. Further, he drew attention to the decision process regarding the target indication for use, selecting between peripheral and coronary revascularization: "Since SFA (superficial femoral artery) therapies are typically life-enhancing rather than life-sustaining, the regulatory paths and risks associated with developing an unproven technology are greatly reduced compared to coronary indications" (p. F73).

Once the target indication for use is established, we typically hear first the requirements for clinical utility of a finished, sterile, delivered (implanted) stent. These usually include that stents must be a certain strength, must degrade quiescently (i.e., not induce an inflammatory response), and must do their job for a certain minimum period of time. Also, one has to include objectives surrounding deliverability of the stent, such as crossing profile, branch vessel occlusion, tracking ability, ability to overexpand to ensure proper apposition without strut failure, and so on. These statements of clinical utility are only the beginning. Sooner rather than later, one also needs to embrace the concept that we have to be able to make the stent in a commercial and cost-effective manner.

As we explore the current approaches from the perspective of a design envelope, let us start with the methodology of stent delivery. The stent must traverse an artery and then the lesion and, when appropriately positioned, somehow be deployed, expanding radially from the crimped state. The stent must become larger than the initial vessel diameter, remodeling the plaque burden, to reduce the blockage, thus opening the flow path (revascularization). This can be achieved by either self-expanding, balloon delivery, or a combination of partial self-expansion with final balloon delivery. With balloon expansion or assisted expansion, it is the angioplasty balloon that is doing the work of vessel and lesion dilation. This stent delivery decision directs subsequent stent architecture, polymer choice, and manufacturing.

Current Approaches

The publishing of the findings of late stent thrombosis in DES-implanted patients presented a new clear clinical need, igniting enthusiasm to drive investment in a new technology platform to replace current DESs. A bioresorbable stent platform seeks to mitigate the issues surrounding the current DESs as well as enable vascular restoration therapy [9].

With the emphasis now on fully bioresorbable stents for revascularization, it would be easy to forget the role of a permanent stent for the exclusion of aneurysms and their possible polymeric platforms. The clinical jobs are quite different. Revascularization can be viewed as the opening of a closed (stenosed) or restricted vessel to restore blood flow, whereas exclusion therapy

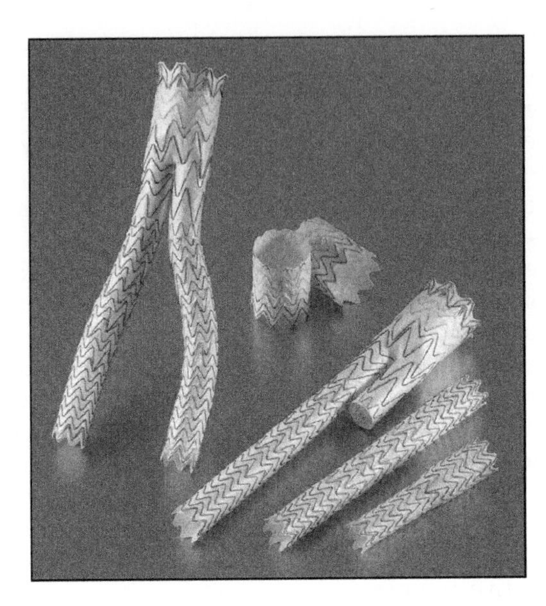

FIGURE 5.4
Covered stent graft for AAA repair. (Reprinted public domain photo from "Covered Stent Graft," Wikipedia, accessed July 20, 2011.)

intervenes in an artery that has a bulging, weakened wall threatening to rupture. These types of stent have an inner and outer covering over the support structure, as shown in Figure 5.4. Currently, these are self-expanding structures and when in place seal both proximal and distal to the threatened area and provide for a new blood conduit. With the pressure now relieved from the damaged wall section, this portion of the artery wall will eventually reduce and conform to the stent's outer profile. Most of these support structures are currently made from shape memory nitinol wire construct covered with either PET mesh or fluoropolymer membrane derived from vascular graft technology. It remains to be shown that biodurable shape memory polymers [21] have a clinical preference. It has yet to be demonstrated if the damaged artery wall from a reduced aneurysm will remodel itself to fully restored healthy function of both the endothelium and the inner elastic lamina. If this were shown, there would be merit to explore a bioresorbable shape memory polymer [22,23] for such a self-expanding stent structure to provide temporary scaffolding and then disappear.

Various examples of current clinical, preclinical, and *in vitro* work with coronary and peripheral revascularization stents are listed in Table 5.3. Some of these are discussed along with the concept of a design envelope and issues of product realization. At this time, the Igaki-Tamai™ stent has 10 years of follow-up in humans and has obtained the CE mark for peripheral indications. The Abbott/BVS stent, with over 2 years of human clinical data, has also received the CE mark, but for coronary indications (allowing for continued clinical trials). Reva Medical has reported on its initial 25-patient

TABLE 5.3

Examples of Current Work with Coronary and Peripheral Revascularization Stents

Current Clinical, Preclinical, and *In Vitro* Work	
Igaki-Tamai	PLLA filament-based construct
Abbott/BVS	Laser-cut, extruded and oriented PLLA tube
Reva Medical	Laser-cut, molded tyrosine polycarbonate sheet
Bioabsorbable Therapeutics Inc. (BTI)	Polyanhydride ester based on salicylic acid
OrbusNeich Medical	Laser-cut, extruded-tube PLLA/PDLA/CL copolymer blend
Arterial Remodeling Technologies (ART)	Molded amorphous PLDLA
Cordis (J&J)	Laser-cut, solvent-cast tube, PLGA85:15/PCL-PLG (Monocryl) blend
Tepha	PLLA/PHB peripheral stent
Additional or Alternate Material Concepts	
Mnemoscience (Aporo Biomedical)	Bioresorbable, self-expanding, shape memory polymer
Alternate Abbott Polymers	Phase-separated star block copolymers [47,48]
Bezwada Biomedical	NSAID-functionalized polymer backbone (e.g., naproxen or salicylic acid)

Note: PLDLA, poly L-co-D,L-lactide; PLGA, poly L-lactide-co-glycotide.

clinical trial experiences and further design optimization. Last, in July 2009, Bioabsorbable Therapeutics completed a 12-month follow-up of its 11-patient first-in-man trial.

Self-Expanding Stents

A fully self-expanding stent is manufactured at its deployed size and then collapsed around a guide catheter. A sheath restrains the stent while it is being delivered and is withdrawn once the stent is positioned for deployment. Either elastic recoil or the response to an applied stimulus like heat to a shape memory polymer is the mechanism for expansion. Polymer creep or stress relaxation while constrained in the protective delivery sheath can diminish the ability to self-expand. A semi-self-expanding stent is manufactured like a fully self-expanding stent, either at its deployed size or at a partial deployed size. When the protective sheath is withdrawn, the stent partially opens and then is fully deployed with the assistance of a balloon catheter. Self-expanding and semi-self-expanding designs, requiring sheathed delivery, are sometimes thought to be more difficult to track, especially in the coronary arteries, potentially somewhat limiting their clinical utility to predominantly peripheral indications.

The Igaki-Tamai stent is considered semi-self-expanding because of the extended length of time it takes to self-expand at physiologic conditions. Therefore to obtain full expansion within a reasonable time frame (e.g., less than 30 seconds), the stent is allowed to self-expand partially and is further assisted into place using a balloon catheter employing heated contrast dye as the expansion fluid. The contrast dye is heated to above the T_g of the polymer (in initial clinical trials, heated to 80°C) and the balloon catheter inflated to 6–14 atmospheres, holding for about 30 seconds [24], then cooling back to 37°C. In later trials, this was reduced to 13 seconds at 50°C to minimize heat injury to the vessel, and the cycle was repeated until there was equilibrium and good apposition to the vascular wall [1].

Many self-expanding stent architectures are braided constructs similar to the metallic Wallstent and the original Stack and Clark PLLA stent. The Igaki-Tamai design presents a marked departure with a zigzag architecture that reduces the filament overlaps and resulting irritation and intimal injury on expansion. The reduced filament overlap also probably reduces the stent profile and thrombogenicity. Both the Igaki-Tamai and the original Stack-Clark stents are based on higher molecular weight (e.g., >2 IV) PLLA spun into monofilament and drawn to impart molecular orientation, paracrystallinity, and crystallinity to enhance the base polymer's mechanical properties. This especially reduced the polymer elongation and increased tensile strength and modulus, enabling self-expansion, good hoop strength, and low creep. Using higher molecular weight PLLA resulted in noticeably quiescent degradation and resorption.

In 2007, the Igaki-Tamai stent was the first bioresorbable stent to receive a CE mark for peripheral indications. In 2009, a new version called the Remedy™ was introduced with a slightly different architecture. The Igaki-Tamai stent was constructed of zigzag elements connected by fabricated bars, whereas the new Remedy appears fabricated with three filaments forming the zigzag elements with a few overlaps in lieu of hard fabricated connections.

Regardless of the construct architecture, both stents are manufactured from similar high-strength, higher molecular weight PLLA filaments. Manufacturing and processing methods present significant challenges over conventional lower molecular weight polymers. One may consider gel spinning over melt spinning to avoid thermal degradation. However, this presents its own set of challenges to remove the solvent. As with solvent casting, there are questions regarding potential differences in the morphology from gel-spun samples and those prepared from a melt process [25] and any resulting microstructure from extracting the solvent. In addition, different postspinning processing, such as secondary orientation and heat treatment (sometimes incorrectly referred to as "annealing") may have to be considered [26]. These process steps to induce orientation and crystallinity are critical to filament constructs to impart sufficient elastic recoil for deployment and then once deployed to be able to resist both acute stent recoil and longer-term creep [27].

The orientation imparted during processing is not stable and can relax over time. Further, this relaxation can be accelerated by sterilization temperatures. Accordingly, special low-temperature ethylene oxide (EtO) sterilization cycles are often utilized, as are freezing of parts that are to be exposed to various radiation sources (e.g., E-beam sterilization). This is also a problem for shelf life and shipping of a commercial product, in particular for self-expanding stents that are stored constrained in their delivery sheath. The orientation can be somewhat stabilized by imparting crystallization that acts as a physical cross-link. The polymer specifications may also be influenced by the choice of filament-manufacturing process. For example, PLLA selected for melt spinning may employ a different polymerization initiator, or chain transfer agent, to impart better thermal stability for processing not necessary for a solvent process. This in turn could also influence the hydrophobicity of the polymer, its degradation kinetics, and so on. The postpolymerization extraction of unreacted residual monomer and the solvent used to carry the catalyst is also crucial for melt processing stability. Improving processing stability preserves the molecular weight for initial mechanical property integrity and reduces monomer and oligomers resulting from thermal degradation that would accelerate the stent degradation kinetics [16].

In addition to the polylactides with clinical experience discussed previously, a new class of bioresorbable shape memory polymers has been proposed for self-expanding stents by Mnemoscience, a spin-out from work originally performed at the Massachusetts Institute of Technology [22,23].

Balloon-Delivered Stents

A balloon-delivered stent presents a whole new field of manufacturing and performance issues. To begin, the stent is manufactured at some size larger than the deflated balloon catheter; it is then crimped onto the balloon. Various design techniques are employed to keep the stent in its proper location on the balloon while it is being delivered down a guide catheter and finally traversing an artery. Typically, a stent is cut from a tube, or a tubular stent is constructed from cut sheet.

There have been a few attempts at injection molding either blanks for further cutting or even a completed stent, as in Cordis/TESco stent (Figure 5.2). Injection molding a fully formed stent presents significant issues with the melt viscosity of the higher molecular weight polymer needed for mechanical properties and biocompatibility. Yoklavich and colleagues [15] reported that the injection-molded struts were about 0.013 inch thick, almost twice the thickness currently typically considered viable for clinical utility. Not only is there the difficulty of getting the polymer to flow into thin-wall sections without degrading it, but also there is the problem of multiple flow front knit lines leading to strut failure.

In 2009, Lafont and coworkers [28] reported on Arterial Remodeling Technologies' program to develop a balloon-delivered "molded" stent platform based on a poly-L-DL-lactide. They reported on a 6-month follow-up on iliac rabbit arteries, using a 6F balloon-delivered stent manufactured with a proprietary molding and memory-shaping process. Midwest Plastics reported an attempt at injection molding a tubular blank for laser cutting. Even molding a blank without molding a finished strut pattern is challenging, with problems such as core pin shift or bending resulting in a nonuniform wall unacceptable for laser cutting.

Many balloon-expanded stent designs, versus self-expanding stents, seem to be at greater risk for strut crazing and fracture when stresses are high during both crimping and expansion deployment. Herein is the challenge in manufacturing: to balance the morphology and microstructure developed during processing for radial strength properties while preserving sufficient elongation and a fracture mechanism that averts strut failure. "Stent fracture will lead to premature radial strength loss, vessel recoil, tissue irritation, and inflammation independent of the material biocompatibility" [20, p. F75]. Further, clinical utility is greatly diminished if a stent cannot be stretched (i.e., overdilated) to match the dimension of the target vessel or comply with either calcified or eccentric lesions without stent or strut fracture. Even with the advancement of QCA to measure the lesion for appropriate stent size selection, calibration errors can lead to underestimation of the target lesion diameter and result in the need to overdilate the stent. It should be noted that underexpansion of a stent could also cause one not to develop the optimal mechanical properties in some stent design/material combinations, resulting in excessive stent recoil and poor apposition.

Stents Fabricated from Sheet

The Reva Medical stent has attempted to mitigate some of these issues by using a different approach to design and construction. It is manufactured by cutting sheet made from an amorphous tyrosine (desaminotyrosyltyrosine ethyl ester) polycarbonate. A unique ratcheting design causes the stent struts to slide and then lock from recoil as it is expanded, minimizing the high-strain points that exist in most strut designs cut from a tube blank. Its mechanical properties and degradation kinetics have been shown to be similar to PLLA [29]. Iodine molecules have even been incorporated into the backbone of the polymer to impart radiopacity. The first-generation REVA stent was evaluated in the 25-patient RESORB clinical trial. The trial data demonstrated the need for "further polymer and design optimization" [30, p. F56] for improved performance under real load conditions. The first REVA ratchet lock design has been replaced with the more flexible helical slide-and-lock ReZolve stent [3], manufactured from a tyrosine polycarbonate slightly modified to improve cyclic or fatigue loading [30].

The embracing of tyrosine polycarbonate by Reva Medical for its stent represents one of the challenges, or risks, in polymer selection as well as the potential opportunity. Typically, one looks for well-established, validated, commercial-scale polymerizations to avoid surprises going into clinical trials and scale-up. The family of tyrosine polycarbonates has seen limited commercial applications in devices, the REVA stent being the most notable, but has had more applications in drug delivery coatings. However, the value of the opportunity to capture a unique polymer to differentiate the product line and the ability to modify the polymer backbone or pendant groups to adapt to the evolving understanding of performance requirements are also significant. I understand that the scale-up of the polymerization had its challenges. Having a unique polymer platform may have significant advantages but needs to be weighed against the risk of manufacturing scale-up taking longer and being more costly than expected, as well as the possibility of a restricted or limited material source.

Stents Fabricated from Tubes

Fabricating a stent by laser cutting a tube follows the dominant manufacturing and design concepts of the most popular BMS and metal DES platforms. Both stainless steel and cobalt-chrome have well-understood structures and properties and are available in tubes drawn to precise uniform wall sections. Laser cutting of metals has progressed such that beam widths are narrower for smaller kerfs, and pulse rates are ever faster, allowing for significantly less heat-affected zone and cleaner cuts. Even with these improvements, laser-cut metal stents still typically require electropolishing and other treatments to clean the surface.

Laser cutting of polymer stents is different from the cutting of metals. Metal ablation is mainly by vaporization of the metal due to heat. Polymer ablation also involves chain scission and vaporization, not just melting. To reduce thermal damage and improve cutting efficiency, the output wavelength of eximer lasers can be selected or tuned to match the ultraviolet (UV) absorption spectra of the polymer. Coupling a tuned laser with very high pulse rates has significantly improved cut edge quality, which in metals was frequently dealt with by secondary operations that are not available with polymers. Polymer struts are typically thicker than metal to compensate for lower mechanical properties; thus it takes several more passes with the laser to complete the stent cut pattern.

These new lasers have shorter focal lengths, leading to them to be less forgiving. This has been problematic for manufacturing teams as metal tubing for stents has much tighter wall section and diameter tolerances than can be readily achieved with most polymer tube manufacturing. So if the polymer tube wall section varies too much, it can fall out of the focal range of the laser. Traditional methods for polymer tubing manufacturing, as well as fixture and inspection methods, needed to be reinvented, leading development teams to embark on customized processes to achieve desired quality and properties. As with any polymer cutting, it has been suggested that the molecular weight is reduced at the cut edge [31]. It has yet to be demonstrated if this significantly affects either initial stent mechanical properties or degradation kinetics.

When stents are cut from a tube, one needs to consider the state of expansion of the cut form prior to crimping or loading onto a delivery balloon catheter. This decision occurs early in the development cycle and can easily entrap the development team in one direction. Your extremes are to have a cut pattern in the crimped state or at an overdilated state; however, reality would probably be somewhere in between. For example, a stent may be laser cut from a tube about 2.0-mm diameter then crimped onto a much smaller 4F or 5F delivery balloon catheter to have a final crossing profile of 6F but a target expansion out to maybe 3.5-mm diameter. An alternate approach might be to laser cut the stent from a tube that is the same diameter as the final target expansion; in the first example, this is about 3.5-mm diameter.

The amounts of strain that the stent struts undergo both in crimping and expansion must be taken into account with materials and strut design. Just dealing with the ability to "fold" the stent struts down into a crimped position can be a challenge, as can keeping them in place. It is reasonable to plan to stretch the stent into final apposition to the artery wall. This can preclude cutting in the final deployed diameter as it may not be able to fold back down onto the balloon from this stretched configuration. This all influences the morphology, that is, the degree of crystallinity or orientation that may be required for stent strength as well as the toughness of the polymer system to withstand subsequent crimping and expansion without strut failure or extensive recoil and creep.

The introduction of strain-induced orientation and crystallization during crimping and expansion may be crucial to performance. When manufacturing the stent tube blank for cutting, the degree of orientation or crystallinity at each stage of manufacture and stent delivery must be well understood. The ability of a stent to be overdilated to ensure good apposition, or to comply with a difficult lesion, is critical to clinical success and utility. Strut cracking can occur if the development and manufacturing teams do not plan for sufficient elongation or compliance in the stent material or design. Manufacturing high-tolerance tubing from high molecular weight bioresorbable polymers with just the right orientation and morphology to meet this objective is no small task.

A tube blank for laser cutting can be manufactured by melt extrusion, injection molding, gel extrusion, dip coating, or spray coating. The last three introduce solvents into the process that at some point need to be extracted. This can be a challenging step. As indicated previously, it has been demonstrated that traces of chloroform remained in cast samples even after several years under a vacuum process. The effect at the cellular level is not clear. Earlier studies such as the early Cleveland Clinic trials that attempted to expose any adverse inflammatory reaction from residual solvent have been questioned. Vipul Dave and colleagues [13] reported solvent dip-coating tubes for stent blanks from PLG (85:15) copolymer blended with polycaprolactone (PCL)-PLG copolymer (Monocryl). They reported using supercritical CO_2 extraction to mitigate the solvent from tube casting.

As mentioned previously, there are questions regarding potential differences in the morphology of solvent-cast polymer versus that obtained from melt processing as well as the phase domain stability of solvent-cast materials [25]. It is not clear if this type of processing is beneficial. For example, some copolymers that do not crystallize from the melt have been shown to develop significant crystallinity cast from solution. In addition, layering or laminating effects from dip or spray coating a tube may need to be better understood. The impact strength of PLLA is reported to become higher by the addition of rubbery biodegradable polymers such as PCL [32]. Similarly, the addition of the soft and elastomeric PCL-PGA copolymer in this blend with stiff PLG increases 85:15 increases the blend's ductility to allow the stent structure to deploy and remain open following balloon catheter removal. The PLGA copolymer was selected with a 2.2–2.4 IV for mechanical performance and absorption time. One of the benefits of this solvent process is the ability to easily add both a radiopacier such as barium sulfate and the anti-proliferative sirolimus (rapamycin) into the bulk of the stent structure without resorting to intense thermal compounding that might otherwise compromise the polymer or active agent.

Bioabsorbable Therapeutics has been working with another unique polymer in an attempt to provide therapeutic moieties from polymer breakdown. Their polymer is a polyanhydride ester based on salicylic acid and adipic acid anhydride and is intended to provide anti-inflammatory properties as the polymer degrades. It is also radiopaque. Even though the stents used in the first-in-man trials included a coating that contained the anti-proliferative sirolimus, insufficient neointimal suppression was reported [3,33]. The first-generation design had a large 8F crossing profile and a 65% occlusion ratio; it has been replaced with a second-generation 6F design with thinner struts. Bezwada Biomedical has also proposed additional unique polymers with nonsteroidal anti-inflammatory drug- (NSAID) functionalized polymer backbones based on, for example, naproxen [34] or salicylic acid [35]. The therapeutic utility and the processing/mechanical requirements for stents of these proposed materials have yet to be determined. The mass of these polymers required to release a therapeutic bolus from the backbone of the polymer will have to be carefully considered and could greatly influence the stent design parameters. The release kinetics of the therapeutic moiety may also be governed by the degradation mechanism of the polymer backbone in combination with a number of other factors that influence drug delivery kinetics (e.g., surface area, molecular free volume, etc.), complicating designing for therapeutic efficacy. In addition, the mechanical performance life cycle will need to be determined in conjunction with changes to the polymer bulk related to the release of the therapeutic moiety.

Melt extrusion of a tube profile appears to be the dominant manufacturing method of blanks for laser cutting. As mentioned, there has been some attempt to injection mold tubing blanks for laser cutting; however, this approach has not met with reported success, and the conventional approaches to micromolding, for example, have not yet demonstrated that they can be adapted to the high molecular weight polymers required for this application. Extruding tubing with these bioresorbable polymers typically excludes conventional thin-walled tubing techniques such as underwater vacuum sizing. We have found that the critical wall section control required for both stent fabrication and uniform stent deployment is considerably tighter than typically practiced, even for what is conventionally considered high-tolerance tubing, leading to customized and usually proprietary extrusion processes.

James Oberhauser [18] presented compelling reinforcement to the previous statements here about the pivotal importance of polymer processing for successful outcome. The Abbott/BVS Absorb™ stent program confronted the less-than-optimal mechanical properties, reported in more generalized resources, by concentrating on the property improvements from polymer orientation and crystalline morphology as demonstrated in applications such as fibers, angioplasty balloons, biaxially oriented film, and stretch blow-molded containers [26,36]. This was accomplished by extruding a tube thicker than the final strut and then stretch blow molding to develop its orientation and crystallinity [18]. The Absorb stent utilizes high molecular weight PLLA as the primary stent structure. Selection of an appropriate polymer is a significant factor toward determining the success or failure of the stent design. This is not just simply specifying a certain molecular weight PLLA. As the polymer will undergo melt extrusion and then further thermal/mechanical processes, the molecular weight not only needs to be called out but also other factors that influence processability.

As mentioned previously, polymerization catalyst, initiators, condition parameters, extraction, and even grinding can have an impact on the thermal processability of the polymer. Yuan and coworkers [37] reported up to about 20% loss just in grinding PLLA small enough to feed in a small extruder. Molecular weight losses from chain scission make the polymer even more unstable in a subsequent molding or extrusion process. There are myriad details surrounding the polymer preparation and extrusion process itself that influence the quality and properties of the stent blank. Further, Oberhauser detailed the attention given to the polymer crystal nucleation and propagation as well as to both crystalline orientation and oriented amorphous (paracrystalline) domains to impart significant increases to the strength and modulus over the bulk unoriented polymer properties. However, there is a risk of applying significant orientation and strain-induced crystallization to a polymer that already has inherently low elongation [20]. Additional strain imparted during crimping or expansion can result in strut failure, particularly where strut cut patterns change directions across oriented polymer chains. Glauser and colleagues [38] discussed crack counts for deployed stents, which suggested further process or materials development may be required. The initial Absorb trial precipitated a stent redesign to provide, for

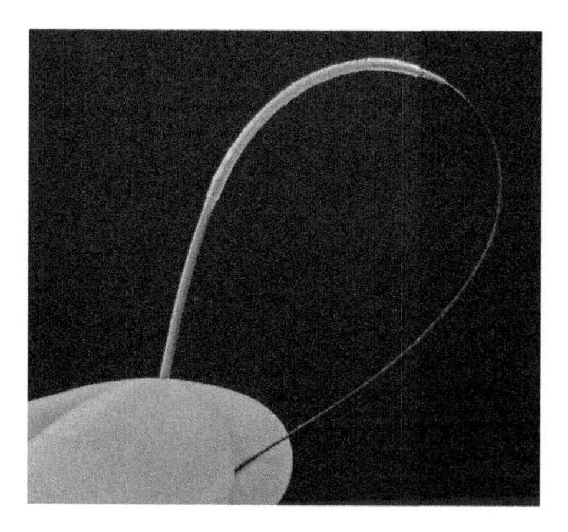

FIGURE 5.5
OrbusNeich R stent crimped on a 6F delivery catheter. (Courtesy of OrbusNeich, Fort Lauderdale, FL. With permission.)

example, more uniform support to the artery wall and higher radial strength without changing the polymer or strut thickness [39].

Robert Cottone [19] has reported on OrbusNeich Medical Incorporated's unique hybrid polymer [40,41] balloon-delivered stent platform (Figure 5.5). It is a platform that combines three technologies: a hybrid material, a novel stent design, and partitioned coatings for both drug delivery and endothelial progenitor cell capture. The hybrid material and stent design are the focus of the present discussion as they represent the stent "platform," a particular approach that "provides a marriage between the polymer material backbone formulations and the mechanical and structural aspects of the stent's design" [42, p. F66]. This stent is fabricated by laser cutting a tube extruded in a proprietary process. The hybrid material is a blend of three lactide polymers used together to address different critical performance criteria during the various stages of the material/stent life cycle, each with known pharmacokinetics: PLLA, poly-D-lactide (PDLA), and a lactide e-caprolactone or trimethylene-carbonate copolymer. The unique blend is suggested to enable polymer mechanics and crystalline orientation at various stages of manufacture and deployment and to present a balance of strength and compliance. It is a polymorphic and polyphasic system in which stereocomplexation between PLLA and PDLA is said to enhance the tensile properties of blends compared to those of the nonblended PLLA or PDLA [43]. The increased properties of these blends may also be attributed to dense chain packing in the amorphous regions due to a strong interaction between the L- and D-unit sequences. Multiple crystal forms are suggested through various stages, whether postextrusion, postprocessing, or strain induced during stent crimping and delivery. It is probably that the microstructure formed by stereocomplexation gelation during initial processing increases the number of spherulites per unit mass to enhance the tensile properties of these blends

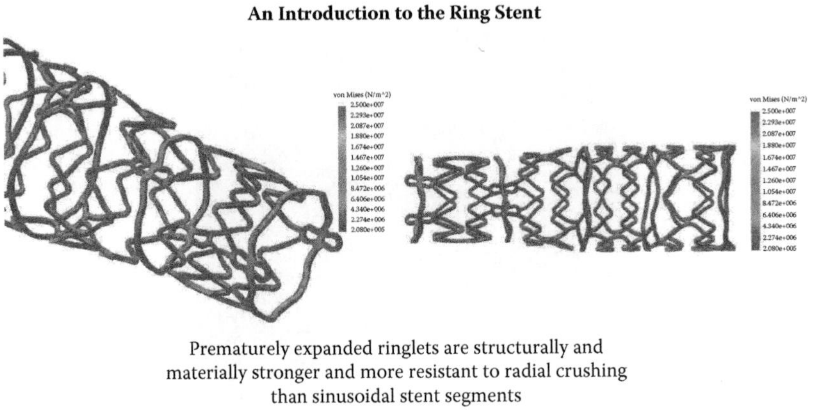

An Introduction to the Ring Stent

Prematurely expanded ringlets are structurally and materially stronger and more resistant to radial crushing than sinusoidal stent segments

FIGURE 5.6 (see color insert)
Finite element analysis (FEA) introduction to the OrbusNeich ring stent. Prematurely expanded ringlets are structurally and materially stronger and more resistant to radial crushing than sinusoidal stent segments. (Courtesy of OrbusNeich, Fort Lauderdale, FL. With permission.)

[43] and is followed by further stereocomplex growth and epitaxial homoenantiomer crystallization. Designed-in molecular free volume probably enables enough polymer chain mobility to provide flexibility and elongation while enhancing molecular orientation and strain-induced crystallization during crimp mounting on a delivery balloon and when stretched at physiologic conditions during deployment. The OrbusNeich program employs a stretched ringlet design to improve strength and recoil resistance, shown in Figures 5.6 and 5.7, which, in combination with the cross-moiety crystallization in the polymer blend, increases resistance to creep [40–42]. The balance of polymer microstructures and stent design appears to present both radial strength and stent strut crack resistance critical to clinical utility.

Van der Giessen and coworkers [44] stated that polyhydroxybutyrate (PHB) and polyhydroxybutyrate valerate (PHBV) are not well-suited materials for immediate and extended blood contact. However, Grabow and coworkers [45] demonstrated promising results with a blend of PLLA with high-elongation poly-4-hydroxybutyrate (P4HB) in porcine iliac arteries. This approach appears built on their work to improve performance of DES coatings by blending poly-D-L-lactide (PDLLA) with P4HB, especially addressing the coating surface quality and mechanical integrity poststent expansion. Their prior work with a PLLA stent prototype prompted "improvements to the expansion behavior of the stent and its *in vivo* biocompatibility" by blending the PLLA with P4HB [45, p. 747]. The differences in biocompatibility of polyhydroxyalkanoates reported by Grabow and Van der Giessen's teams may well stem from dramatic improvements in the genetic-engineered fermentation process for monomer production as earlier PHB polymers were noted for cell debris that promoted extensive inflammatory responses.

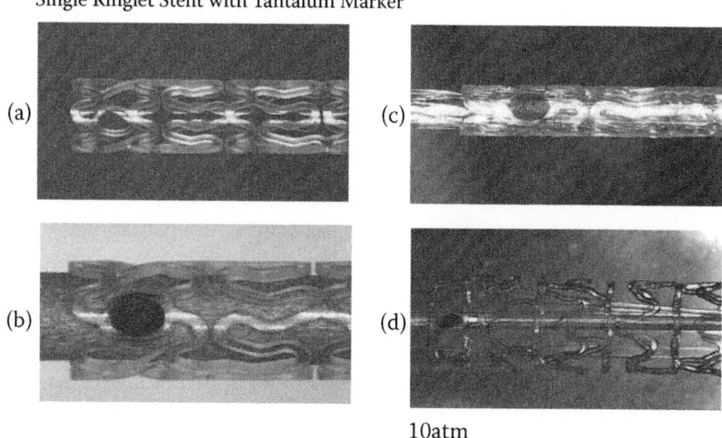

FIGURE 5.7 (see color insert)
OrbusNeich stent: (a) as cut, (b) as cut with marker dot, (c) crimped on balloon, (d) deployed at 10 atmospheres. (Courtesy of OrbusNeich, Fort Lauderdale, FL. With permission.)

Conclusions

The vision of leaders in interventional cardiology is now clear. The mandate is to develop a fully bioresorbable stent platform that performs mechanically and clinically equivalent to the current DESs—and then disappears, resulting in vascular restoration therapy. The rationale for a bioresorbable stent is to

- Eliminate the chronic presence of a foreign body and allow for "complete healing" or vascular restoration therapy
  - Limiting the need for anticoagulation/antiplatelet therapy with no late adverse events
  - Providing opportunity for reintervention therapy
- Provide for drug elution
  - With greater drug loading possible
  - With greater flexibility in elution characteristics
- Provide improved compatibility with imaging technologies
- Enable broader development of percutaneous local therapeutics for the treatment or prevention of vascular diseases

Undoubtedly, there will be additional polymers, designs, and development programs for fully bioresorbable endovascular stent platforms. Ultimately, fully bioresorbable stents may replace permanent stents, and even though the feasibility and safety of some systems has been established, there remain important issues and improvements before they become both clinically and commercially viable to enjoy widespread clinical use [46].*

References

1. Onuma, Y., S. Garg, T. Okamura, et al. 2009. Ten-year follow-up of the IGAKI-TAMAI stent: a posthumous tribute to the scientific work of Dr. Hideo Tamai. *EuroIntervention Supplement* 5:F109–F111.
2. Zidar, J.P., A.M. Lincoff, R.S. Stack. 1994. Biodegradable stents. In *Textbook of Interventional Cardiology*, 2nd ed., ed. E. J. Topol, 787–802. New York: Saunders.
3. Onuma, Y., P.W. Serruys. 2011. Bioresorbable scaffold: the advent of a new era in percutaneous coronary and peripheral revascularization. *Circulation* 123:779–797.
4. Labinaz, M., J. Carter, M. Dossenbach, M. Sketch. 1996. New device therapy for coronary artery disease (revisited). *New Developments in Medicine and Drug Therapy* Sep/Dec.
5. Costa, M.A., M. Sabate, W.J. van der Giessen, et al. 1999. Late coronary occlusion after intracoronary brachytherapy. *Circulation* 100:789–792.
6. Sousa, J.E., M.A. Costa, A. Abizaid, et al. 2001. Lack of neointimal proliferation after implantation of sirolimus-coated stents in human coronary arteries: a quantitative coronary angiography and three-dimensional intravascular ultrasound study. *Circulation* 103:192–195.
7. Virmani, R., G. Guagliumi, A. Farb, et al. 2004. Localized hypersensitivity and late coronary thrombosis secondary to a sirolimus-eluting stent: should we be cautious? *Circulation* 109:701–705.
8. Joner, M., A.V. Finn, A. Farb, et al. 2006. Pathology of drug-eluting stents in humans: delayed healing and late thrombotic risk. *Journal of the American College of Cardiology* 48:193–202.
9. Wykrzykowska, J., Y. Onuma, P.W. Serruys. 2009. Vascular restoration therapy: the fourth revolution in interventional cardiology and the ultimate "Rosy" prophecy. *EuroIntervention Supplement* 5:F7–F8.
10. Murphy, J.G., R.S. Schwartz, W.D. Edwards, et al. 1992. Percuntaneous polymeric stents in porcine coronary arteries: initial experience with polyethylene terephthalate stents. *Circulation* 86:1596–1604.
11. van der Giessen, W.J., C.J. Slager, E.J. Gussenhoven, et al. 1993. Mechanical features and *in vivo* imaging of a polymer stent. *International Journal of Cardiac Imaging* 9:219–226.
12. Tamai, H., K. Igaki, T. Tsuji, et al. 1999. A biodegradable poly-l-lactic acid coronary stent in porcine coronary artery. *Journal of Interventional Cardiology* 12:443–450.

* Details of the preclinical and clinical trials, introduced in the above text, may be found in the listed references.

13. Dave, V., D. Overaker, R. Donovan, R. Falotico. 2009. Polymer, process and design elements of a balloon expandable bioabsorbable drug eluting stent. Presentation at the annual meeting of the Society for Biomaterials, San Antonio, TX, April 22–25.
14. Lincoff, A.M., J.G. Furst, S.G. Ellis, et al. 1997. Sustained local delivery of dexamethasone by a novel intravascular eluting stent to prevent restenosis in the porcine coronary injury model. *Journal of the American College of Cardiology* 29:808–816.
15. Yoklavich, M.F., G.L. Thatcher, H.F. Sasken. 1996. Vessel healing response to bioabsorbable implant. Proceedings from the Fifth World Biomaterials Congress, Toronto, May 29–June 2.
16. Thatcher, G. L. 2009. Product realization: the processing of bioabsorbable polymers. In *Degradable Polymers for Skeletal Implants,* ed. P.I.J.M. Wuisman and T.H. Smit, 93–122. New York: Nova Science.
17. Oberhauser, J.P., S. Hossainy, R.J. Rapoza. 2009. Design principles and performance of bioresorbable polymeric vascular scaffolds. *EuroIntervention Supplement* 5:F15–F22.
18. Oberhauser, J. 2011. Engineering bioresorbable polymers into vascular scaffolds: an application in interventional cardiology. Presentation at the MD&M West Conference, Anaheim, CA, February 7–10.
19. Cottone, R J. 2010. Fully absorbable vascular scaffold with combination CD34 ab cell capture and abluminal sirolimus eluting coating. Presentation at the Transcatheter Cardiovascular Therapeutics, Washington, DC, September 21–25.
20. Berglund, J., Y. Guo, J.N. Wilcox. 2009. Challenges related to development of bioabsorbable vascular stents. *EuroIntervention Supplement* 5:F72–F79.
21. Toensmeier, P.A. 2005. Shape memory polymers reshape product design. *Plastics Engineering* (March): 10–11.
22. Venkatraman, S.S., L.P. Tan, J.F.D. Joso, Y.C.F. Boey, X. Wang. 2006. Biodegradable stents with elastic memory. *Biomaterials* 27:1573–1578.
23. Lendlein, A., P. Simon, K. Kratz, B. Schnitter. Stents for use in the non-vascular field, which comprise an SMP material. U.S. Patent Application Number 2007, 0129784, filed June 9, 2004, issued June 7, 2007.
24. Tsuji, T., H. Tamai, K. Igaki, et al. 2001. Biodegradable polymeric stents. *Current Cardiology Reports* 3:10–17.
25. Manson, J.A., L.H. Sperling. 1976. Diblock and triblock copolymers: effect of solvent casting on morphology. In *Polymer Blends and Composites,* 141–142. New York: Plenum Press.
26. Ghosh, S., N. Vasanthan. 2006. Structure development of poly(L-lactic acid) fibers processed at various spinning conditions. *Journal of Applied Polymer Science* 101:1210–1216.
27. Zilberman, M., K.D. Nelson, R.C. Eberhart. 2005. Mechanical properties and *in vitro* degradation of bioresorbable fibers and expandable fiber-based stents. *Journal of Biomedical Material Research-A Part B* 74B (2):792–799.
28. Lafont, A., E. Durand. 2009. A.R.T.: concept of a bioresorbable stent without drug elution. *EuroIntervention Supplement* 5:F83–F87.
29. Tovar, N., S. Bourke, M. Jaffe, et al. 2010. A comparison of degradable synthetic polymer fibers for anterior cruciate ligament reconstruction. *Journal of Biomedical Material Research Part A* 93(2):738–747.

30. Pollman, M.J. 2009. Engineering a bioresorbable stent: REVA programme update. *EuroIntervention Supplement* 5:F54–F57.
31. Crugnola, A.M., E.L. Radin, R.M. Rose, I.L. Paul, S.R. Simon, M.B. Berry. 1976. Ultrahigh molecular weight polyethylene as used in articular prostheses (a molecular weight distribution study). *Journal of Applied Polymer Science* 20:809–812.
32. Grijpma, D.W., R.D.A. van Hofslot, H. Supèr, A.J. Nijenhuis, A.J. Pennings. 1994. Rubber toughing of poly(lactide) by blending and block copolymerization. *Polymer Engineering Science* 34(22): 1674–1684.
33. Jabara, R., L. Pendyala, S. Geva, J. Chen, N. Chronos, K. Robinson. 2009. Novel fully bioabsorbable salicylate-based sirolimus-eluting stent. *EuroIntervention Supplement* 5:F58–F64.
34. Bezwada, R.S. 2007. Absorbable poly naproxen. Presentation at the annual meeting of the Society for Biomaterials, Chicago, April 18–21.
35. Bezwada, R.S. 2007. Absorbable polymers from functionalized salicylic acid. Presentation at the annual meeting of the Society for Biomaterials, Chicago, April 18–21.
36. Yu, L., H. Liu, F. Xie, L. Chen, X. Li. 2008. Effect of annealing and orientation on microstructures and mechanical properties of polylactic acid. *Polymer Engineering and Science* 48(4):634–641.
37. Yuan, X., A.F.T. Mak, K.W. Kwok, B.K.O. Yung, K. Yao. 2001. Characterization of poly(L-lactic acid) fibers produced by melt spinning. *Journal of Applied Polymer Science* 81:251–260.
38. Glauser, T., V.J. Gueriguian, B. Steichen, J. Oberhauser, M. Gada, L. Kleiner. Controlling crystalline morphology of a bioabsorbable stent. International Patent Application Number WO 2011/031872 A2, filed September 9, 2010, publication March 17, 2011.
39. Onuma, Y., N. Piazza, J.A. Ormiston, P.W. Serruys. 2009. Everolimus-eluting bioabsorbable stent—Abbot Vascular programme. *EuroIntervention Supplement* 5:F98–F102.
40. Thatcher, G.L., R.J. Cottone. Bioabsorbable polymeric composition for a medical device. U.S. Patent Number US7846361 B2, filed July 20, 2007, issued December 7, 2010.
41. Thatcher, G.L., R.J. Cottone. Bioabsorbable polymeric composition for a medical device. U.S. Patent Number US7897224 B2, filed July 22, 2009, issued March 1, 2011.
42. Cottone, R.J., G.L. Thatcher, S.P. Parker, et al. 2009. OrbusNeich fully absorbable coronary stent platform incorporating dual partitioned coatings. *EuroIntervention Supplement* 5:F65–F71.
43. Tsuji, H., Y. Ikada. 1999. Stereocomplex formation between enantiomeric poly(lactic acid)s. 11. Mechanical properties and morphology of solution-cast films. *Polymer* 40(24):6699–6708.
44. van der Giessen, W.J., A.M. Lincoff, R.S. Schwartz, et al. 1996. Marked inflammatory sequelae to implantation of biodegradable and nonbiodegradable polymers in porcine coronary arteries. *Circulation* 94:1690–1697.
45. Grabow, N., D.P. Martin, K. Schmitz, K. Sternberg. 2009. Absorbable polymer stent technologies for vascular regeneration. *Journal of Chemical Technology and Biotechnology* 85(6):744–751.
46. Cottone, R. 2008. Bioabsorbable R stent design concepts. Presentation at the Transcatheter Cardiovascular Therapeutics Conference, Washington, DC, October.

47. Wang, Y. Implantable medical devices fabricated from block copolymers. U.S. Patent Application Number 11/864729, filed September 28, 2007, issued June 7, 2011.
48. Wang, Y., D.C. Gale, V.J. Gueriguian. Implantable medical devices fabricated from polymers with radiopaque groups. U.S. Patent Application Number 11/799354, filed April 30, 2007, issued October 30, 2008.

Recommended Reading

Arterial Remodeling Technologies. 2010. Bioresorbable stent. http://www.art-stent.com/index.php (accessed June 29, 2011).

Brugaletta, S., H.M. Garcia-Garcia, R. Diletti, et al. 2011. Comparison between the first and second generation bioresorbable vascular scaffolds: a six month virtual histology study. *EuroIntervention* 6:1110–1116.

Buchbinder, M. 2010. Biodegradable stents: future or fancy. Presentation at China Interventional Therapeutics Conference, Beijing, March 31–April 3.

Colombo, A., E. Karvouni. 2000. Biodegradable stents: fulfilling the mission and stepping away. *Circulation* 102:371–373.

DiMario, C., F. Borgia. 2009. Assimilating the current clinical data of fully bioabsorbable stents. *EuroIntervention Supplement* 5:F103–F108.

Douglas, F.L., S. Acharya, B.L. Davis, et al. 2011. Value-driven engineering for U.S. global competitiveness: a call for a national platform to advance value-driven engineering. http://www.abiakron.org/Data/Sites/1/pdf/abiawhitepaper6-14-11.pdf.

Farooq, V., Y. Onuma, M. Radu, et al. 2011. Optical coherence tomography (OCT) of overlapping bioresorbable scaffolds: from bench-work to clinical application. *EuroIntervention* 2011 (January):1–13. http://www.pcronline.com/eurointervention/ahead_of_print/32_04/index.php?ind=1.

Fourné, F. 1999. *Synthetic Fibers: Machines and Equipment, Manufacture, Properties: Handbook for Plant Engineers, Machine Design, and Operation*. Munich, Germany: Hanser.

Ge, J. 2007. Limus-eluting stents with poly-L-lactic acid coating. *Asia Pacific Cardiology* 1:42–43.

Guo, Q., Z. Lu, Y. Zhang, S. Li, J. Yang. 2011. *In vivo* study on the histocompatibility and degradation behavior of biodegradable poly(trimethylene carbonate-co-D,L-lactide). *Acta Biochim Biophys Sin* 43(6):433–440.

Hietala, E., U. Salminen, A. Stahls, et al. 2001. Biodegradation of the copolymeric polylactide stent. *Journal of Vascular Research* 38: 361–369.

Jamiolkowski, D.D. 2011. Satisfying product requirements with absorbable polyesters. Presentation at the MD&M West Conference, Anaheim, CA, February 7–10.

Lendlein, A., R. Langer. 2002. Biodegradable, elastic shape-memory polymers for potential biomedical applications. *Science* 296(5573):1673–1676.

Ormiston, J.A., P.W.S. Serruys. 2009. Bioabsorbable coronary stents. *Circulation: Cardiovascular Interventions* 2:255–260.

Salemi, T. 2007. Can stents pull off a disappearing act? *Start-Up* 12(1).

Schmitz, K., D. Behrend, K. Sternberg, et al. Polymeric, degradable drug-eluting stents and coatings. U.S. Patent No. 7618448, filed February 6, 2007, issued November 17, 2009.

Scholz, C. 2009. The molecular structure of degradable polymers. In *Degradable Polymers for Skeletal Implants*, ed. P.I.J.M. Wuisman and T.H. Smit, 3–20. New York: Nova Science.

Serracino-Inglott, F. 2008. Endovascular aneurysm repair—technical aspects. http://www.stent-graft.com/id2.html.

Shalaby, S.W., K.J.L. Burg. 2004. *Absorbable and Biodegradable Polymers*. Boca Raton, FL: CRC Press.

Soares, J.S., J.E. Moore Jr., K.R. Rajagopal. 2007. Theoretical modeling of cyclically loaded, biodegradable cylinders. In *Modeling of Biological Materials*, ed. F. Mollica, L. Preziosi, and K.R. Rajagopal, 125–177. Boston: Birkhäuser Boston.

Soares, J.S., J.E. Moore Jr., K.R. Rajagopal. 2008. Constitutive framework for biodegradable polymers with applications to biodegradable stents. *ASAIO Journal* 54: 295–301.

Soares, J.S., J.E. Moore Jr., K.R. Rajagopal. 2009. Mechanics of deformation-induced degradation of poly(L-lactic acid) endovascular stents. Proceedings of the ASME Summer Bioengineering Conference, Lake Tahoe, CA, June 17–21.

Su, S., R.Y.N. Chao, C.L. Landau, et al. 2003. Expandable bioresorbable endovascular stent. I. Fabrication and properties. *Annals of Biomedical Engineering* 31:667–677.

Tsuji, H. 2009. Poly(lactide)s and their copolymers: physical properties and hydrolytic degradation. In *Degradable Polymers for Skeletal Implants*, ed. P.I.J.M. Wuisman and T.H. Smit, 41–70. New York: Nova Science.

Vert, M. 2009. Bioabsorbable polymers in medicine: an overview. *EuroIntervention Supplement* 5:F9–F14.

Waksman, R. 2006. Biodegradable stents: they do their job and disappear. *Journal of Interventional Radiology* 18(2):70–74.

6

Nitric Oxide Delivery for Prevention of Restenosis

Elizabeth A. Lipke, Lakeshia J. Taite, and Jennifer L. West

CONTENTS

Introduction

Cardiovascular disease (CVD) is the number one cause of death in the United States each year. Over 50% of CVD deaths are caused by coronary heart disease (CHD), making it the single largest killer of both women and men in the United States. More than half a million Americans die from CHD each year, and the yearly cost of CHD is $142 billion (American Heart Association 2004). Since its introduction in the late 1970s, percutaneous coronary intervention (PCI), formerly known as percutaneous transluminal coronary angioplasty (PTCA), has been used as a treatment for CHD (Bult 2000). The procedure involves the inflation of a balloon attached to a catheter in the stenosed vessel to compress the occluding plaque. Restenosis, the reocclusion of blood vessels after the use of PCI, is a serious clinical concern in the treatment of coronary artery disease, affecting 20–50% of all PCI patients within 6 months of the procedure (Bult 2000), necessitating repeat procedures, increasing patient morbidity, and causing higher medical costs (Schwartz et al. 1992a). Each year, over 600,000 percutaneous coronary interventional procedures are performed in the United States to treat CHD (American Heart Association 2011); more than 50% of these procedures involve the placement of a stent, and the average cost per procedure is approximately $28,500 (American Heart Association 2004). There is no clinically effective strategy to date to prevent restenosis.

Restenosis

Restenosis is characterized as a healing response following the injury caused by PCI that occurs over a period of 3–6 months. Vessel injury during vascular procedures triggers a cascade of events that leads to the eventual restenosis (Libby et al. 1992; Eltchaninoff et al. 1998; Bhatia et al. 2004) (Figure 6.1); the need to improve current methods drives biomedical research in this area, including the development of new materials for next-generation stents and localized drug delivery.

During balloon expansion, occlusive plaque is compressed against the vessel wall. Elastic recoil of the artery causes fractional loss of the expansion instantly (Bult 2000). Beginning immediately after the initial injury, endothelial disruption, and the resulting lack of nitric oxide (NO) production, encourages platelet adhesion and aggregation (Bauters and Isner 2000). This stimulates the release of mitogenic substances, including platelet-derived growth factor (PDGF), which has been implicated in the migration and proliferation of smooth muscle cells (SMCs) into the lumen, leading to formation of a neointima (Bauters and Isner 1997; Costa and Simon 2005). Other mechanisms associated with the restenotic cascade include the activation of

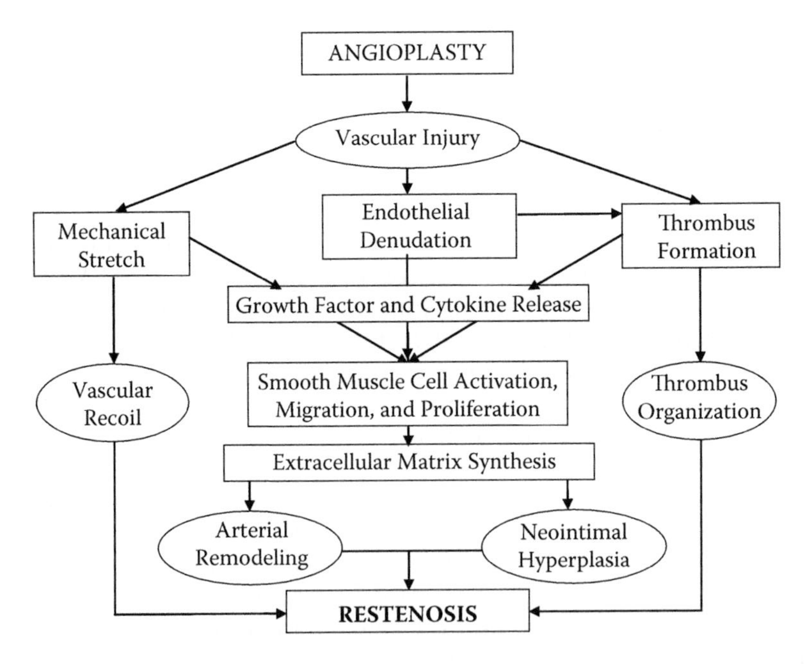

FIGURE 6.1
Following balloon angioplasty, a cascade of events occurs, leading to the eventual restenosis or reocclusion of the vessel. Both mechanical and molecular components contribute to producing this undesirable response, which is considered an overreaction of the body's natural healing mechanisms.

mitogens, including basic fibroblast growth factor (bFGF), PDGF, and transforming growth factor beta (TGF-β) through direct injury to subendothelial smooth muscle, which also leads to smooth muscle activation (Bult 2000; Tanabe et al. 2004; Khan et al. 2007). As SMCs proliferate and migrate into the injured area, they deposit matrix proteins that form an occlusive scar tissue in a process termed *neointimal hyperplasia* (Bauters and Isner 1997). Over 3 to 6 months, constrictive vessel remodeling by adventitial myofibroblasts leads to additional loss in lumen diameter. Complete or partial vessel reendothelialization generally takes longer than 3 months; reendothelialization is associated with suspension of SMC proliferation (Allaire and Clowes 1997).

With the placement of a stent, acute recoil and long-term negative remodeling are limited by the force of the stent pressing against the vessel wall; however, the increased injury and inflammation caused by the stent over the long term can lead to a higher proliferative response than is seen with balloon angioplasty alone (Fattori and Piva 2003; Beyar 2004; Grewe et al. 2000). In addition, more pronounced long-term endothelial dysfunction has been observed in vessels receiving stents as compared to balloon angioplasty alone (van Beusekom et al. 1998). The majority of in-stent restenosis consists of extracellular matrix (ECM) components, proteoglycans, and collagen, with only 11% composed of cells, and the deeper the penetration of the stent struts into the medial layer, the greater the degree of neointima formation (Fattori and Piva 2003).

Limiting injury to the vessel is difficult due to the degree of balloon expansion necessary to reopen the artery; when a vessel that is 90% occluded is properly dilated, the vessel undergoes a 10-fold expansion (Schwartz et al. 2004). Although modern stent designs result in less vessel injury due to overexpansion than earlier wire stents (Schwartz et al. 1992b), there is a substantial amount of unavoidable injury to the vessel that occurs with both angioplasty alone and stenting procedures. In an attempt to control the vascular response to this injury, drug-eluting stents (DESs) have been developed to provide localized drug delivery to halt excessive neointimal growth and preserve lumen diameter. In 2006, 76% of stent procedures employed DESs as opposed to bare metal stents (American Heart Association 2011).

DES Devices

Although DES devices have the potential to reduce restenosis rates, particularly among high-risk patients, such as diabetics, DES devices have their own drawbacks. The polymer coatings used for drug delivery can elicit an increased inflammatory response, and in comparison to bare stents, slower or incomplete healing has been observed (Virmani et al. 2003; Stampfl et al. 2009). The drugs incorporated into DESs include sirolimus (rapamycin), which is an immunosuppressive agent with anti-inflammatory and antiproliferative effects, and derivatives of taxol, including paclitaxel, which polymerize microtubules, preventing cell migration and proliferation (Hiatt et al. 2002; Bhatia et al. 2004). In addition to inhibiting the undesirable SMC proliferation and migration that cause neointimal hyperplasia, these compounds inhibit the highly desirable endothelial cell (EC) proliferation and migration that is necessary for vessel reendothelialization and healing. Thus there is significant need for therapeutic approaches that inhibit SMC proliferation and migration while encouraging proliferation and migration of ECs.

Nitric Oxide Therapy

Nitric oxide (NO) is an important regulator of vascular cellular proliferation capable of promoting EC growth and inhibiting the proliferation of SMCs in the medial layer of the vessel (Kuo and Schroeder 1995). NO also reduces platelet adhesion and aggregation (Kuo and Schroeder 1995). ECs constitutively produce NO from L-arginine using the enzyme nitric oxide synthase (NOS). As shown in Figure 6.2, NOS catalyzes the five-electron oxidation of the terminal guanido nitrogen of L-arginine to form L-citrulline and NO; molecular oxygen and nicotinamide adenine dinucleotide phosphate (NADPH) are cosubstrates in the reaction, and redox cofactors include enzyme-bound heme, flavin adenine dinucleotide (FAD), flavin mononucleotide (FMN), and tetrahydrobiopterin (Fukuto and Mayer 1996; Michel and Feron 1997). The cellular

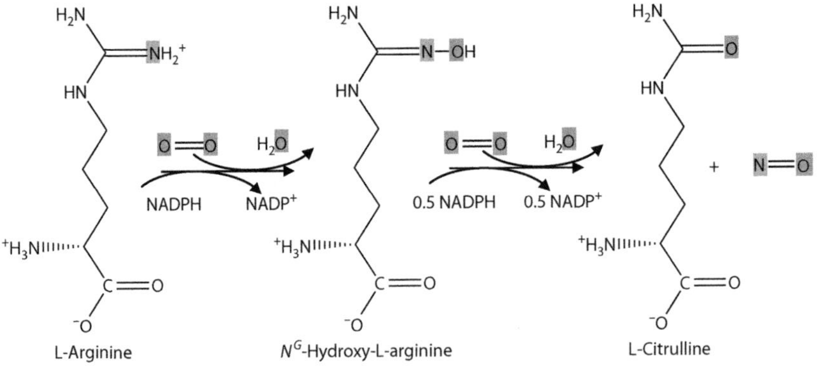

FIGURE 6.2
Nitric oxide synthase (NOS) catalyzes the conversion of L-arginine to L-citrulline and NO. Nicotinamide adenine dinucleotide phosphate (NADPH) acts as a source of electrons for oxygen reduction-activation. First, one oxygen is incorporated to form an enzyme-bound intermediate, N^G-hydroxy-L-arginine, through a two-electron oxidation. Then, NOS mediates a three-electron oxidation of the intermediate, inserting a second oxygen to form L-citrulline and NO.

effects of NO are predominantly mediated through its binding to soluble guanylyl cyclase and resultant production of cyclic guanosine monophosphate (cGMP) (Friebe and Koesling 2003). This signaling pathway turns on cGMP-dependent protein kinases, cGMP-gated ion channels, and cGMP-regulated phosphodiesterases (Ahern et al. 2002; Friebe and Koesling 2003), which leads to alterations in cell function. NO signaling through the cGMP pathway results in both acute and chronic responses, including changes in vascular muscle cell contraction, platelet aggregation, and gene expression. When ECs are lost or damaged during vascular interventional procedures, NO production is locally disrupted, contributing to a local environment conducive to platelet adhesion and aggregation as well as SMC proliferation and migration.

The effects of NO in the vascular system make it a promising therapeutic candidate for the prevention of restenosis following balloon angioplasty. NO is able to inhibit adhesion molecule activation and expression, platelet adhesion and aggregation, leukocyte adhesion, and SMC proliferation and migration, all of which contribute to the restenosis cascade (Vallance and Chan 2001; Vural and Bayazit 2001). In addition, NO stimulates EC proliferation, which could aid in the repair of the damaged endothelium (Heydrick 2000); EC loss alone has been shown to trigger intimal hyperplasia, and regrowth of the endothelium has been associated with downregulation of SMC proliferation (Allaire and Clowes 1997).

Appropriate delivery of NO has been challenging. NO concentrations must be well controlled due to toxicity issues at high concentrations (Dimmeler and Zeiher 2000). In addition, localized NO delivery is highly preferable compared to systemic delivery, as NO exerts effects on many cell types throughout the body (Kuo and Schroeder 1995), thus raising possibilities for side effects. Upregulation of NO production by endogenous NOS has been attempted by the administration of L-arginine and NOS potentiators. Supplemental L-arginine has been shown to inhibit neointima formation in the rat carotid artery model and the hypercholesterolemic rabbit model of balloon angioplasty (Le Tourneau et al. 1999; Vermeersch et al. 2001), although short-term high-dose administration of L-arginine has been shown not to reduce restenosis rates significantly in humans (Shiraki et al. 2004). Since NOS capacity can be impaired if there is significant loss of endothelium, exogenous delivery may be preferable. Due to its small size and hydrophobicity, NO can easily cross cell membranes, facilitating intracellular delivery. However, the half-life of NO *in vivo* is only a few seconds (Loscalzo 2000). Thus NO donors, compounds that react under physiological conditions to generate NO, are generally employed for NO-based therapeutics requiring sustained delivery.

NO donors fall into a number of different chemical classes, including organic nitrates, organic nitrites, ferrous nitro complexes, sydnonimines, nucleophile adducts, and *S*-nitrosothiols (Bauer et al. 1995). Although pharmacological tolerance limits the long-term usefulness of organic nitrates, this has not been shown to be a problem for other classes of NO donors (Bauer et al. 1995), including the *S*-nitrosothiol and diazeniumdiolate NO donors.

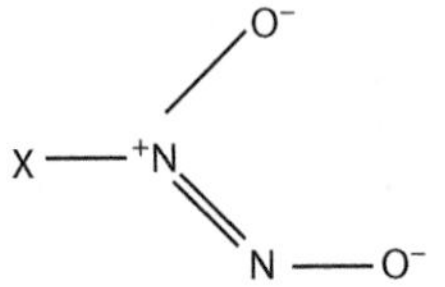

FIGURE 6.3
Structure of diazeniumdiolate compounds; X is a nucleophilic group.

S-Nitrosothiols are formed by reactions of thiols with oxidized derivatives of NO and are of the form RSNO, where R may be a host of compounds (Leopold and Loscalzo 2000). *S*-Nitrosothiols exist in the body as stores of bioavailable NO, decomposing to generate NO and form disulfide bonds. A number of widely used naturally occurring and synthetic *S*-nitrosothiols have been characterized, including *S*-nitrosocysteine, *S*-glutathione, and *S*-nitroso-*N*-acetyl-d,L-penicillamine; these have been utilized widely in studies to investigate the physiologic and pathophysiologic effects of NO (Williams 1999). The cysteine-containing donor SPM-5185 has been shown to accelerate recovery of damaged endothelium and inhibit vascular SMC proliferation following vascular injury in a rat carotid experimental model (Guo et al. 1994). It has also been suggested that cysteine-modified polymers may show improved hemocompatibility through *S*-transnitrosation with endogenous NO (Duan and Lewis 2002).

Diazeniumdiolates, also called NONOates, are compounds containing the structural unit shown in Figure 6.3, where X is a nucleophilic residue, most often an amine (Fitzhugh and Keefer 2000). The anionic portions of these compounds spontaneously decompose in aqueous solution to release NO, leaving the amine molecule as a by-product (Hrabie et al. 1993). Rates of dissociation depend on the structure of the NO donor as well as pH (Keefer et al. 1996; Davies et al. 2001). NO release is acid catalyzed (Keefer et al. 1996). Complexes of this nature are especially useful in NO delivery to biological systems due to their structural diversity, dependable rates of NO release, and chemistry that may facilitate targeting of NO to specific sites of interest (Saavedra et al. 2000; Keefer 2003). Several therapeutic applications of these donors have been reported. Diazeniumdiolates formed from spermine (SPER/NO) or diethylamine have shown significant antiplatelet effects (Diodati et al. 1993). Perivascular application of polymer gels loaded with SPER/NO have been used to reduce the onset of restenosis after experimental balloon injury to the iliofemoral artery of a rat (Kaul et al. 2000) and in decreasing neointimal lesions in rabbits (Yin and Dusting 1997).

Because of the necessity for localization of NO therapy, it may be desirable to modify materials with NO donor groups directly. Such materials could be utilized as stent coatings, perivascular delivery depots, or coatings applied to the luminal surface of the damaged vessel wall. Several studies have demonstrated improved blood compatibility of polymers modified with diazeniumdiolate species (Smith et al. 1996; Mowery et al. 2000; Bohl and West 2000;

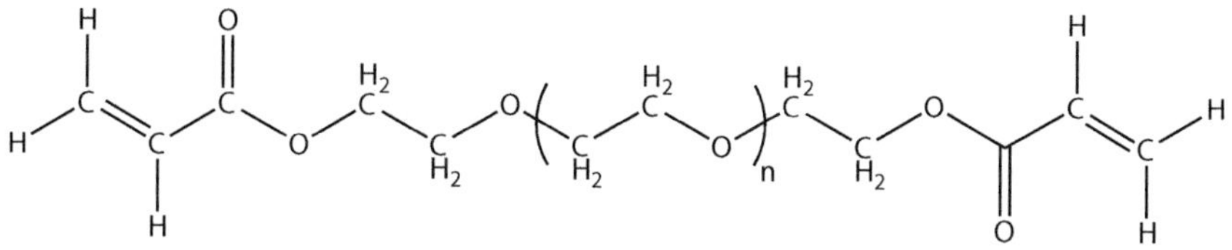

FIGURE 6.4
The chemical structure of poly(ethylene glycol) diacrylate. Addition reactions of the acrylate termini allow cross-linking to form hydrogel materials. Other compounds with acrylate termini can be immobilized within the hydrogel structure during cross-linking.

Zhang et al. 2002; Jun et al. 2005; Taite et al. 2008; Kushwaha et al. 2010; Zhao et al. 2010) or nitrosothiols (Bohl and West 2000; Seabra et al. 2008). Polyethylene glycol (PEG) diacrylate (Figure 6.4) hydrogels with covalently immobilized diazeniumdiolate complexes have been shown to provide NO release for over 60 days and to reduce restenosis in a rat balloon injury model significantly (Masters et al. 2005; Lipke and West 2005). Interfacial photopolymerization has been utilized to generate thin (<50 mm) coatings on the luminal surface of balloon-injured vessels (Hill-West et al. 1994; West and Hubbell 1996); this may be translated to NO-releasing derivatives for a more clinically relevant deployment. Materials for these applications may also be modified with peptides that facilitate adhesion of ECs but not platelets or SMCs. This has been accomplished by modification with the laminin-derived peptide YIGSR combined with NO donor groups (Taite et al. 2008).

A number of studies have also explored the possibility of using gene therapy to reduce restenosis following vascular injury by increasing NOS expression (Chen et al. 2002); transfection with NOS immediately following balloon injury has resulted in reductions in neointima formation in the rat carotid balloon injury model, rabbit carotid injury model, and porcine coronary balloon injury model (von der Leyen et al. 1995; Chen et al. 1998; Janssens et al. 1998; Varenne et al. 1998; Cooney et al. 2007). There has been less response to gene therapy with NOS at time points several days postinjury and no regression of neointima formation has been shown to occur in response to later therapy (Chen et al. 2002), indicating the importance of timing of therapy. Technologies are currently being developed to utilize stents for local gene delivery. Promising approaches include coating stents with DNA-loaded nanoparticles (Zhu et al. 2010), hydrogel coatings (Zhong et al. 2009), and surface immobilization of viruses (Fishbein et al. 2006, 2008).

Conclusions

Even after decades of research, balloon angioplasty fails in 20–40% of cases due to restenosis within the first 6 months (Libby et al. 1992; Eltchaninoff et al.

1998; Bhatia et al. 2004); the need to improve current methods drives biomedical research in this area, including the development of new materials for next-generation stents and localized drug delivery. NO is a particularly attractive therapeutic strategy due to its ability to decrease platelet adhesion and aggregation simultaneously as well as SMC proliferation while increasing desirable EC proliferation and migration. Clinically successful therapy for restenosis is likely to require a multiprong strategy, potentially delivering multiple therapeutic agents, exerting mechanical actions, and controlling cell-material interactions.

References

Ahern, G.P., Klyachko, V.A., and Jackson, M.B. 2002. cGMP and S-nitrosylation: two routes for modulation of neuronal excitability by NO. *Trends Neurosci* 25:510–17.

Allaire, E., and Clowes, A.W. 1997. Endothelial cell injury in cardiovascular surgery: the intimal hyperplastic response. *Ann Thorac Surg* 63:582–91.

American Heart Association. 2004. *Heart Disease and Stroke Statistics—2005 Update*. Dallas, TX: American Heart Association.

American Heart Association. 2011. *Heart Disease and Stroke Statistics—2011 Update*. Dallas, TX: American Heart Association.

Bauer, J.A., Booth, B.P., and Fung, H.L. 1995. Nitric oxide donors: biochemical pharmacology and therapeutics. *Adv Pharmacol* 34:361–81.

Bauters, C., and Isner, J.M. 1997. The biology of restenosis. *Prog Cardiovasc Dis* 40:107–16.

Beyar, R. 2004. Novel approaches to reduce restenosis. *Ann N Y Acad Sci* 1015:367–78.

Bhatia, V., Bhatia, R., and Dhindsa, M. 2004. Drug-eluting stents: new era and new concerns. *Postgrad Med J* 80:13–18.

Bohl, K.S., and West, J.L. 2000. Nitric oxide-generating polymers reduce platelet adhesion and smooth muscle cell proliferation. *Biomaterials* 21:2273–78.

Bult, H. 2000. Restenosis: a challenge for pharmacology. *Trends Pharmacol Sci Technol* 21:274–79.

Chen, A.F., Ren, J., and Miao, C.Y. 2002. Nitric oxide synthase gene therapy for cardiovascular disease. *Jpn J Pharmacol* 89:327–36.

Chen, L., Daum, G., Forough, R., et al. 1998. Overexpression of human endothelial nitric oxide synthase in rat vascular smooth muscle cells and in balloon-injured carotid artery. *Circ Res* 82:862–70.

Cooney, R., Hynes, S.O., Sharif, F., Howard, L., and O'Brien T. 2007. Effect of gene delivery of NOS isoforms on intimal hyperplasia and endothelial regeneration after balloon injury. *Gene Ther* 14:396–404.

Costa, M.A., and Simon, D. I. 2005. Molecular basis of restenosis and drug eluting stents. *Circulation* 111:2257–73.

Davies, K.M., Wink, D.A., Saavedra, J.E., et al. 2001. Chemistry of the diazeniumdiolates. 2. Kinetics and mechanism of dissociation to nitric oxide in aqueous solution. *J Am Chem Soc* 123(23): 5471–81.

Dimmeler, S., and Zeiher, A. 2000. Cytotoxicity, apoptosis, and nitric oxide. In *Nitric Oxide and the Cardiovascular System*, ed. J.A. Vita. Totowa, NJ: Humana Press, pp. 69–83.

Diodati, J.G., Quyyumi, A.A., Hussain, N., and Keefer, L.K. 1993. Complexes of nitric oxide with nucleophiles as agents for the controlled biological release of nitric oxide: antiplatelet effect. *Thromb Haemost* 70:654–58.

Duan, X., and Lewis, R.S. 2002. Improved haemocompatibility of cysteine-modified polymers via endogenous nitric oxide. *Biomaterials* 23:1197–203.

Eltchaninoff, H., Koning, R., Tron, C., Gupta, V., and Cribier, A. 1998. Balloon angioplasty for the treatment of coronary in-stent restenosis: immediate results and 6-month angiographic recurrent restenosis rate. *J Am Coll Cardiol* 32:980–84.

Fattori, R., and Piva, T. 2003. Drug-eluting stents in vascular intervention. *Lancet* 361:247–49.

Fishbein, I., Alferiev, I., Bakay, M., et al. 2008. Local delivery of gene vectors from bare-metal stents by use of a biodegradable synthetic complex inhibits in-stent restenosis in rat carotid arteries. *Circulation* 117:2096–103.

Fishbein, I., Alferiev, I.S., Nyanquile, O., et al. 2006. Bisphosphonate-mediated gene vector delivery from the metal surfaces of stents. *Proc Natl Acad Sci U S A* 103:159–64.

Fitzhugh, A.L., and Keefer, L.K. 2000. Diazeniumdiolates: pro- and antioxidant applications of the NONOates. *Free Radic Biol Med* 28:1463–69.

Friebe, A., and Koesling, D. 2003. Regulation of nitric oxide-sensitive guanylyl cyclase. *Circ Res* 93:96–105.

Fukuto, J.M., and Mayer, B. 1996. The enzymology of nitric oxide synthase. In *Methods in Nitric Oxide Research*, ed. M. Feelisch and J.S. Stamler. Chichester, UK: Wiley, pp. 147–60.

Grewe, P.H., Deneke, T., Machraoui, A., Barmeyer, J., and Muller, K.M. 2000. Acute and chronic response to coronary stent implantation. *J Am Coll Cardiol* 35:157–63.

Guo, J., Siegfried, M., and Lefer, A. 1994. Endothelial preserving actions of a nitric oxide donor in carotid arterial intimal injury. *Meth Find Exp Clin Pharmacol* 16:347–54.

Heydrick, S. 2000. Cellular signal transduction and nitric oxide. In *Nitric Oxide and the Cardiovascular System*, ed. J. Loscalzo and J A. Vita. Totowa, NJ: Humana Press, pp. 33–49.

Hiatt, B.L., Ikeno, F., Yeung, A.C., and Carter, A.J. 2002. Drug-eluting stents for the prevention of restenosis: in quest for the Holy Grail. *Catheter Cardiovasc Interv* 55:409–17.

Hill-West, J.L., Chowdhury, S.M., Slepian, M.J., and Hubbell, J.A. 1994. Inhibition of thrombosis and intimal thickening by *in situ* photopolymerization of thin hydrogel barriers. *Proc Natl Acad Sci U S A* 91:5967–71.

Hrabie, J.A., Klose, J.R., Wink, D.A., and Keefer, L.K. 1993. New nitric oxide-releasing zwitterions derived from polyamines. *J Org Chem* 58:1472–76.

Janssens, S., Flaherty, D.Z., Nong, O., et al. 1998. Human endothelial nitric oxide synthase gene transfer inhibits vascular smooth muscle cell proliferation and neointima formation after balloon injury in rats. *Circulation* 97:1274–81.

Jun, H.W., Taite, L.J., and West, J.L. 2005. Nitric oxide-producing polyurethanes. *Biomacromolecules* 6:838–44.

Kaul, S., Cercek, B., Rengstrom, J., et al. 2000. Polymeric-based perivascular delivery of a nitric oxide donor inhibits intimal thickening after balloon denudation arterial injury. *J Am Coll Cardiol* 35:493–501.

Keefer, L.K. 2003. Progress toward clinical application of the nitric oxide-releasing diazeniumdiolates. *Annu Rev Pharmacol Toxicol* 43:585–607.

Keefer, L.K., Nims, R.W., Davies, K.M., and Wink, D.A. 1996. NONOates as nitric oxide donors: convenient nitric oxide dosage forms. *Methods Enzymol* 268:281–93.

Khan, R., Argots, A., and Bobik, A. 2007. Understanding the role of transforming growth factor-beta1 in intimal thickening after vascular injury. *Cardiovasc Res* 74:223–34.

Kuo, P.C., and Schroeder, R.A. 1995. The emerging multifaceted roles of nitric oxide. *Ann Surg* 221(3):220–35.

Kushwaha, M., Anderson, J.M., Bosworth, C.A., et al. 2010. A nitric oxide releasing, self assembled peptide amphiphile matrix that mimics native endothelium for coating implantable cardiovascular devices. *Biomaterials* 31:1502–8.

Leopold, J.A., and Loscalzo, J. 2000. Clinical importance of understanding vascular biology. *Cardiol Rev* 8:115–23.

Le Tourneau, T., Van Belle, E., Corseaux, D., et al. 1999. Role of nitric oxide in restenosis after experimental balloon angioplasty in the hypercholesterolemic rabbit: effects on neointimal hyperplasia and vascular remodeling. *J Am Coll Cardiol* 33: 876–82.

Libby, P., Schwartz D., Brogi, E., Tanaka, H., and Clinton, S. K. 1992. A cascade model for restenosis. A special case of atherosclerosis progression. *Circulation* 86(6 Suppl):III47–52.

Lipke, E.A., and West, J.L. 2005. Localized delivery of nitric oxide from hydrogels inhibits neointima formation in a rat carotid balloon injury model. *Acta Biomater* 1:597–606.

Loscalzo, J., and Welch, G. 1995. Nitric oxide and its role in the cardiovascular system. *Prog Cardiovasc Dis* 38:87–104.

Masters, K.S., Lipke, E.A., Rice, E.E., et al. 2005. Nitric oxide-generating hydrogels inhibit neointima formation. *J Biomater Sci Polym Ed* 16:659–72.

Michel, T., and Feron, O. 1997. Nitric oxide synthases: which, where, how, and why? *J Clin Invest* 100:2146–52.

Mowery, K.A., Schoenfisch, M.H., Saavedra, J.E., Keefer, L.K., and Meyerhoff, M.E. 2000. Preparation and characterization of hydrophobic polymeric films that are thromboresistant via nitric oxide release. *Biomaterials* 21:9–21.

Saavedra, J.E., Mooradian, D.L., Mowery, K.A., et al. 2000. Conversion of a polysaccharide to nitric oxide-releasing form. Dual-mechanism anticoagulant activity of diazeniumdiolated heparin. *Bioorg Med Chem Lett* 10:751–53.

Schwartz, R.S., Chronos, N.A., and Virmani, R. 2004. Preclinical restenosis models and drug-eluting stents: still important, still much to learn. *J Am Coll Cardiol* 44:1373–85.

Schwartz, R.S., Holmes, D.R., Jr., and Topol, E.J. 1992a. The restenosis paradigm revisited: an alternative proposal for cellular mechanisms. *J Am Coll Cardiol* 20:1284–93.

Schwartz, R.S., Huber, K.C., Murphy J.G., et al. 1992b. Restenosis and the proportional neointimal response to coronary artery injury: results in a porcine model. *J Am Coll Cardiol* 19:267–74.

Seabra, A.B., da Silva, R., de Souza, G.F., and de Oliveira, M.G. 2008. Antithrombogenic polynitrosated polyester/poly(methyl methacrylate) blend for the coating of blood-contacting surfaces. *Artif Organs* 32:262–67.

Shiraki, T., Takamura, T., Kajiyama, A., Oka, T., and Saito, D. 2004. Effect of short-term administration of high dose L-arginine on restenosis after percutaneous transluminal coronary angioplasty. *J Cardiol* 44:13–20.

Smith, D.J., Chakravarthy, D., Pulfer, S., et al. 1996. Nitric oxide-releasing polymers containing the [N(O)NO]-group. *J Med Chem* 39:1148–56.

Stampfl, U., Radeleff, B., Sommer, C., et al. 2009. Paclitaxel-induced arterial wall toxicity and inflammation: long-term tissue response in a minipig model. *J Vasc Interv Radiol* 20:1608–16.

Taite, L.J., Yang, P., Jun, H.W., and West, J.L. 2008. Nitric oxide-releasing polyurethane-PEG copolymer containing the YIGSR peptide promotes endothelialization with decreased platelet adhesion. *J Biomed Mater Res B Appl Biomater* 84:108–16.

Tanabe, K., Regar, E., Lee, C.H., et al. 2004. Local drug delivery using coated stents: new developments and future perspectives. *Curr Pharm Des* 10:357–67.

Vallance, P., and Chan, N. 2001. Endothelial function and nitric oxide: clinical relevance. *Heart* 85:342–50.

van Beusekom, H.M., Whelan, D.M., Hofma, S.H., et al. 1998. Long-term endothelial dysfunction is more pronounced after stenting than after balloon angioplasty in porcine coronary arteries. *J Am Coll Cardiol* 32:1109–17.

Varenne, O., Pislaru, S., Gillijns, H., et al. 1998. Local adenovirus-mediated transfer of human endothelial nitric oxide synthase reduces luminal narrowing after coronary angioplasty in pigs. *Circulation* 98:919–26.

Vermeersch, P., Nong, Z., Stabile, E., et al. 2001. L-Arginine administration reduces neointima formation after stent injury in rats by a nitric oxide-mediated mechanism. *Arterioscler Thromb Vasc Biol* 21:1604–9.

Virmani, R., Kolodgie, F.D., Farb, A., and Lafont, A. 2003. Drug eluting stents: are human and animal studies comparable? *Heart* 89:133–38.

von der Leyen, H.E., Gibbons, G.H., Morishita, R., et al. 1995. Gene therapy inhibiting neointimal vascular lesion: *in vivo* transfer of endothelial cell nitric oxide synthase gene. *Proc Natl Acad Sci U S A* 92(4):1137–41.

Vural, K. M., and Bayazit, M. 2001. Nitric oxide: implications for vascular and endovascular surgery. *Eur J Vasc Endovasc Surg* 22:285–93.

West, J.L., and Hubbell, J.A 1996. Separation of the arterial wall from blood contact using hydrogel barriers reduces intimal thickening after balloon injury in the rat: the roles of medial and luminal factors in arterial healing. *Proc Natl Acad Sci U S A* 93:13188–93.

Williams, D. 1999. The chemistry of S-nitrosothiols. *Acc Chem Res* 32:869–76.

Yin, Z.L., and Dusting, G.J. 1997. A nitric oxide donor (spermine-NONOate) prevents the formation of neointima in rabbit carotid artery. *Clin Exp Pharmacol Physiol* 24:436–38.

Zhang, H., Annich, G.M., Miskulin, J., et al. 2002. Nitric oxide releasing silicone rubbers with improved blood compatibility: preparation, characterization, and *in vivo* evaluation. *Biomaterials* 23:1485–94.

Zhao, H., Serrano, M.C., Popowich, D.A., Kibbe, M.R., and Ameer, G.A. 2010. Biodegradable nitric oxide-releasing poly(diol citrate) elastomers. *J Biomed Mater Res A* 93:356–63.

Zhong, H., Matsui, O., Xu, K., et al. 2009. Gene transduction into aortic wall using plasmid-loaded cationized gelatin hydrogel-coated polyester stent graft. *J Vasc Surg* 50:1433–43.

Zhu, D., Jin, X., Leng, X., et al. 2010. Local gene delivered chitosan via endovascular stents coated with dodecylated chitosan-plasmid DNA nanoparticles. *Int J Nanomed* 6:1095–102.

7

Clinical Uses and Applications of Ureteral Stents

Ben H. Chew, Ryan F. Paterson, and Dirk Lange

CONTENTS

Introduction

The *Merriam-Webster Dictionary* describes the term *stent* as a tube that is inserted into the lumen of an anatomical vessel to keep a previously blocked passageway open; it is named after Dr. Charles Thomas Stent, a dentist who in 1885 coined the term (Ring 2001). Dr. Stent invented a dental compression compound that was later used by a plastic surgeon to mold (or "splint") tissue over a facial fracture. The more common current meaning for a stent is a tube that relieves obstructions in diseases such as coronary artery disease. In urology, a stent is a tube that facilitates urinary drainage from the kidney through the ureter into the bladder (Figure 7.1). Obstruction of the ureter and kidney occurs most commonly from kidney stones, which affect 10% of the population. Ureteral stents are placed to allow urine to bypass the obstructing stone and relieve pain until the stone can be treated definitively. Ureteral stents are

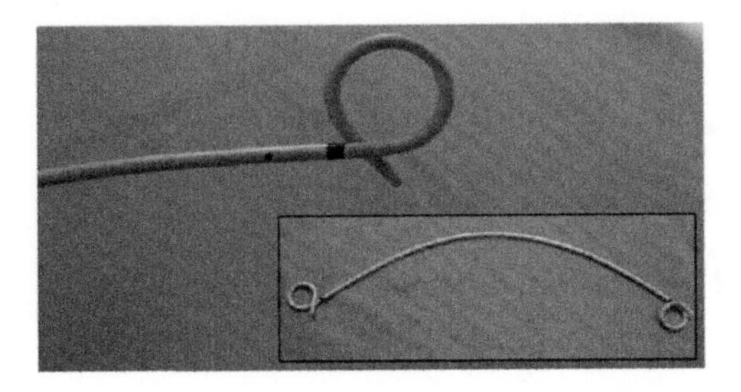

FIGURE 7.1
A typical double pigtail ureteral stent. The material is typically made of polyurethane or other plastic materials. The pigtail curl on either end helps maintain its position in the bladder and kidney so that the stent will not migrate. Note the side holes along the stent to allow drainage of urine into the lumen. The black markers help the surgeon determine where the stent will coil when placing it under visual endoscopic guidance.

also placed after a kidney stone has been treated surgically. Ureteral stents are not the complete answer to ureteral obstruction, however, and patients require definitive management of the original obstructing source. Unfortunately, ureteral stents themselves can be the source of pain and infection for the patient. This chapter outlines the clinical uses of ureteral stents and their limitations.

Causes of Urinary Obstruction

Obstruction of the ureter and kidney results in pain when urine cannot fully drain from the kidney into the bladder. Causes are classified as those that are intraluminal or within the lumen of the ureter compared to those that are extraluminal. Extraluminal causes are less common and include compression of the ureter from an external source such as enlarged lymphatic nodes secondary to cancer; adjacent tumors or cancer; other inflammatory processes such as endometriosis, retroperitoneal fibrosis, or radiation therapy; and physiologically enlarged organs such as an enlarged uterus during pregnancy. Intramural causes or things that can obstruct the inner lumen of the ureter include stones (the most common cause); blood clots; tissue such as tumors of the lining of the ureter (known as transitional cell carcinoma); and other tissue, such as sloughed epithelial cells from a severe infection or in diabetic patients. Rarely, benign tissue outgrowths of the epithelial cells of the ureter may also cause obstruction but are difficult to discern from malignant tumors on radiologic investigations. These causes can all result in blockage of the ureter and failure to drain urine completely, resulting in swelling of the kidney, also known as *hydronephrosis*. With stagnant urine in place, this can result in bacterial growth and systemic infection.

Infected Obstructed Kidneys

If an obstructed kidney is infected, the surgical principle is to provide drainage of that kidney to give an outlet for bacteria from the infection to exit the body. A ureteral stent would provide the necessary drainage to abate the infection and allow antibiotics to fight the portion that has spilled into the systemic circulation. Antibiotics alone would not be useful without draining what is essentially an abscess of infected urine. Another alternative to placing a ureteral stent is to insert a tube externally through the back directly into the kidney to drain the infected urine, a tool known as a nephrostomy tube. Nephrostomy tubes are fraught with complications: First, inserting one involves using a needle that is guided by ultrasound or x-ray fluoroscopy into the kidney, followed by dilation to 8 to 12 French (F), which can result in bleeding. Second, an externalized tube provides easy access for bacteria on the skin to migrate onto the material into the kidney, resulting in a urinary tract infection and possibly a systemic infection. Last, these tubes are cumbersome and painful and can be inadvertently dislodged. Even under the best circumstances, they must be replaced every 6–8 weeks to avoid infection and encrustation forming on the material.

Ureteral Stents and Kidney Stones

Kidney stones are the most common cause of blockage of the ureter and kidney necessitating treatment. Stones 5 mm and less have a high likelihood (>55%) of passing on their own without any intervention (Ohkawa et al. 1993; Skolarikos et al. 2010). Patients who have a fever (indicating a systemic infection and potential blockage of the kidney), severely decreased renal function as measured by serum creatinine, or unrelenting pain that is uncontrollable by oral analgesics must undergo immediate decompression of the blocked kidney. Patients without these indications may be managed conservatively and given analgesics or medical expulsive therapy such as an a-blocker to relax ureteral smooth muscle, which has been shown to hasten the spontaneous passage of stones (Lamb et al. 2011). Urgent decompression can be performed by placing a ureteral stent to provide urinary drainage.

If a stent is not required immediately and the patient continues to have intermittent pain and discomfort, then a stent may be placed at that time prior to definitive therapy for the stone, or therapy can be undertaken first and if necessary, a stent placed at the end of the procedure. Methods such as extracorporeal shock wave lithotripsy, which involves the generation of an acoustic shock wave that is then focused to fragment the stone within the patient's body, is one of the most commonly utilized methods of treating kidney stones. It is noninvasive and typically requires only intravenous sedation as opposed to a general anesthetic. Furthermore, with no incisions made in the body, patients may go home the same day. The overall success rates for completely fragmenting and eliminating stones with shock wave lithotripsy ranges up to 82% (Pedro et al. 2008).

For stones made of a harder composition or for those patients whose stones do not fragment with shock wave lithotripsy, endoscopic surgery under general anesthesia can be performed with a success rate of greater than 90% (Youssef et al. 2009; Watterson et al. 2002). A semirigid metal or flexible fiberoptic endoscope is passed through the urethra into the bladder and directly into the ureter up to the level of the stone. The flexible endoscope can reach practically every area of the kidney and provides the surgeon with good control for maneuvering by direct visualization.

A variety of instruments can be used to treat the stone, ranging from a basket retrieval device made of nickel-titanium (nitinol) to a flexible quartz glass fiber inserted through the endoscope and delivering energy from a holmium:YAG (yttrium-aluminum-garnet) laser, which effectively heats the stone to its melting point and fragments the stone (Razvi et al. 1996; Teichman 2002). The stone can be fragmented and the pieces can be retrieved using a nitinol basket device, or the stones can be fragmented into very small pieces that are left to pass spontaneously.

Once the surgeon has finished the surgical procedure, a ureteral stent is often left in place for a variety of reasons. If the procedure has been performed without any complication, a stent is often left in place to (a) provide urinary drainage as the ureteral tissues typically become edematous and block urinary flow following the introduction of the endoscope and treating the stone and (b) facilitate urinary drainage while the small stone fragments pass through the ureter. Furthermore, ureteral stents result in ureteral dilation, which then facilitates the passage of larger stone fragments (Cetti, Biers, and Keoghane 2011). If a complication occurs, such as perforation of the ureter or kidney, urine can leak, causing a collection, pain, and infection or even a permanent fistula. This is typically treated by inserting a ureteral stent (Kramolowsky 1987). By allowing the urine to bypass the perforation, this allows the ureteral wall to heal without urine constantly flushing through it. The majority of stents are used in the treatment of kidney stones, which is a common disease.

Ureteral Reconstruction

Urologic surgeons often have to reconstruct the ureter for a variety of reasons—damage from trauma (i.e., penetrating trauma such as a gunshot wound or tearing forces during deceleration injuries from a motor vehicle accident); surgical misadventure (e.g., accidental injury to the ureter during surgery to adjacent organs such as the rectum, prostate, or uterus); or planned reconstruction for a defect in the ureter or removal of the bladder for cancer. In these instances, the term *stent* takes on its other meaning, which is to "splint" or "stint" an anastomosis. By allowing urine to drain through the middle of the stent rather than extravasate through the anastomosis, this facilitates healing of the ureter at the anastomosis.

Method of Implanting a Ureteral Stent

There are two methods of inserting a ureteral stent, and the most common method popular with surgeons is termed a retrograde approach. The term *retrograde* refers to the fact that it is going against (hence "retro") the natural flow of urine (i.e., it is inserted through the bladder into the kidney). A special endoscope named a cystoscope is inserted into the bladder, and a 0.035-inch or 0.038-inch diameter Teflon-coated guide wire is inserted through the cystoscope into the ureter under direct visual guidance. Typically, fluoroscopy is used concurrently to visualize the proximal end of the guide wire and to confirm that it has reached the kidney. The ureteral stent, which ranges in size from 4.7F, 5F, 6F, 7F, to 8F, is then railroaded over the guide wire in a Seldinger fashion and inserted through the cystoscope. Once the proximal end has reached the kidney, the guide wire is slightly withdrawn, allowing the stent to recoil into its pigtail curl, which helps retain its position (Figure 7.2). A marker at the bladder portion helps the surgeon determine where the bottom curl will sit, and once the guide wire is fully removed, the bottom pigtail curl will hold its position in the bladder, not allowing the stent to migrate in either direction. This is done while monitoring the stent position under fluoroscopy. The cystoscope is then removed, and the stent procedure is complete. Alternatively, once the guide wire has been placed into the kidney, the cystoscope can be removed and the remainder of the procedure can be performed while visualizing it under fluoroscopy. The stent and guide wires are radiopaque, allowing this procedure to be performed solely using fluoroscopy.

Antegrade ureteral stenting is typically performed by interventional radiologists puncturing the kidney with a needle, feeding a guide wire, and inserting the stent in an "antegrade" fashion, or in the direction that urine flows—from top to bottom. This is done under fluoroscopy or ultrasound guidance and is typically performed if the surgeon cannot access the ureter retrogradely.

The last method of implantation is done during a nonendoscopic surgical procedure such as when the bladder is removed for cancer. When an open

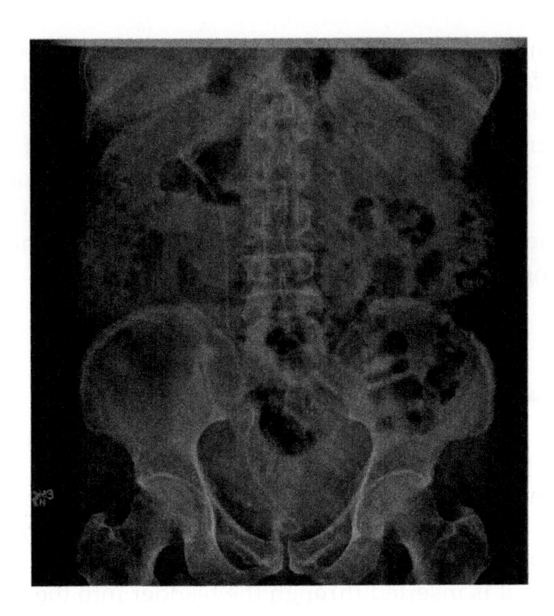

FIGURE 7.2
An x-ray of a patient with an indwelling ureteral stent in the right kidney. Note there is a stone adjacent to the stent just above the curl in the bladder. All ureteral stents have a compound to make them radiopaque so that they may be monitored using x-ray.

incision has been made and the ureter is to be anastomosed to a loop of bowel brought out to the skin as a stoma to drain the urine (known as an ileal conduit), the stent is simply inserted into the open end of the cut ureter through the open incision.

External Causes of Ureteral Obstruction

There are many things external to the ureter that may cause blockage, including endometriosis, a pregnant uterus, or retroperitoneal fibrosis. Physician-induced causes include radiation for pelvic malignancies (such as endometrial cancer or prostate cancer) and surgery involving various organs, including vascular surgery, hysterectomy, colorectal surgery, or endoscopic ureteral surgery for kidney stones. A recognized ureteral injury or ligation typically requires surgery and reconstruction; a partial ureteral injury or tear is first treated by inserting a ureteral stent to splint the damaged ureter while it heals and to ensure urine drains into the bladder during this process. If surgical reconstruction is required, a ureteral stent is often placed at that time to splint the anastomosis, whether it is reconnecting ureter to ureter or ureter to bladder/bowel to fix the damaged ureteral portion. Once the healing of the anastomosis or damaged ureter has occurred, the stent has served its purpose and may be removed.

Duration of Stenting

The duration of time that a stent is left indwelling depends on its purpose. If placed after endoscopic ureteroscopy, it may be removed any time after 48 hours to 4 weeks. There is no proscribed time for stents in every situation, but the time varies from surgeon to surgeon and is generally based on opinion rather than Level 1 medical evidence. Generally for reconstruction, stents are left in for longer periods of time, ranging anywhere from 2 to 8 weeks. Of course, the longer a stent remains indwelling, the greater the risk of complications. The most common complications associated with indwelling ureteral stents include encrustation, bacterial biofilm formation, and pain. Despite the fact that ureteral stents are designed to relieve symptoms associated with ureteral obstruction, their presence in the ureter is associated with a number of complications.

Ureteral Stent Complications

Stent Encrustation and Biofilm Formation

It has long been speculated that stent encrustation and bacterial biofilm formation occur as a result of a urinary conditioning film that deposits on the stent surface. It has previously been shown that shortly after insertion of a ureteral device, urinary components begin depositing and covering its surface. Canales and colleagues identified conditioning film components on the surface of ureteral stents with and without encrustation (Canales et al. 2009). They identified that immunoglobulins and Tamm-Horsfall protein nonselectively bind to the stent surface during the early indwelling stages and hypothesized that their positively charged histones and nuclear DNA-condensing proteins promoted encrustation (Canales et al. 2009).

Similarly, we have compared urinary conditioning film components on stents between patients as well as between stents made of different materials (unpublished data). This study did not find any significant differences in the most common conditioning film components between stents and patients, suggesting that the major components of conditioning films are the same between patients. These conditioning film components included several cytokeratins associated with the urogenital tract, hemoglobin, Tamm-Horsfall protein, fibrinogen, apolipoprotein, serum albumin, and S100A9. Relating the identification of these conditioning film components back to stent-associated complications, bacteria have receptor molecules called adhesins on their surface that are able to interact with the majority of the components facilitating bacterial adhesion, colonization, and biofilm formation. In addition to this, calcium-binding proteins such as Tamm-Horsfall protein, serum albumin, and S100A9 may form a nidus for stent encrustation. Stent surface coatings and drug-eluting stents that are designed to prevent encrustation and infection are likely rendered ineffective by bacterial biofilm formation, which covers the entire surface of the stent. Furthermore, the buildup of biofilm can clog the lumen of the stent, resulting in inadequate urinary flow and increasing the pressure on the kidney.

Bacteria and encrustation can act independently from one another to cause stent-associated complications, making use of the conditioning film component to bind bacteria as well as urinary ions, which can lead to further encrustation. Aside from this, certain types of bacteria have also been associated with triggering encrustation within the urinary tract. These bacterial species produce urease, an enzyme that is able to break down urea, one of the major components in urine, to produce ammonia. The buildup of ammonia gathers free hydrogen ions and leads to an increase in urinary pH, which leads to the precipitation of magnesium ammonium phosphate and calcium apatite crystals. Given the interaction of calcium and magnesium with proteins of the conditioning film, encrustation of the indwelling stent can occur. Aside from bacterial-induced urinary alkalization, several medical conditions may lead to an increase in urinary pH that in the absence of bacteria triggers precipitation of urinary ions that in the presence of the conditioning film will cause encrustation.

Prevention of conditioning film deposition and bacterial adhesion are important targets that should be considered for future stent biomaterial design. Although prevention of conditioning film formation will be a big step in preventing encrustation, it may not eliminate bacterial adhesion as bacteria contain several factors on their surface that will allow them to interact with biomaterials in the absence of specific binding partners via ionic and hydrophobic interactions. Finding a biomaterial that resists both encrustation and bacterial adhesion is one of the largest challenges.

Stent-Associated Discomfort

The most common complication of an indwelling ureteral stent is pain experienced by the patient. Over 80% of patients with a ureteral stent experience pain and discomfort (Joshi et al. 2003). Much speculation has gone into the cause of the discomfort, and the exact causes are unknown, but one theory is that it is the result of uroepithelial irritation during stent movement within the ureter as the patient goes about day-to-day activities. A previous study showed that the ureteral stent moves within the ureter, kidney, and bladder when the patient moves and may cause discomfort (Chew et al. 2007). This movement is likely attributed to the fact that ureteral JJ stents are not anchored in place: The pigtail curls in the bladder and kidney are designed to prevent migration of the stent but allow the stent to slide and move. Using an *in vitro* stent-induced injury model, we showed that the irritation of urothelial cells by a ureteral stent piece triggered the secretion of vast amounts of proinflammatory cytokines (Elwood et al. 2009), which may be a cause of stent-associated pain felt by the patient. El Nahes and colleagues identified additional factors that contribute to stent-associated symptoms, including crossing of the lower coil to the other side of the bladder, calyceal position of the upper coil, stent length, and larger stent diameter (El-Nahas et al. 2006). Certainly, stents that have a lot of excess material in the bladder may cause more mucosal irritation of the bladder and have been shown to result in more patient discomfort.

In addition to irritating the uroepithelium, indwelling ureteral stents have been shown to affect the rate of ureteral peristalsis, which is the contraction of muscles surrounding the ureter that facilitate and drive urinary flow. Several studies have shown that ureteral stents prevent ureteral peristalsis, which causes back pressure on the kidney due to decreased urinary flow down the ureter (Venkatesh et al. 2005; Kinn and Lykkeskov-Andersen 2002; Patel and Kellett 1996). This back pressure may be an additional cause for patient discomfort. The decrease and disruption of ureteral peristalsis can also be attributed to the shape and location of the ureteral stent—the renal curl sits in the renal pelvis and may disrupt the pacemaker of ureteral peristalsis, which is located in the renal pelvis (Constantinou 1974; Constantinou and Djurhuus 1981; Lang, Davidson, and Exintaris 2002; Mendelsohn 2004). Contact between the stent and the renal pelvis is believed to throw off the pacemaker, disrupting the rhythmic muscular contractions responsible for driving urinary flow into the bladder. Without these contractions, the renal pelvis becomes swollen or hydronephrotic and is thought to cause significant patient symptoms. Similarly, the diameter of the stent has also been shown to affect peristalsis as smaller-diameter stents have less contact with the ureteral wall compared to larger-diameter stents (Venkatesh et al. 2005; Natalin et al. 2009). The prevention of stent symptoms needs to address the overall structure of the stent and minimize the degree of urothelial irritation and disruption of peristaltic activity.

Conclusions

Ureteral stents are used in many facets of urology, including the treatment of kidney stone disease, ureteral obstruction from extrinsic causes, and in reconstructive surgery. While they provide good urinary drainage of the kidney, problems include patient discomfort, encrustation of the stent, and stent-related urinary tract infections. Novel coatings, newer materials, drug-eluting materials, and newer designs are being attempted to reduce these problems in a commonly used urologic tool.

References

Canales, B.K., Higgins, L., Markowski, T., et al. 2009. Presence of five conditioning film proteins are highly associated with early stent encrustation. *Journal of Endourology* 23:1437–42.

Cetti, R.J., Biers, S., and Keoghane, S.R. 2011. The difficult ureter: what is the incidence of pre-stenting? *Annals of the Royal College of Surgeons of England* 93:31–33.

Chew, B.H., Knudsen, B.E. Nott, L., et al. 2007. Pilot study of ureteral movement in stented patients: first step in understanding dynamic ureteral anatomy to improve stent comfort. *Journal of Endourology/Endourological Society* 21:1069–75.

Constantinou, C.E. 1974. Renal pelvic pacemaker control of ureteral peristaltic rate. *The American Journal of Physiology* 226:1413–19.

Constantinou, C.E., and Djurhuus, J.C. 1981. Pyeloureteral dynamics in the intact and chronically obstructed multicalyceal kidney. *The American Journal of Physiology* 241:R398–R411.

El-Nahas, A.R., El-Assmy, A.M., Shoma, A.M., et al. 2006. Self-retaining ureteral stents: analysis of factors responsible for patients' discomfort. *Journal of Endourology/Endourological Society* 20:33–37.

Elwood, C.N., Lange, D., Nadeau, R., et al. 2009. Novel *in vitro* model for studying ureteric stent-induced cell injury. *BJU International* 105:1318–23.

Joshi, H.B., Stainthorpe, A., MacDonagh, R.P., et al. 2003. Indwelling ureteral stents: evaluation of symptoms, quality of life and utility. *The Journal of Urology* 169:1065–69; discussion 1069.

Kinn, A.C., and Lykkeskov-Andersen, H. 2002. Impact on ureteral peristalsis in a stented ureter. An experimental study in the pig. *Urological Research* 30:213–18.

Kramolowsky, E.V. 1987. Ureteral perforation during ureterorenoscopy: treatment and management. *The Journal of Urology* 138:36–38.

Lamb, A.D., Vowler, S.L, Johnston, R., Dunn, N., and Wiseman, O.J. 2011. Meta-analysis showing the beneficial effect of alpha-blockers on ureteric stent discomfort. *BJU International* Mar 31. doi: 10.1111/j.1464-410X.2011.10170.x. [Epub ahead of print].

Lang, R.J., Davidson, M.E., and Exintaris, B. 2002. Pyeloureteral motility and ureteral peristalsis: essential role of sensory nerves and endogenous prostaglandins. *Experimental Physiology* 87:129–46.

Mendelsohn, C. 2004. Functional obstruction: the renal pelvis rules. *The Journal of Clinical Investigation* 113:957–59.

Natalin, R.A., Hruby, G.W., Okhunov, Z., et al. 2009. Pilot study evaluating ureteric physiological changes with a novel "ribbon stent" design using electromyographic and giant magnetoresistive sensors. *BJU International* 103:1128–31.

Ohkawa, M., Tokunaga, S., Nakashima, T., et al. 1993. Spontaneous passage of upper urinary tract calculi in relation to composition. *Urologia Internationalis* 50:153–58.

Patel, U., and Kellett, M.J. 1996. Ureteric drainage and peristalsis after stenting studied using colour Doppler ultrasound. *British Journal of Urology* 77:530–35.

Pedro, R.N., Lee, C., Weiland, D., et al. 2008. Eighteen-year experience with the Medstone STS lithotripter: safety, efficacy, and evolving practice patterns. *Journal of Endourology/Endourological Society* 22:1417–21.

Razvi, H.A., Denstedt, J.D., Chun, S.S., and Sales, J.L. 1996. Intracorporeal lithotripsy with the holmium:YAG laser. *The Journal of Urology* 156:912–14.

Ring, M.E. 2001. How a dentist's name became a synonym for a life-saving device: the story of Dr. Charles Stent. *Journal of the History of Dentistry* 49:77–80.

Skolarikos, A., Laguna, M.P., Alivizatos, G., Kural, A.R., and de la Rosette, J.J. 2010. The role for active monitoring in urinary stones: a systematic review. *Journal of Endourology/Endourological Society* 24:923–30.

Teichman, J.M. 2002. Laser lithotripsy. *Current Opinion in Urology* 12:305–9.

Venkatesh, R., Landman, J., Minor, S.D., et al. 2005. Impact of a double-pigtail stent on ureteral peristalsis in the porcine model: initial studies using a novel implantable magnetic sensor. *Journal of Endourology/Endourological Society* 19:170–76.

Watterson, J.D., Girvan, A.R. Beiko, D.T., et al. 2002. Ureteroscopy and holmium:YAG laser lithotripsy: an emerging definitive management strategy for symptomatic ureteral calculi in pregnancy. *Urology* 60:383–87.

Youssef, R.F., El-Nahas, A.R., El-Assmy, A., et al. 2009. Shock wave lithotripsy versus semirigid ureteroscopy for proximal ureteral calculi (<20 mm): a comparative matched-pair study. *Urology* 73:1184–87.

8

Intravaginal Drug Delivery

Jason M. Olbrich, Georgios T. Hilas, and Waleed S. W. Shalaby

CONTENTS

Introduction

Women's health issues continue to generate considerable interest. In recent years, we have seen an escalation in cesarean deliveries in the United States, reaching 30% of all deliveries, less-invasive modalities for nonhormonal contraception and abnormal uterine bleeding, increased awareness for and management of sexually transmitted diseases, availability of vaccines to prevent HPV (human papilloma virus) transmission (the etiology of cervical dyplasia and cancer), as well as increased options to treat urinary incontinence (stress and mixed incontinence), pelvic prolapse, menopause, and gynecologic cancers. While oral, intravenous, and transdermal routes of drug administration have been heavily leveraged, intravaginal drug delivery has made only modest strides. Interestingly, there are many instances for which intravaginal drug delivery may be more suitable and efficacious. For example, it has been postulated and observed that therapeutic targeting to the reproductive tract may be more efficient through the intravaginal route. Therefore, elevated drug levels may be achieved at a fraction of the systemic dose and toxicity. The rich vascular supply of the vaginal, paravaginal, and parametrial tissues represents a rapid portal of entry when systemic drug levels are also desired without the first-pass hepatic metabolism seen with oral drug delivery.

While there is great potential to improve on existing modalities to treat women's health-related issues, a number of important questions need to be addressed before the true potential of this route of administration can be utilized. As in many areas of applied science, a multidisciplinary approach often yields the most efficient, yet practical, results. This review examines a number of areas pertinent to intravaginal drug administration and the development of systems to deliver agents via this route. Current examples of intravaginal drug delivery are also reviewed in an effort to highlight areas for future investigation.

Anatomy and Physiology of the Vagina

Key Histological Features

The vagina is a fibromuscular tube that exists in a relaxed state. The walls are suspended by their attachment to the paravaginal lateral connective tissue and the arcus tendineus (Nichols and Randall 1996). Grossly, the vagina possesses many rugal folds. While the pattern varies dramatically, the folds provide a certain degree of distensibility. The vagina is lined by stratified squamous epithelium rich in glycogen during the reproductive years. The surface of the vaginal wall is made up of numerous microridges that run longitudinally or in circles (Hafez 1975). It is believed that the morphology and pattern of the microridges affect the firmness of the epithelium (Schuchner et al. 1974).

The epithelium is comprised of five layers (Witkin 1993; Burgos and De Vargas-Linares 1978). The first three layers are the superficial, transitional, and intermediate layers. Deep to these layers reside the parabasal and basal layers. Traversing along the vaginal epithelium is a system of intercellular channels. It is believed that this network provides a route for transport of macromolecules, fluids, and cells from the basal lamina to the vaginal lumen. Furthermore, transport may also proceed in the opposite direction, which would have unique implications for high molecular weight agents, including peptide drugs. The basal lamina contains macrophages, lymphocytes, plasma cells, Langerhan's cells, eosinophils, and mast cells. Lymphocytes reside predominantly in the intermediate, parabasal, and basal layers. During infection, these cells can migrate into the intercellular channels toward the epithelial surface. In menopause, the vagina undergoes an alteration in the pattern of the rugae with associated decreased epithelial thickness, glycogen deposition, and cell size. The microridges become irregular with increased cell fragmentation (Steger and Hafez 1978). Beneath the epithelium resides a thin layer of elastic fibers, followed by a well-developed fibromuscular layer. The latter is described as a muscular meshwork of smooth muscle oriented longitudinally in the innermost aspect while becoming more circularly arranged peripherally (Smout et al. 1969). External to the muscular layer is a fibrous capsule that contains large venous plexuses as well as elastic fibers.

Vaginal Anatomy

The overall shape of the vaginal canal and its distensibility are limited by the elasticity of the vaginal wall and its proximity to other pelvic organs. The introitus of the vagina is located between the urethra and symphysis superiorly and the rectum posteriorly. In the upright position, the vagina is directed obliquely upward and backward at approximately a 45° angle to the horizontal axis. The vagina has a convex curve, resulting in an almost-horizontal axis of the upper two-thirds of the vagina. The anterior and posterior walls of the vagina are slack and remain in contact with each other. The lateral walls of the vagina are fairly rigid and defined by the anatomical pelvic support. The lower third of the vagina is supported by connection with fibers of the pelvic and urogenital diaphragms. The middle third receives its main support from the lateral and inferior segments of the cardinal ligament. The upper third, however, rests mainly on the rectum, which overlies the pubococcygei of the levator plate (Nichols and Randall 1996). It maintains its position over the levator plate through lateral attachments to the upper cardinal ligaments (von Peham and Americh 1934). Because the lateral walls remain separated, cross sections of the vagina take on a classic H-shaped appearance (Nichols and Randall 1996).

The dimensions of the vagina vary considerably, depending on both sexual arousal and reproductive stage. In a normal reproductive-age woman, the anterior wall of the vagina measures 6 to 8 cm long, while the posterior wall is up to 14 cm long (Pendergrass et al. 1996; Forsberg 1996; Weber et al. 1995). Since the cervix is incorporated in the anterior vaginal wall, the length of the anterior vagina plus cervix approximates the length of the posterior wall.

The shape of the vagina also varies considerably among women. Common features of the vagina include a posterior widening around and behind the cervix, with posterior fornices being quite deep in some subjects. Anterior to the cervix, the caliper of the vagina is constricted, especially near the introitus.

Vascular and Lymphatic Systems of the Pelvis

In general, the arteries of the pelvis are bilateral with multiple collateral vessels (Herbst et al. 1992). They enter their respective organ laterally and unite at the midline through multiple anastomoses. The arteries interpenetrate a large venous meshwork to terminate via branching arcades. The venous system of the reproductive organs lies within a meshwork of large veins that form numerous interconnecting venous plexuses. The arterial supply is intimately related as it interpenetrates the venous plexus en route to respective organs (Herbst et al. 1992). Venous drainage of the pelvis begins in small sinusoids leading to adjacent venous plexuses. These venous plexuses, interestingly, communicate with plexuses in the paravaginal tissue, perineum, rectum, and bladder (Nichols and Randall 1996). The veins of the pelvis and perineum are generally thin walled and contain few valves. They drain the pelvic plexuses along the course of their corresponding arterial supply.

A minor contribution to drug absorption and disposition may reside with the lymphatic architecture of the pelvis (Murphy and Krantz 1994). In the vagina, the lymphatic system is divided into three anatomical groups. At the mucosal surface, lymphatics originate from numerous mucosal plexuses that anastomose with deeper muscular plexuses. The superior group of lymphatics joins those of the cervix where they follow the uterine artery either to terminate in the external iliac nodes or anastomose with the uterine/obturator plexus. The middle group of lymphatics drains the greater part of the vagina. These lymphatics follow the vaginal arteries to the hypogastric channels. The inferior group forms anastomoses with the opposite side and travels either upward to connect with the middle group of lymphatics or toward the vulva to drain into the inguinal nodes. Lymphatic drainage of the uterus includes several chains of lymph nodes involving the external iliac chain or lateral sacral nodes.

Vaginal Microbiology

Infectious diseases involving the vagina have received considerable interest in recent years. With the rise in incidence of pelvic inflammatory disease, HPV prevalence in reproductive-age women, adenocarcinoma of the cervix (high-risk HPV associated), and heterosexual HIV transmission in underdeveloped populations, research efforts have focused on both treatment and prophylaxis. Our understanding of the vaginal microbiology has largely resulted from research efforts in bacterial vaginosis. Microbial colonization

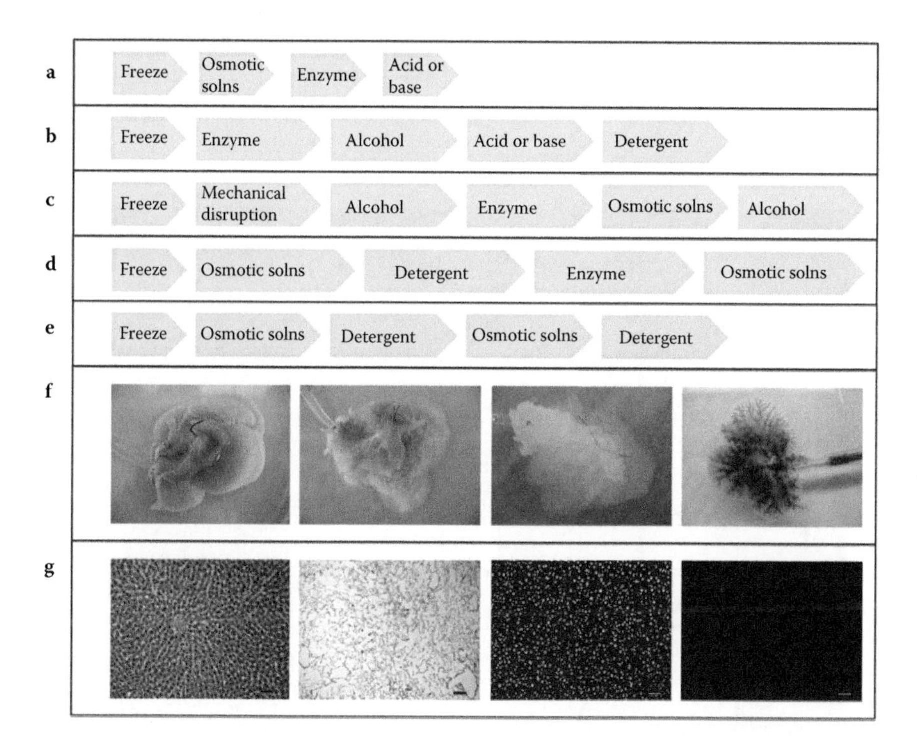

FIGURE 3.4
Example decellularization protocols for (a) thin laminates such as pericardium; (b) thicker laminates such as dermis; (c) fatty, amorphous tissues such as adipose; (d) composite tissues or whole simple organs such as trachea; and (e) whole vital organs such as liver. Arrow lengths represent relative exposure times for each processing step. Rinse steps for agent removal and sterilization methods are not shown to simplify comparison. (f) Representative images of the gross appearance of intact rat liver subjected to decellularization (left to right): before, during, and after decellularization; decellularized liver perfused with blue dye. (g) Representative photomicrographs showing no nuclear staining after whole-organ decellularization (left to right): native rat liver hematoxylin and eosin (H&E); decellularized liver ECM H&E; native rat liver DAPI (4′,6-diamidino-2-phenylindole); liver ECM DAPI. Scale bars are 50 mm. (From Crapo, P.M., Gilbert, T.W., and Badylak, S.F. 2011. An overview of tissue and whole organ decellularization processes. *Biomaterials* 32:3233–43. With permission.)

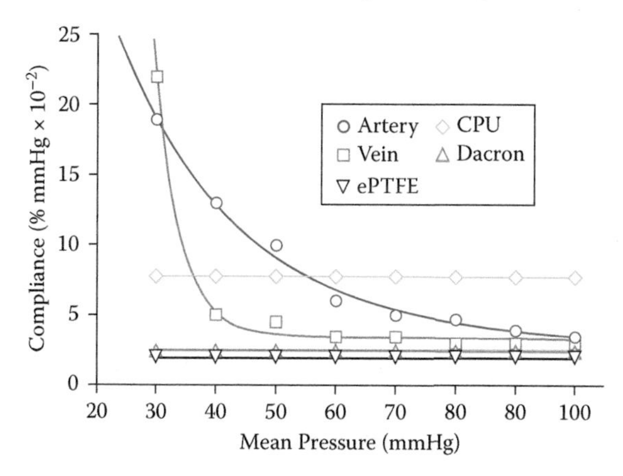

FIGURE 4.5
Modulation of compliance as a function of mean pressure for different vascular conduits. (From Sarkar S., Salacinski H.J., Hamilton G., Seifalian A.M. 2006. The mechanical properties of infrainguinal vascular bypass grafts: their role in influencing patency. *Eur J Vasc Endovasc Surg* 31:627–36. With permission.)

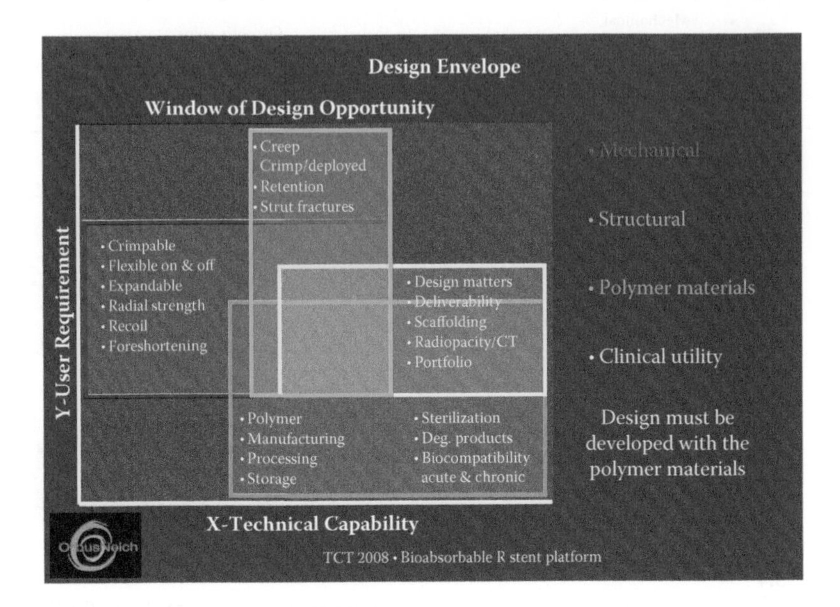

FIGURE 5.3
Design envelope. (Courtesy of Cottone, R. 2008. Bioabsorbable R stent design concepts. Presentation at the Transcatheter Cardiovascular Therapeutics Conference, Washington, DC, October. With permission.)

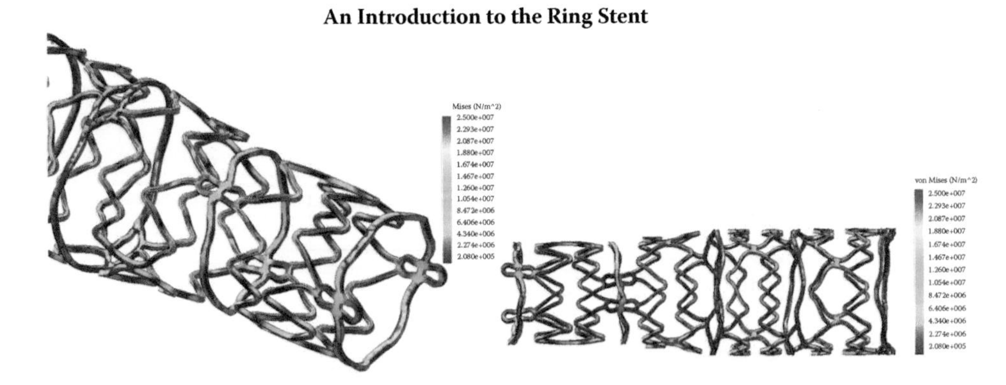

FIGURE 5.6
Finite element analysis (FEA) introduction to the OrbusNeich ring stent. Prematurely expanded ringlets are structurally and materially stronger and more resistant to radial crushing than sinusoidal stent segments. (Courtesy of OrbusNeich, Fort Lauderdale, FL. With permission.)

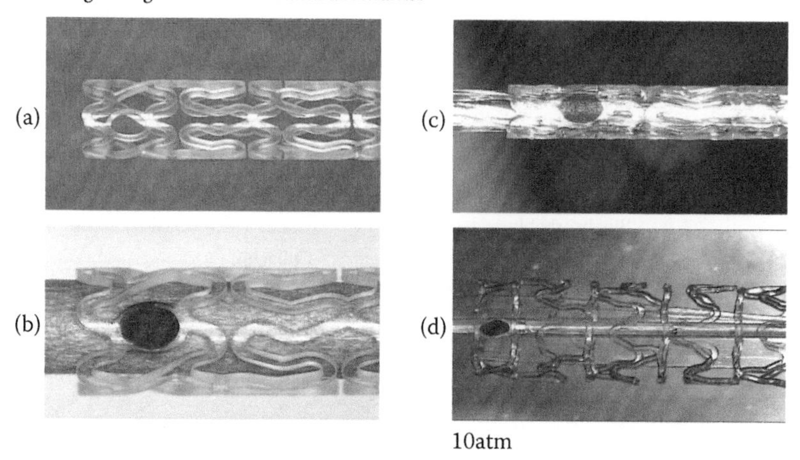

FIGURE 5.7
OrbusNeich stent: (a) as cut, (b) as cut with marker dot, (c) crimped on balloon, (d) deployed at 10 atmospheres. (Courtesy of OrbusNeich, Fort Lauderdale, FL. With permission.)

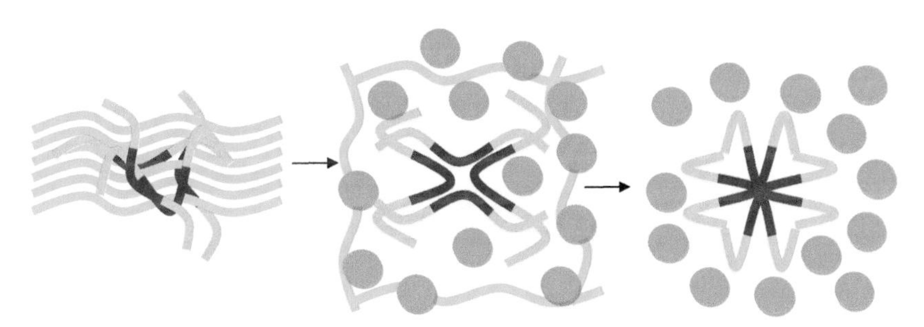

FIGURE 8.5
Progression of *in situ* gelation of amphiphilic polymer system such as the OC series of polymers. Green is the original injection solvent, red represents the hydrophobic portion of the chains, orange the hydrophilic portions, and blue water molecules.

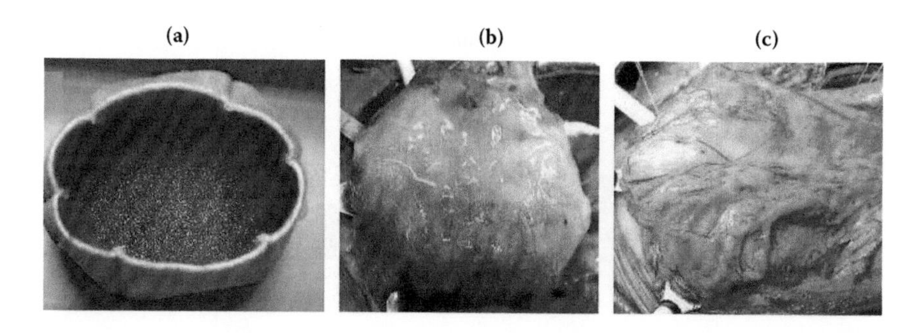

FIGURE 9.3
Construction of engineered bladder: (a) scaffold seeded with cells; (b) engineered bladder anastomosed to native bladder with running 4-0 polyglycolic sutures; (c) implant covered with fibrin glue and omentum.

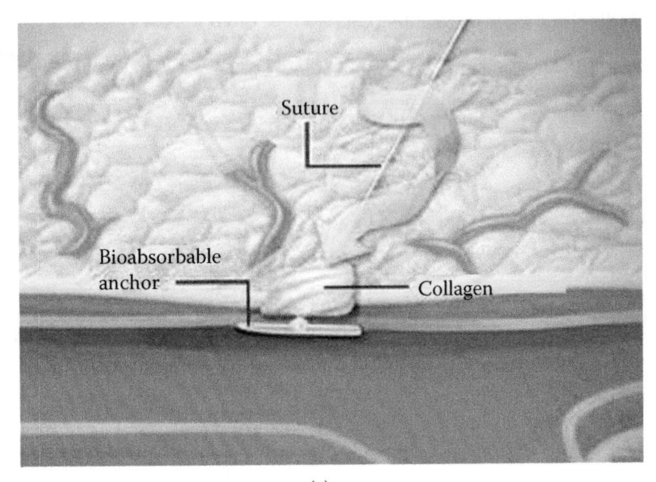

(a)

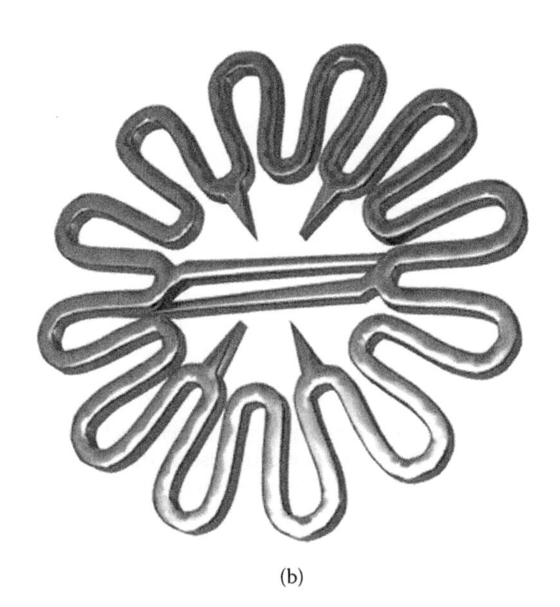

(b)

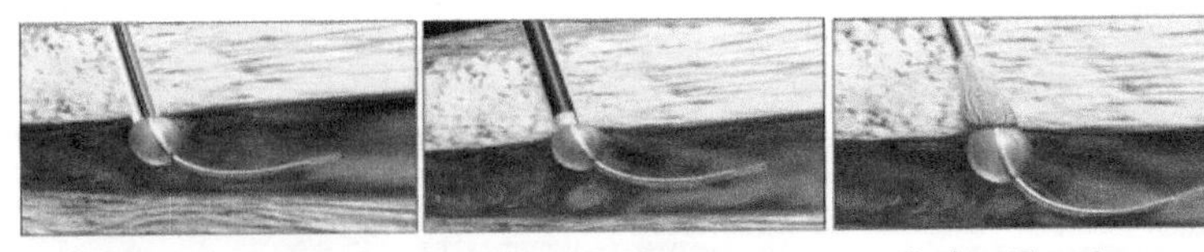

(c)

FIGURE 10.3
(a) Angio-Seal™ after implantation; (b) StarClose™ clip; (c) steps involved with the implantation of the Mynx™ sealant system.

involves multiple species of organisms that are uniform in neither growth requirements nor metabolic end products (Larsen 1993). The vagina contains 109 bacterial colony-forming units/gram of secretions (Sweet 1995). Isolates include a variety of aerobic and anaerobic bacteria, yeast, viruses, and parasites. An extensive review of these organisms was discussed by Sweet and Gibbs (Sweet 1995).

The microecology of the vagina is characterized by a dynamic equilibrium of host-microbe and endogenous-exogenous microbe interactions (Larsen 1993). Thus, synergistic or antagonistic effects arise depending on the nature of a physiological stress on the microecology. Metabolic end products have long been considered significant flora-controlling substances. They may serve as a growth substrate for one species of bacteria or inhibit growth of others. For example, lactic acid produced by lactobacilli is well recognized for its ability to control bacterial growth in the adult vagina through regulation of pH between 4.0 and 5.0 (Eschenbach et al. 1989). For this reason, only acid-tolerant species are permitted to grow. Hydrogen peroxide has also been postulated as an alternative explanation for the growth-controlling success of certain lactobacilli strains (Eschenbach et al. 1989). Other agents may also serve to control bacterial colonization. It is believed that antibacterial toxins, such as gliotoxin and hemolysin from *Gardnerella vaginalis*, as well as bacteriocins exert antagonistic effects (Larsen 1993; Cohen et al. 1985). Another aspect of the vaginal microenvironment that controls bacterial colonization is the low oxidation-reduction potential. Studies have shown that anaerobic bacteria outnumber facultative species by a factor of 10 (Bartlett et al. 1977). Investigators believe that the low redox potential is related to the presence of obligate anaerobes and facultative organisms in addition to oxygen-consuming organisms such as staphylococci, streptococci, and *Escherichia coli*.

The microbial environment of the vagina is also influenced by age, sexual activity, contraceptive use, antibiotics, and childbirth. At birth, maternal estrogen facilitates vaginal colonization by lactobacilli. However, lactobacilli disappear over the course of several weeks as the estrogen effect diminishes. Lactobacilli later dominate the vaginal flora with the onset of puberty and thereafter during the reproductive years (Larsen 1993). Lactobacillus colonization declines during menopause. From these observations, it appears that lactobacillus colonization is largely influenced by estrogenic effects. It should be noted, however, that control of vaginal colonization is still not well understood. Much of the debate is focused on whether the production of metabolic substrates that are used by lactobacilli are solely influenced by estrogen. Estrogen is believed to promote glycogen deposition in the vaginal epithelium. While most lactobacilli utilize glycogen through fermentation to yield lactic acid, studies have shown that some lactobacilli are not capable of utilizing glycogen. Furthermore, glycogen deposition does not change between pre- and postmenopausal women (Larsen 1993). Despite the specific mechanisms involved, it is generally agreed that estrogen stimulation plays an important role in the normal colonization of the vagina.

Sexual intercourse also leads to changes in the vagina. This occurs through the introduction of sexually transmitted pathogens such as *Neisseria gonorrheae, Chlamydia trachomatis,* and herpesvirus. The use of intrauterine devices for contraception has been found to increase the number of anaerobic bacteria in the cervix. It is believed that this increases the risk for bacterial vaginosis (Mardh 1991; Houkkamaa et al. 1986). Furthermore, the use of diaphragms in conjunction with spermicide has been associated with recurrent urinary tract infections through vaginal colonization by *E. coli* (Fihn et al. 1985). Interestingly, oral contraceptives have a minimal effect on the vaginal environment (Mardh 1991).

The effects of parenteral antibiotics on vaginal flora have been well studied (Spence et al. 1980; Lossick et al. 1986; Krieger, Tam, and Stevens 1988). Short-term prophylactic use of antibiotics, such as penicillin or cefazolin, has been shown to have little effect, while longer courses increase the presence of *Pseudomonas* or enterococci.

During pregnancy, there is a progressive increase in lactobacillus colonization as well as the prevalence of yeast (Larsen and Galask 1980). Whether a synergism exists between yeast and lactobacilli or other vaginal flora has yet to be determined (Larsen 1993). After delivery, the vaginal flora undergo a dramatic change, with the prevalence of anaerobic species. It is postulated that anaerobic colonization is related to birth trauma, the presence of lochia and suture materials, and hormonal changes (Sweet 1995). The vaginal flora, however, is restored to a normal distribution by the sixth week postpartum.

In summary, it should be emphasized that the ecosystem of the vagina represents an array of organisms that are in a dynamic equilibrium, undergoing shifts in population density in response to exogenous and endogenous influences. The net response either benefits the host by minimizing colonization of exogenous microorganisms or produces undesirable lower or upper genital tract infections.

Intravaginal Drug Delivery

Intravaginal drug delivery can be utilized for topical, local, or systemic effects. Topical administration has been used in the treatment of bacterial or fungal infections, atrophic vaginitis, and vaginal intraepithelial neoplasia. In terms of local therapy, vaginal drug administration has been used to treat stress urinary incontinence, labor induction, medical abortions, and infertility. The advantage of this route is the large surface area for drug absorption and ease of administration. To date, there have been few studies to examine the mechanisms that control vaginal drug absorption and distribution. Models for drug absorption have stemmed from early studies in mice and rabbits that have not been validated in humans. Furthermore, recent findings in reproductive medicine and gynecologic oncology raise many questions regarding the mechanism of drug distribution after vaginal absorption.

Drug Absorption

The large surface area of the vaginal epithelium combined with the rich vascular supply make it an ideal route for drug administration. Contributions by Benziger and colleagues and Aref and coworkers have extensively reviewed the various classes of drugs and chemical agents that undergo vaginal absorption (Benziger and Edelson 1983; Aref et al. 1978). The mechanisms involved in vaginal drug absorption obey many of the basic concepts developed from gastrointestinal drug absorption (Hsu et al. 1983; Yotsuyanagi et al. 1975; Hwang et al. 1976, 1977a, 1977b; Ho et al. 1976). Absorption depends on the physicochemical properties of the drug in terms of molecular weight, dissolution characteristics, and ionization properties. Absorption may proceed either by simple diffusion or by active transport. Many drugs, however, are weakly acidic or basic. Therefore, the equilibrium dissociation constant of the drug, the microenvironment pH of the delivery vehicle, and the vaginal pH will have an important influence on the extent of drug absorption.

The pH-partition hypothesis was developed based on the observations that biologic membranes were predominantly lipophilic and that drug penetration occurs mainly in the undissociated form (Jollow and Brodie 1972). It was believed that drug transport by passive diffusion favored the fraction of undissociated drug at a given pH. In biological systems, however, this was found to be partly applicable given the observations that appreciable amounts of ionized drug partitioned across lipophilic membranes. It was determined that ionic and nonionic species were also transported across the aqueous channels of biologic membranes (Stehle and Higuchi 1967; Suzuki et al. 1970; Ho et al. 1972). These observations led to a diffusion model for drug absorption. The model incorporated a simple aqueous boundary layer in series with the biologic membrane. The membrane was composed of lipophilic regions in parallel with aqueous pores (Figure 8.1).

This model was later applied to vaginal drug absorption and tested in rabbits. Under steady-state conditions, drug diffusion across the vaginal mucosa may be described by Fick's law:

$$-dM/dt = D_m SK/\mathrm{h}\,(C_v - C_p) \tag{8.1}$$

where M is the amount of drug in the vagina at time t, D_m is the diffusivity in the vaginal membrane, S is the surface area, K is the partition coefficient between the aqueous medium of the vagina and the vaginal epithelium, h is the thickness of the vaginal epithelium, and C_v and C_p are the drug concentrations in the vagina and plasma, respectively. If the vaginal drug concentration is kept high relative to the plasma concentration, then sink conditions are met, and C_p is omitted from Equation 8.1.

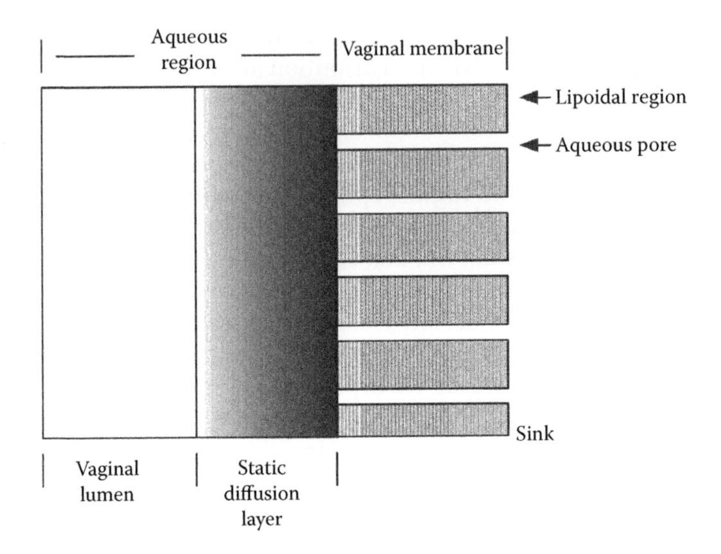

FIGURE 8.1
Model of drug absorption from the vagina.

$$-dM/dt = D_m SKC_v/h \tag{8.2}$$

This equation can be rearranged to describe the permeability of drug across the vaginal epithelium:

$$P_v = -V/C_v(dC_v/dt) \tag{8.3}$$

where V is the volume of the vaginal compartment, and P_v is the permeability coefficient (cm/second) for drug passage from vagina to plasma. It should be noted that certain stimulating hormones such as estrogen will increase the thickness of the vaginal epithelium and thus alter drug permeability (Hsu et al. 1983). Drug flux across mucosal membranes is described as follows:

$$J = P_{app}C_v \tag{8.4}$$

where J is the flux, and C_v represents total drug concentration in the vagina. The apparent permeability coefficient is given by

$$P_{app} = (1/P_{aq} + 1/P_m)^{-1} \tag{8.5}$$

in which P_{aq} is the permeability coefficient of drug in the aqueous boundary layer (static diffusion layer in Figure 8.1), and P_m is the effective permeability coefficient for drug in the lipophilic and aqueous regions of the membrane. The flux may be written in terms of concentration in the vagina

C_v by combining it with a term for vaginal volume V and surface area S as follows:

$$J = -V/S(dC_v/dt) \tag{8.6}$$

Since rate of drug loss from the vagina can be written as

$$dC_v/dt = -K_aC_v \tag{8.7}$$

then Equation 8.7 may be substituted into Equation 8.6, yielding

$$J = V/S(K_aC_v) \tag{8.8}$$

where K_a is the absorption rate constant (s^{-1}) of drug across the vaginal epithelium. The absorption rate constant may then be expressed as follows by combining Equations 8.4 and 8.5 with Equation 8.8.

$$K_a = (S/V)(P_{aq})/(1 + P_{aq}/P_m) \tag{8.9}$$

Thus, drug absorption from the vagina will be influenced by the relative permeability of drug in the aqueous boundary layer and vaginal membrane. These relative permeabilities will depend on the dissolution characteristics of the drug, the pH of the vagina as it affects drug dissociation, drug lipophilicity, and drug size.

Drug Disposition after Vaginal Administration

As mentioned, vaginal drug administration can be utilized to produce high local or systemic drug levels (Nahoul et al. 1993; Casson et al. 1996). For drugs with low oral bioavailability, the vaginal route is ideal since hepatic first-pass metabolism is bypassed. The administration of estradiol and micronized progesterone provides excellent examples of how relative bioavailability can be improved through intravaginal administration (Simon 1995; Johnston 1996; Heimer 1987). Rigg and colleagues studied systemic levels of 17b-estradiol and conjugated estrogens using vaginal creams (Rigg et al. 1978). A 2-mg dose produced detectable levels of estradiol within 15 minutes, with peak concentrations reached at 4 hours. Circulating levels of estradiol were dose dependent, with peak concentrations that were 7 and 45 times the mean basal level after 0.2-mg and 2-mg doses, respectively. Administration of conjugated estrogens, in contrast, resulted in a slower rise in serum levels with lower peak concentrations. Drug levels were first detected 3 hours after administration, with peak concentrations that were 2.5 times the basal level. Similar data have been reported elsewhere (Martin et al. 1979; Deutsch et al. 1981). Heimer and coworkers compared the systemic levels of estriol after oral and vaginal administration (Heimer and Englund 1984). They showed that the

24-hour levels as measured by the area under the concentration versus time curve (AUC) were nearly equivalent when 1 mg of vaginally administered estriol was compared to a 10-mg oral dose. Furthermore, estriol levels after 21 days of intravaginal dosing were still equivalent to the 10-mg oral dose despite a mature vaginal epithelium.

Chakmakjian and coworkers studied the bioavailability of micronized progesterone after different routes of administration (Chakmakjian and Zachariah 1987). Micronized progesterone levels were measured after 50- to 200-mg doses were given sublingually, orally, vaginally, and rectally. Peak levels were observed within 1 hour after sublingual administration and between 2 to 3 hours for the other routes. Interestingly, 24-hour serum levels after vaginal and rectal dosing were found to be nearly 2 to 2.5 times that of the oral route. AUC calculations for the first 8 hours showed that the rectal route had the largest relative bioavailability (169.9 cm^2), followed by the vaginal (96 cm^2), sublingual (95 cm^2), and oral (76.9 cm^2) routes, respectively. The authors postulated that the large difference between the vaginal and rectal routes was due to drug loss from the vagina. Similar studies using different delivery vehicles reported improved bioavailability, presumably by minimizing vaginal drug loss (Nahoul et al. 1993; Devroey et al. 1990).

It is evident from these studies that vaginal drug administration can be utilized to achieve significant systemic levels for certain agents. However, poorly understood phenomena are the high local levels observed throughout the reproductive system that were not reproducible through intravenous or oral routes of administration. Studies by Miles and colleagues compared endometrial tissue levels of progesterone after vaginal and intramuscular administration (Miles et al. 1994). Twenty functionally agonadal women aged 25 to 54 were enrolled in the study. All subjects underwent an estrogen and progesterone simulated replacement cycle. On day 16 of the estrogen replacement cycle, patients either received vaginally administered micronized progesterone capsules (200 mg) every 6 hours or intramuscular progesterone (50 mg) twice daily. Endometrial sampling with a pipelle endocurette was performed on day 21 of the simulated cycle. Samples were then assayed for progesterone concentration as well as estrogen and progesterone receptor content. Serum progesterone levels by cycle day 21 were 221.89 + 18.78 nmol/L after intramuscular injection and 37.83 + 3.82 nmol/L after intravaginal administration. However, endometrial concentrations were 4.45 + 1.27 after intramuscular versus 36.56 + 8.27 nmol/L vaginally. Thus, an eightfold increase in endometrial levels was achieved despite serum concentrations that were nearly sixfold less. This study clearly illustrated the significant local drug effect after vaginal administration.

Mizutani and colleagues determined danazol levels in the ovary, uterus, and serum after vaginal administration (Mizutani et al. 1995). Patients making up the study were women with regular menstrual cycles, ages 23 to 43, who underwent a total abdominal hysterectomy and unilateral oophorectomy after drug administration. The patients were divided into three groups; group I received a danazol suppository (100 mg) in the posterior vaginal fornix at 4, 12, or 36 hours prior to surgery; group II individuals were instructed to administer a danazol suppository (100 mg) vaginally daily for 30 days prior to surgery; group III received a danazol capsule (200 mg) by mouth twice daily for 30 days prior to surgery. A single vaginal administration of danazol resulted in significant uptake in the ovary and uterus within 4 hours. The highest levels were observed in the ovary. Danazol levels decreased in concentration from the ovary, endometrium, myometrium of the cervix, to the myometrium of the uterine corpus. Peak levels ranged from 10 ng/mg of tissue to nearly 80 ng/mg of tissue. Drug levels decreased rapidly to one-fourth the peak levels after 12 hours. In contrast, serum danazol concentrations were always less than 1 ng/mL. Danazol concentrations in the ovary and uterus after daily vaginal administration were two to three times greater than after the single-dose regimen and comparable to daily oral dosing. However, serum levels after vaginal administration were less than 5% of those of oral dosing. The authors postulated that vaginally and orally administered danazol reached the ovary and uterus by different routes. They proposed that the venous plexus or lymphatic system of the reproductive organs was the probable route by which drugs distributed after vaginal administration.

Similar findings have been observed using a human *ex vivo* uterine perfusion model (Bulletti et al. 1997). In this study, uterine specimens were obtained immediately after abdominal hysterectomy for early-stage cervical cancer or uterine prolapse. A mixture of tritiated and unlabeled progesterone was applied to the cuff of vaginal tissue removed with the uterus (Bulletti et al. 1997). ^{3}H and ^{14}C radioactivity were measured in the uterine tissue following a 12-hour perfusion period. Progesterone concentrations were 185 + 155 ng/100 mg of tissue and 254 + 305 ng/100 mg of tissue in the endometrium and myometrium, respectively. Autoradiography performed 4 hours after perfusion showed a uniform capture of radioactivity by the endometrium. In the myometrium, however, radioactive tracer accumulated within or proximal to the vascular casts. The authors suggested that this may reflect arterial-to-venous counterperfusion. It should be noted the this study sample was small, and the model, although rigorously tested, may not have accurately reflected perfusion physiology (Bulletti et al. 1986, 1988). Nonetheless, the findings provide additional support for local drug distribution following vaginal absorption.

Fujii and coworkers studied the distribution and effects of intravaginal cisplatin for the treatment of cervical cancer (Fujii et al. 1995). Four patients with cervical cancer ranging from stage Ib to stage IIa were preoperatively treated with 20-mg cisplatin suppositories. Doses were administered every other day for a total of seven doses. Serum levels obtained 12 hours after the last dose ranged from 0.17 to 0.57 mg/mL. Postoperative tissue samples showed significant drug levels in the cervix (55.4 mg/mL average), vagina (13.13 mg/mL), endometrium (3.17 mg/mL), uterine wall (0.64 mg/mL), and ovary (0.57 mg/mL). Lymph node groups sampled showed average drug levels in the parametrium (1.14 mg/mL), obturator (0.34 mg/mL), inguinal (0.28 mg/mL), external iliac (0.51 mg/mL), internal iliac (0.42 mg/mL), and common iliac (0.54 mg/mL) areas. Para-aortic node levels were too low to detect. Posttreatment colposcopy showed a disappearance of bleeding and reduction of tumor outgrowth. Microscopically, the authors observed degeneration and necrosis of cancer nests from the surface to approximately 2 mm. The interesting feature of this study was significant levels of cisplatin in the reproductive tissues and lymphatic groups sampled.

Mechanisms of Pelvic Drug Distribution

Pelvic drug distribution after vaginal administration may be dependent on a number of mechanisms. It is possible that drug may distribute topically in an antegrade or retrograde manner within the vaginal canal. This could account for drug loss through the introitus as well as distribution to the upper reproductive structures. Following vaginal absorption, simple diffusion across parenchymal and interstitial structures may contribute to local distribution as well. However, growing evidence suggests that the predominant route of drug distribution occurs after vaginal absorption. Studies by Chakmakjian and coworkers (Chakmakjian and Zachariah 1987), Miles and colleagues (1994), and Mizutani and coworkers (1995) showed that vaginal drug absorption leads to elevated levels of drug in the upper reproductive structures within 4 to 6 hours. Conventionally, venous flow is a unidirectional process favoring systemic transport rather than redistribution to proximal pelvic structures. The data presented raise the possibility that another mechanism may be involved that distributes drug to the upper reproductive organs. Retrograde transport through the endocervical canal, uterine cavity, and fallopian tubes may be partially responsible. However, it may not adequately describe the relatively rapid kinetics of drug uptake observed in tissues such as the ovaries.

A mechanism that may explain these findings involves the exchange of drug between venous and arterial segments of capillaries known as countercurrent exchange. The countercurrent exchange model has been described in the uterine adnexa, kidney, and small intestine (Lundgren and Haglund 1978; Dan-Axel Hallback et al. 1978; Bendz et al. 1982b). The model is dependent on the close association between venous and arterial limbs in a vascular loop. It was originally proposed as an autocrine modality for the ovary (Bendz 1977; Bendz et al. 1978, 1982a; Halket et al. 1985; Einer-Jensen et al. 1989). It was postulated that a certain area of ovarian tissue was responsible for secreting factors into efferent venules that could be directly transferred to an arterial branch supplying another region of the ovary. The authors speculated that this may account for the influence of prostaglandins on the corpus luteum.

Bendz and colleagues tested this hypothesis in the human adnexa during a total abdominal hysterectomy (Bendz et al. 1979). The study was designed to test whether krypton-85 could be transferred from the utero-ovarian vein to the ipsilateral ovary. In five of the eight women studied, an ipsilateral increase in ovarian radioactivity was detected within 60 seconds. Maximum radioactivity was measured within 2 to 4 minutes. The authors noted that two of the eight patients who did not demonstrate ovarian radioactivity developed hematomas around the punctured vein, suggesting experimental error. Similar findings were noted using ^{13}C-labeled progesterone (Halket et al. 1985). Einer-Jensen and coworkers even speculated that this mechanism may exist between lymphatic and arterial vessels as well (Einer-Jensen et al. 1989).

These studies raise the intriguing possibility that drug distribution to upper reproductive tissues may be due to countercurrent exchange. After vaginal absorption, it is conceivable that drug initially distributes along the reproductive tract via exchange between venous plexuses. Countercurrent exchange may then occur between adjacent arterial vessels, leading to drug transport to respective reproductive organs. The studies cited to support this mechanism were small in number and limited to the utero-ovarian vasculature. However, it is one of the few models that can account for the rapid kinetics of drug distribution to pelvic organs after vaginal absorption. Clearly, further investigation is needed to support this hypothesis.

Pharmacokinetic Modeling of Vaginal Drug Absorption

From the studies mentioned, drug disposition following vaginal absorption appears to be kinetically distinct from the general systemic circulation. The disproportionate levels observed within the reproductive tissues indicated that conventional single-compartment kinetic modeling may not accurately reflect drug disposition. Therefore, it is proposed that drug disposition within the pelvic structures be treated as a kinetically unique compartment that is in equilibrium with the systemic circulation or central compartment. With this in mind, drug disposition would be treated in terms of a multicompartment pharmacokinetic model in which drug input occurs in a peripheral compartment (i.e., pelvic compartment) (Gibaldi and Perrier 2007). The difference in kinetic modeling is the mode of drug entry and initial disposition. After vaginal drug absorption, high local drug concentrations are achieved within the pelvic compartment, which is in equilibrium with the systemic circulation. Figure 8.2 represents a multicompartment pharmacokinetic model that may be used to describe the distribution and elimination of drug after vaginal absorption (Gibaldi and Perrier 2007).

Here, the pelvic organs are treated as a separate kinetic compartment (X_p) that is in equilibrium with central compartment (X_c). In this model, the central compartment refers to the systemic circulation. The compartment designated as X_t represents the summation of all peripheral tissues that are poorly perfused. The extent to which drug distributes into poorly perfused tissues depends on the physicochemical properties of the drug and may be omitted under certain circumstances. It is included in this discussion so

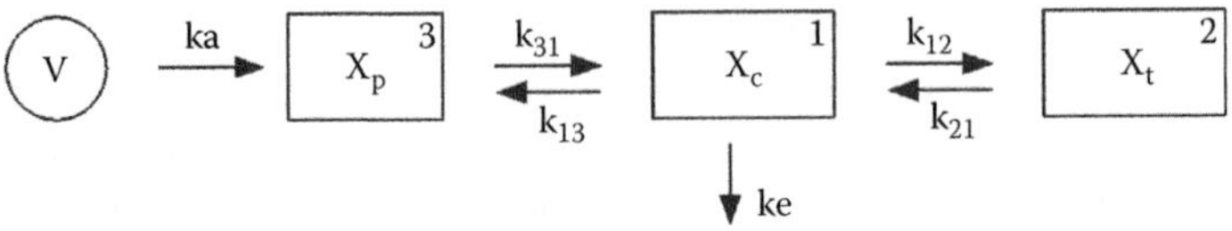

FIGURE 8.2
Multicompartment model lists the various rate constants of absorption from the vagina (k_a), intercompartmental rate constants between the pelvic and central (k_{31}, k_{13}) and central and peripheral compartments (k_{12}, k_{21}), and a general elimination rate constant from the central compartment (k_e). The last describes both urinary excretion and hepatic metabolism.

that a general expression may be derived. The kinetic model presented in Figure 8.2 may be solved using general equations for linear mammillary models when drug is administered into a peripheral compartment such as the vagina (X_p) (Vaughan and Trainor 1975). The method for solving linear mammillary models requires the use of general input and disposition functions, a method for solving partial fractions to obtain Laplace transforms, and a multiple-dosing function. The input function denotes the mode of drug entry into the body, which in this case represents the vaginal route. The disposition function describes everything that happens to the drug in terms of distribution and elimination (Gibaldi and Perrier 2007). The product of the input and disposition function yields the Laplace transform of the equation that describes the time course of drug in a model compartment. Equation 8.10 has been derived to describe the Laplace transform for the disposition function of the central compartment when drug input occurs into a peripheral compartment (Vaughan and Trainor 1975):

$$\left(d_{s1}\right)_q = \frac{k_{q1}\prod_{\substack{j=2\\ j\neq q}}^{n}\left(S+E_j\right)}{\prod_{j=1}^{n}\left(S+E_j\right)-\prod_{j=2}^{n}k_{1j}k_{j1}\prod_{\substack{m=2\\ m\neq j}}\left(S+E_m\right)} \tag{8.10}$$

In Equation 8.10, $(d_{s1})_q$ represents the disposition function in the central compartment X_c (i.e., systemic circulation) for drug input from the vagina; P is the continued product, where any term is defined as equal to 1; k_{ij}, k_{ji}, and k_{q1} are the intercompartment transfer rate constants; E_j and E_m are the sum of exit rate constants out of compartments j or m, respectively. Equation 8.11 denotes the product of the input and disposition functions, which yields the Laplace transform for the amount of drug in the central compartment.

$$\left(a_{s1}\right)_q = in_s\left(d_{s1}\right)_q \tag{8.11}$$

The *ins* term is the input function, which is given as

$$\left(in\right)_s = \frac{k_a X_o}{S + k_a} \tag{8.12}$$

Equation 8.12 denotes any first-order absorption rate process, which in this case refers to vaginal drug absorption. Equation 8.11 can then be rewritten to yield the following expression:

$$\left(a_{s1}\right)_q = \frac{k_a k_{31} X_o \left(S + E_2\right)\left(S + E_3\right)}{\left(S + k_a\right)\left(S + \lambda_1\right)\left(S + \lambda_2\right)\left(S + \lambda_3\right)} \tag{8.13}$$

The anti-Laplace of the resulting transform may be solved by a general partial fraction theorem for obtaining inverse Laplace transforms. Therefore, the general expression denoting drug amount in the central compartment after vaginal drug absorption is given by

$$X_c = A_{1e}^{-\lambda_1 t} + A_{2e}^{-\lambda_2 t} + A_{3e}^{-\lambda_3 t} \tag{8.14}$$

The values for individual coefficients $A_{1,2,3}$ and the constants $l_{1,2,3}$ can be obtained graphically from drug concentration-time profiles. The amount of drug in the pelvic compartment may also be calculated in a similar fashion, yielding the following equation:

$$X_p = A_{1e}^{!-\lambda_1 t} + A_{2e}^{!-\lambda_2 t} + A_{3e}^{!-\lambda_3 t} + A^{!}_{4\left(e^{-k_{31}t} - e^{-k_a t}\right)} \tag{8.15}$$

In short, these equations represent general expressions to describe drug disposition in the body following vaginal drug absorption. The purpose for including such a discussion is to show that local distribution in the pelvis can be treated as if in a kinetically unique compartment when drug is administered vaginally. The rationale behind this mathematical treatment is based on the clinical observations noted by the investigators. It is obvious, however, that a more rigorous line of studies is needed to characterize drug disposition better. It is hoped that these mathematical derivations may better describe the kinetics involved with vaginal drug administration.

Current Trends in Intravaginal Drug Delivery

Labor Induction

Spontaneous labor and delivery involve a sequence of events that includes softening, or ripening, and effacement of the cervix. Labor induction is indicated when there is evidence of preeclampsia, diabetes, heart disease, or fetal-placental insufficiency. Prolonged labor in the context of an unfavorable cervix can increase the likelihood of numerous maternal and fetal complications, such as infection, fetal distress/demise, the need for operative delivery, and postpartum hemorrhage. Pharmacological intervention is often implemented in an effort to "ripen" the cervix to facilitate vaginal delivery. Numerous studies dating to the 1970s have documented the successful use of prostaglandins for labor induction through intracervical or intravaginal routes of administration. In recent years, dinoprostone (a synthetic prostaglandin E2) has been used for cervical ripening via vaginal administration. Early efforts utilized glycerol ester-based formulations to deliver dinoprostone (Liggins 1979; Shepherd et al. 1979; MacKenzie et al. 1981). Currently, methylcellulose-based materials (Norchi et al. 1993; Smith et al. 1996) and polyethylene oxide-based hydrogels (Norchi et al. 1993; Smith et al. 1994, 1996; Taylor et al. 1990; McNeill and Graham 1984; Embrey et al. 1980, 1986; Graham and McNeill 1984) have been formulated for cervical ripening. Early concerns for these devices were related to dose dumping and ease of removal. While a burst release of drug in the early phase is difficult to avoid, signs and symptoms of toxicity have been less significant with current devices. The success of this system has largely been due to incorporating drug into hydrogel delivery systems, in which release is swelling controlled and more predictable. In terms of retrieval, Cervidil™ (a polyethylene oxide/urethane-based hydrogel) is incorporated within a polyester net that can be used to remove the device should signs or symptoms of hyperstimulation result. It is expected that future delivery systems for labor induction will utilize both newer agents and polymeric systems. Although considerable interest has been placed on labor induction, it bears mention that other areas in obstetrics may benefit from intravaginal therapeutics. These include the management of preterm labor with intravaginal tocolytic agents or through administration of antibiotics in the context of preterm rupture of membranes to prolong intrauterine gestational time. Labor augmentation in the latent period of stage 1 may be another phase of labor that could benefit from intravaginal therapeutics.

Hormone Replacement Therapy

Hormone replacement has received considerable attention and controversy in recent years. However, there is little dispute that estrogen therapy will continue to be widely utilized for vaginal and urogenital atrophy. Hormone replacement therapy can be achieved by many routes of administration, the most common of which are oral and transdermal. Vaginal estrogen creams have been in existence for many years. Stumpf and coworkers were some of the early investigators to disperse estradiol homogeneously into polysiloxane vaginal rings for this purpose (Stumpf et al. 1982). These delivery systems were capable of maintaining estradiol levels ranging from 109 to 159 pg/mL for 3 months in postmenopausal volunteers. Serum levels could also be adjusted based on the loading dose of estradiol and surface area of the device (Stumpf 1986). Estring™ and other similar devices were later designed with an inner core or reservoir of estradiol and an outer polysiloxane sheath for diffusion-controlled release. Stable serum levels have been achieved for up to 3 months (Schmidt et al. 1994; Nachtigall 1995; Smith et al. 1993; Bachmann 1995).

Contraception

The development of new hormonal contraceptive modalities has been an ongoing effort for over 40 years. Oral, injectable, and implantable contraceptives have all been widely used with exceptional efficacy. Intravaginal hormonal contraception was initially investigated by Mishell and coworkers using medroxyprogesterone (Mishell et al. 1970). Medroxyprogesterone was homogeneously dispersed in cylindrical rings prepared from polysiloxane. Over a 28-day cycle, an absence of the midcycle leutinizing hormone (LH) surge was observed. Endometrial biopsies taken were consistent with progestational effects. Furthermore, removal of the device resulted in prompt withdrawal bleeding.

Similar designs have also been developed for 90-day clinical trials (Burton et al. 1978). Ballagh and colleagues tested a core-designed vaginal ring containing norethindrone acetate and ethinyl estradiol (Ballagh et al. 1994). Ovulation and breakthrough bleeding were better controlled, with average daily ethinyl estradiol release rates ranging from 30 to 65 mg. However, unacceptably high levels of nausea resulted with the 65-mg daily release rates. Similar rings containing levonorgestrel have also been studied (Landgren et al. 1994a, 1994b). Unlike the preceding ethinyl estradiol vaginal rings, there was greater individual variation in levonorgestrel levels, incomplete suppression of ovulation, and breakthrough bleeding.

As described, many of the birth control methods currently employed require the use of hormones to suppress ovulation. However, there are a number of clinical risks and side effects associated with hormonal contraception, including an increased risk for venous thromboembolism and its association with breast cancer (Mulders et al. 2002). Therefore, an alternative approach would be to develop a nonhormonal contraceptive device with comparable efficacy to the hormone equivalent. A nonhormonal contraceptive ring, Ovaprene™ (Poly-Med Inc., Anderson, SC), has been developed that employs ferrous gluconate, ascorbic acid (vitamin C), and polyglycolide particles as the active contraceptive ingredients (Figure 8.3).

Ferrous gluconate acts by immobilizing the sperm tail through iron-catalyzed lipid peroxidation, ascorbic acid increases the viscosity of the cervical mucus, and the polyglycolide particles function to lower vaginal pH levels and control the release of the previous two components (Aiken et al. 1993; World Health Organization [WHO] 1999; Saxena et al. 2004). The ring itself consists of a silicone matrix (containing the contraceptive ingredients) surrounding a mesh component, which functions as a physical barrier to inhibit

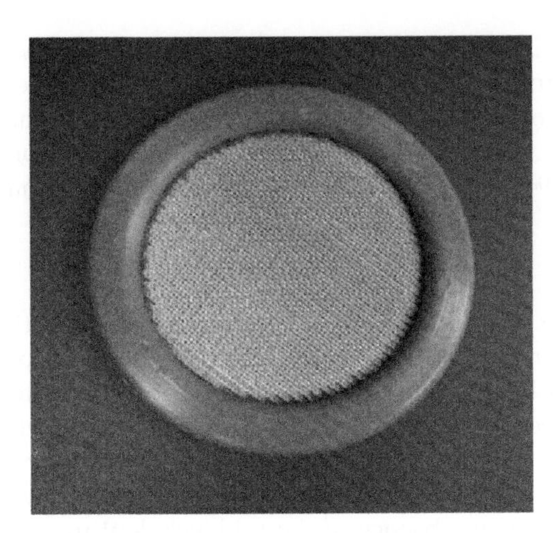

FIGURE 8.3
Ovaprene™ nonhormonal contraceptive device.

the movement of sperm into the cervix. Initial clinical safety and tolerability trials conducted at New York Downtown Hospital showed promise as the rings were well tolerated and accepted (Del Priore et al. 2009). In addition, postcoital testing of female patients from this initial clinical trial revealed nonmobile sperm in the vaginal canal and none in the cervical mucus (Del Priore et al. 2009).

The medical management of abortions and ectopic pregnancies involves two areas of converging study. Randomized trials by Creinin and colleagues utilized oral or intramuscular methotrexate with intravaginal administration of misoprostal to provide safe and efficacious medical abortions (Creinin et al. 1995; Creinin 1996). These studies suggested that oral administration of methotrexate may have improved efficacy while minimizing systemic side effects. It is conceivable that intravaginal methotrexate administration may provide additional advantages in terms of higher local drug levels at lower doses. This could conceivably improve efficacy while further minimizing systemic side effects. Similarly, the medical management of ectopic pregnancies requires the intramuscular administration of methotrexate over one to four doses followed by leucovorin rescue. In this regard, the administration of an intravaginal methotrexate delivery system may be capable of releasing lower doses of drug over a predictable time course to improve efficacy and compliance while decreasing systemic side effects.

Infertility

Progesterone supplementation or replacement is widely implemented for assisted reproductive technology in the treatment of infertility. Oral administration of progesterone leads to extensive intestinal and hepatic metabolism. The standard of treatment for progesterone deficiency is through intramuscular administration, which can be painful. An intravaginal progesterone gel (Crinone™) has been developed. The delivery system is a bioadhesive gel formulation prepared from polycarbophil. The gel is administered once or twice daily, delivering 90 mg of micronized progesterone with each dose. Treatment may be continued for up to 12 weeks until placental autonomy is achieved. The manufacturer (Wyeth-Ayerst Laboratories) purported it elicited less drowsiness as compared to the oral form. This delivery system is also being studied in conjunction with oral estrogen for hormone replacement therapy.

Infectious Diseases

Interest in the administration of intravaginal agents for the treatment and prophylaxis of sexually transmitted diseases and other infections has been considerable. Early efforts in this field focused on treatment modalities for bacterial vaginosis. Bacterial vaginosis is a syndrome in women of reproductive age in which the normal lactobacilli-dominated vaginal microflora are replaced by high concentrations of mixed anaerobic and facultative flora. Typically, this includes *Peptostreptococcus* sp., *G. vaginalis*, *Mycoplasma hominis*, and *Ureaplasma urealyticum* (Hill et al. 1985; Gravett et al. 1986a). It is considered to be the most common vaginal infection and has been associated with an increased risk of preterm labor and delivery (Gravett et al. 1986b); premature rupture of membranes (Lamont et al. 1986); chorioamnionitis (Lamont et al. 1986; Hillier et al. 1988; Eschenbach et al. 1988); and pelvic inflammatory disease (Hillier et al. 1990).

Topical administration of clindamycin or metronidazole has been most successful in the treatment of bacterial vaginosis. Hillier and colleagues studied the efficacy of 0.1% to 2.0% clindamycin creams administered daily for 7 days in nonpregnant women (Hillier et al. 1990). They found that the 2% cream had the greatest effect on bacterial vaginosis-associated flora, with a 94% resolution of bacterial vaginosis both 1 week and 1 month after treatment. Similar findings have been reported elsewhere (Livengood et al. 1990; Hill and Livengood 1994).

The efficacy of intravaginal clindamycin has also been shown to be similar to oral metronidazole (Schmitt et al. 1992). The bioavailability of clindamycin has been shown to be minimal, ranging from 2.7% to 4.7% (Borin et al. 1995). Intravaginal metronidazole has been studied to improve patient compliance and decrease systemic side effects such as seen with the oral regimen. Edelmen and coworkers administered intravaginal sponges containing either 250 mg (twice daily for 2 days) or 1 g (once daily for 3 days) of metronidazole (Edelman and North 1989). While the study was carried out in a small group of women, cure rates of 85% and 92% were noted after 1 week, respectively. Failure rates after 1 month were 42% in the low-dose and

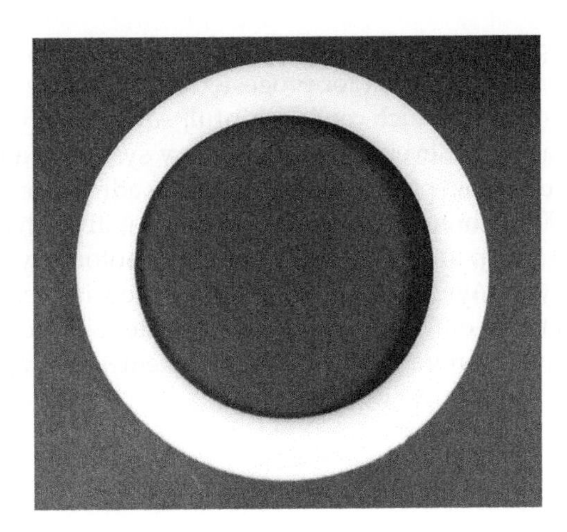

FIGURE 8.4
EVA copolymer ring that can be loaded with drugs to prepare the Bactoprene™ or Mycoprene™ device.

12% in the high-dose group. Systemic side effects such as nausea, headache, and metallic taste were slightly more frequent in patients using the higher-dose sponge. Hillier and colleagues studied the efficacy of 5-g metronidazole gels (0.75%) administered twice daily for 5 days (Hillier et al. 1993). A clinical cure rate of 87% was observed after 9 to 21 days, with a recurrence rate of 15% after 1 month. Furthermore, there were no significant side effects noted in the treatment group. Similar results have been reported in a larger study by Livengood and colleagues (1994). Systemic levels of metronidazole after vaginal administration are significant (Cunningham et al. 1994). The relative bioavailability compared to the oral form is 56%.

Although the use of creams and gels for the treatment of bacterial vaginosis has proved effective, it often requires multiple applications due to the limited residence time and can pose some sanitary issues. Therefore, it would be ideal to have a drug-eluting intravaginal device that can be placed (single application) into the vaginal canal to release the antifungal or antibacterial drug, depending on the type of infection, over a period of 1 week. Currently, two intravaginal ring types are being developed by researchers at Poly-Med, trademarked Bactoprene™ and Mycoprene™ (Figure 8.4).

Each consists of an ethylene vinyl acetate (EVA) copolymer ring matrix that contains the microbicidal drug along with a hydrophilic component to promote drug release. Bactoprene, formulated for the treatment of bacterial vaginosis, is loaded with either metronidazole or clindamycin. Mycoprene, alternatively, is loaded with miconazole and is specifically formulated for the treatment of vaginal yeast infections. *In vitro* inhibition studies (Table 8.1) conducted against the target microbe for each device showed sustained drug delivery at therapeutic levels for at least 5 days. Briefly, the studies involved

TABLE 8.1

Percentage Inhibition of Target Microbe by Mycoprene™ and Bactoprene™

Day	% Inhibition	
	C. albicans[a]	*V. parvula*[b]
1	61.55	90.00
2	78.70	75.50
3	72.75	18.25
4	74.05	29.40
5	70.25	26.05

[a] A model microorganism for studying fungal inhibition.
[b] A model microorganism for studying bacterial inhibition.

incubation of each ring type with growth media that had been inoculated with either *Candida albicans* (to study Mycoprene) or *Veillonella parvula* (to study Bactoprene). After incubation (18–22 hours), optical densities were read on a spectrophotometer at a wavelength of 600 nm and compared to that of the control to obtain a percentage of inhibition. Although still in the research-and-development phase, early test results seemed promising and could lead to a significant advancement for the treatment of bacterial vaginosis.

Current standards in the treatment of sexually transmitted diseases have focused on oral and intravenous administration of antibiotics and antiviral agents. While little has been done in terms of intravaginal treatment strategies, a growing interest in prophylaxis has emerged using vaginal microbicides and antiviral agents. The ultimate goal is to develop a vaginal delivery system that has activity against a broad spectrum of pathogens, including HPV and HIV. A number of compounds have been considered, such as benzalkonium chloride, chlorhexidine, nonoxynol-9, and polymixin B (Lyons and Ito 1995; Pauwels and De Clercq 1996). In terms of HIV transmission, both virucidal agents and biomaterials that prevent HIV adsorption/fusion are being studied (Pauwels and De Clercq 1996). Although this area is still in its infancy, the growing urgency for prevention strategies will quickly attract many investigators from multidisciplinary backgrounds to study this problem. It is clear, however, that the active agent as well as the delivery system will play an equal role in optimizing efficacy.

One such delivery system being developed is the OC system (Poly-Med). This system consists of an amphiphilic copolymer diluted with a solvent to allow for injectability. On injection into the body, the solvent immediately releases from the polymer, allowing for *in situ* formation of a delivery depot. The system is then capable of delivering diffusion-based release of the pharmaceutical payload over a predeterminable period of time. The use of exclusively biodegradable monomers (lactide, glycolide, caprolactone, etc.) in the copolymer formulation also ensures biocompatibility, biodegradability, and,

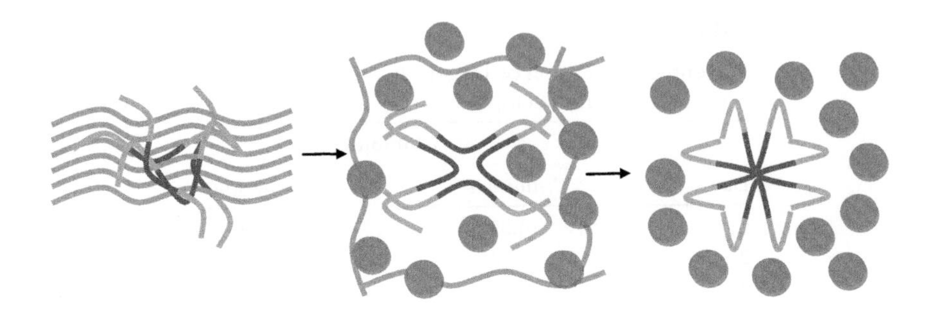

FIGURE 8.5 (see color insert)
Progression of *in situ* gelation of amphiphilic polymer system such as the OC series of polymers. Green is the original injection solvent, red represents the hydrophobic portion of the chains, orange the hydrophilic portions, and blue water molecules.

most important, stabilization of the vaginal flora by maintaining a slightly acidic pH in the microenvironment.

This system varies from other thermogelling treatments in that the mechanism of the sol/gel transition relies on hydrophobic interactions rather than temperature gradients. Due to the amphiphilic nature of the polymer portion of the system, on injection the chains orient themselves to form the release depot. This is postulated to be due to the instant exposure of the hydrophobic and hydrophilic segments to the largely aqueous environment of the human body (Figure 8.5).

On said exposure, the hydrophobic portions of the copolymer chain orient themselves to an inner core, while the hydrophilic portions form the outer regions of the delivery depot. Following this orientation, a multilayer construct is developed through which release of the drug payload, homogeneously distributed within, is achieved mainly through diffusion. This diffusion can then be influenced through modifications to either the hydrophobic or hydrophilic segments of the chains.

The novelty of this platform technology lies in the ability to modulate nearly any of the variables mentioned previously. Release speed, degradation period, and even gel formation speed can be tailored to the exact needs of the individual application. A series of polymers has been developed with minor modifications to allow for a variety of delivery applications. In the area of vaginal delivery, local dimensionally stable delivery of the aforementioned drugs, such as clindamycin or metronidazole, would be highly advantageous to the current paradigm of oral and nonstationary gel delivery. The OC system has been shown to be capable of delivering water-soluble drugs over a variety of periods, as exhibited in Figure 8.6. This modularity allows for the implementation of the system against a wide range of pathogens.

Delivery modalities such as the OC system from Poly-Med provide a look at the future of drug delivery. In the area of localized delivery for treatment of vaginal infections, such controlled-release systems hold great promise for a myriad antibacterial and possibly virucidal activity.

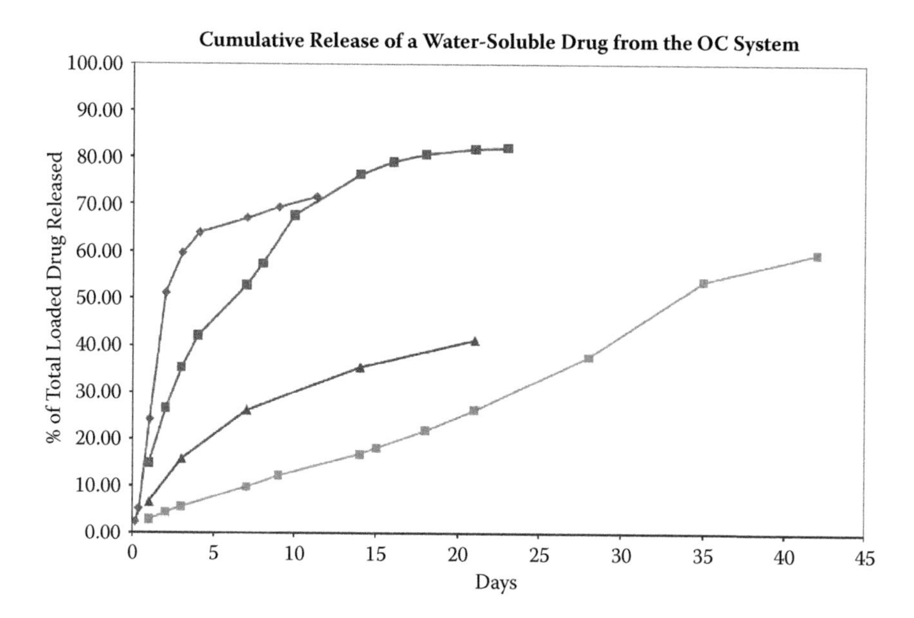

FIGURE 8.6
Examples of modulated release of a water-soluble drug from the OC system. This ability allows a variety of treatment options and methods.

Gynecologic Oncology

Intravaginal administration of chemotherapy has been evaluated for the treatment of vaginal and cervical dysplasias. The rationale is based on the assumption that higher localized levels can be achieved at a fraction of the intravenous dose with minimal systemic side effects. A case report by Bowens-Simpkins and coworkers first described the topical administration of 5-fluorouracil (5-FU) for treatment of multifocal vaginal intraepithelial neoplasia (Bowen-Simpkins and Hull 1975). Twice-daily administration of 5% 5-FU cream for 2 weeks resulted in benign cytological findings for up to a 15-month follow-up period. However, evidence of excoriation and thinning of the vaginal wall were noted 1 month after treatment. This resulted in some dyspareunia for up to 7 months. Similar efficacy and side effects were noted using different 5-FU concentrations (Woodruff et al. 1975) and dosing regimens (Caglar et al. 1981; Kirwan 1985).

Piver and colleagues studied the administration of 20% 5-FU over monthly 5-day courses in patients with postirradiation vaginal carcinoma *in situ* (Piver et al. 1979). Seven of the eight women studied had an initial complete response, with three of the patients developing a recurrence after treatment was stopped. Retreatment, however, resulted in a complete response in two of the three recurrences. The authors noted that most of the patients developed vulvovaginitis, which they claimed was well controlled by sitz baths and analgesics.

HPV-associated lesions of the vulva and vagina have been treated with topical 5-FU as well. Krebs studied prophylactic topical 5-FU following ablative treatment (Krebs 1986). Patients given biweekly doses of 5% 5-FU creams for 6 months developed recurrence in 13% of the cases as compared to 35% in the control group. The authors noted that maintenance therapy was most effective in women with multiple lesions, multiple organ involvement (vulva, vagina, cervix, anus, distal urethra), or a depressed immune system. Similar findings were noted using a once-a-week dosing regimen (Krebs 1987). In terms of toxicity, however, long-term topical administration of 5-FU can lead to chronic ulcerative changes in the vagina. Krebs and coworkers found that the incidence of ulcers was higher in women who used 5-FU for longer than 10 weeks (Krebs and Helmkamp 1991). Associated symptoms included serosanguinous or watery discharge, postcoital spotting or bleeding, irregular bleeding, and pain. Conservative treatment with estrogens or cauterizing agents did not facilitate healing. However, excision of the ulcer with primary closure was found to be curative.

The treatment of cervical intraepithelial neoplasias (CINs) has been studied. Meyskens and coworkers studied the regression of CIN II with topically administered all-*trans*-retinoic acid (RA) (Meyskens et al. 1983, 1994). The device used to deliver RA was a collagen sponge inserted into a cervical cap comprised of a bioadhesive hydrogel (Dorr et al. 1982). The results showed that locally applied RA (daily for 4 days) led to complete histologic regression of CIN II in 43% of the patients. Patients returned at 3 and 6 months for follow-up as well as maintenance treatment consisting of daily RA for 2 days. No treatment effect was observed in cases of severe dysplasia. Side effects included cervical inflammation by colposcopic evaluation, mild vaginal inflammation, and vulvar burning and irritation during initial treatment. Intravaginal administration of interferon gamma has also been studied for the treatment of CIN (Singer et al. 1990; Schneider et al. 1995). In terms of cervical cancer, some investigators have proposed intravaginal administration of cisplatin (Nakayama et al. 1990). However, few case reports exist. Thus, any perceived benefit is purely speculative at this time.

The preceding discussion illustrates the possible benefit of intravaginal chemotherapy in the treatment of vaginal and even cervical dysplasias. Again, the choice of the chemotherapeutic agent and mode of delivery will be equally as important if efficacy is to be optimized.

One of the most exciting areas is HPV vaccination for the prevention of HPV-related urogenital warts and cervical dysplasia.

Future Perspectives: Intravaginal Vaccine Development

HPV as Promoter or Inducer of Cervical Dysplasia and Cancer

It is well recognized that 99.7% of cervical cancers worldwide show molecular evidence of HPV. An understanding and proper modulation of the immune response to HPV is critical in determining the optimal treatment strategies for CIN. Successful prevention or treatment of cervical precursor lesions ultimately depends on the success of the host immune response. Compromised immunity causes a very high rate of recurrence following any treatment modality. HPV is derived from the Papillomaviridae family of DNA viruses, which contains greater than 100 types. HPV types are differentiated by the genetic sequence of the outer capsid protein *L*. HPV is divided into low and high oncogenic risk:

- *Low-risk HPV (6, 11)*: benign genital warts and no oncogenic potential
- *High-risk HPV (16, 18, 26, 31, 33, 35, 39, 45, 51, 52, 56, 58, 59, 68, 73, and W13b)*: causative agent of cervical cancer and its intraepithelial precursors

At the molecular level, the difference between HPV types is that *high-risk can integrate* into the host cell genome. HPV transmission, similar to HIV, typically arises through ulcerative defects in the cervical-vaginal mucosa created by inflammation/infection. Detection of HPV is much slower, with a significant delay in immune response. HPV infection of the basal epithelium produces little viral replication and no cell lysis. Little antigen is available to be detected by immune surveillance. Differentiating squamous epithelial cells have little antigen-presenting capability despite viral replication that results initially in 25 to 50 viral genomes/cell.

Vaccine Development for Cervical Cancer and Dysplasia

Ideally, the primary response should be cell mediated (T cells or natural killer [NK] cells). In most cases, host immune response to most viral infections is usually quite rapid. As a result, antigen-presenting cells (APCs) are activated, releasing local cytokines within 24 to 48 hours of the detection of virus. Thereafter, there is clonal expansion of antigen-specific cytotoxic CD8 and helper CD4 cells within 5 to 7 days. In terms of vaccination, virus-like particles (VLPs) have been prepared from the L1 capsid protein, which self-assembles from the VLPs. As a result, conventional injectable vaccines have been developed to target and prevent HPV transmission across the cervical-vaginal mucosa. Gardasil™ (produced by Merck and Co., Inc.) is an L1 major capsid protein expressed and self-assembled in *Saccharomyces cerevisiae* (yeast) to noninfectious VLPs. The VLPs are adsorbed on an aluminum-containing adjuvant (aluminum hydroxyphosphate) with a 0.5-mL dose containing:

- 20 mg HPV 6 L1 protein
- 40 mg HPV 11 L1 protein
- 40 mg HPV 16 L1 protein
- 20 mg HPV 18 L1 protein

Thus, it is well known as a quadrivalent vaccine designed to target genital warts and up to 80% of HPV-related cervical cancers. Studies have shown efficacy of the vaccine in 5-year follow-ups to be upward of 90% in combating HPV complications (Villa et al. 2006). A more recent addition to the field is that of Cervarix™, GlaxoSmithKline's offering. Cervarix targets HPV 16 and 18 using an aluminum salt plus monophosphoryl lipid A (AS04) adjuvant to boost the immune response. Clinical trials have exhibited efficacies of up to 100% against HPV 16 and 18 as well as potential cross protection against HPV types 31 and 45 (Wang 2007).

While the efficacy has been established, the long-term memory and need for boosters remains a critical question for widespread adoption in the United States and underdeveloped countries. Protection is conferred through immunoglobulin (Ig) G-specific secretion across the cervical-vaginal mucosa. One would postulate that the development or local delivery of the antigen (or VLPs) in the region of transmission may provide a more robust cell-mediated and antibody-mediated response. This would be similar to our experience with the oral polio vaccine as opposed to the injectable form, whereby clonal expansion of APCs from the Peyer's patches leads to a more robust immune response that can also be transported to other mucosal surfaces via the mucosal-associated lymphoid tissue (MALT). It is our contention that vaccine development with intravaginal delivery systems may also be incorporated with other preventive agents or strategies for problems that often coexist with HPV.

Conclusions

The field of intravaginal drug delivery is largely in its infancy compared to other routes of drug administration. We have seen in the discussion that a great deal is yet to be understood. The successful development of intravaginal drug delivery systems will require identifying critical physiological barriers that will control efficacy. Key areas that will require further study include (a) perfusion physiology of the upper and lower reproductive system; (b) mechanisms of drug absorption and drug disposition; (c) control of drug release and duration of action; and (4) development of new biomaterials that will optimize drug efficacy, patient compliance, and safety. While some of these areas may be studied in the lab, many require investigation in suitable animal models and humans. Delineating these areas will be paramount in the successful design of novel intravaginal delivery systems.

While this review was not meant to be exhaustive, its intent was to help define intravaginal drug delivery as a viable route for therapeutics and to elucidate critical areas in this field that are poorly understood. Clearly, the development of this field could have a profound influence on many women's health issues, ranging from obstetrics to gynecologic oncology.

Acknowledgments

We wish to acknowledge the helpful comments of Dr. Shalaby W. Shalaby in the preparation of this chapter.

References

Aiken, R.J., et al. 1993. Relationship between iron-catalyzed lipid peroxidation potential and human sperm function. *J. Reprod. Fertil.* 98:257–65.

Aref, I., El-Sheikha, Z., Hafez, E.S.E. 1978. In *The Human Vagina*, eds. Hafez, E.S.E., Evans, E.T., 179–81. Amsterdam, the Netherlands: Elsevier.

Bachmann, G. 1995. The estradiol vaginal ring—a study of existing clinical data. *Maturitas* 22(Suppl.):S21–29.

Ballagh, S., Mishell, D., Lacarra, M. 1994. A contraceptive vaginal ring releasing norethindrone acetate and ethinyl estradiol. *Contraception* 50:517–33.

Bartlett, J.G., Ondernonk, A.B., Drude, E. 1977. Quantitative bacteriology of the vaginal flora. *J. Infect. Dis.* 136:271–77.

Bendz, A. 1977. The anatomical basis for a possible counter current exchange mechanism in the human adnexa. *Prostaglandins* 13:355–62.

Bendz, A., Einer-Jensen, N., Lundgren, O. Janson, P.O. 1979. Exchange of krypton-85 between blood vessels of the human uterine adnexa. *J. Reprod. Fertil.* 57:137–42.

Bendz, A., Hansson, H.A., Svendsen, P., Wiqvist, N. 1982a. On the extensive contact between the veins and arteries in the human ovarian pedicle. *Acta Physiol. Scand.* 115:179–82.

Bendz, A., Lundgren, O., Hamberger, L. 1982b. Countercurrent exchange of progesterone and antipyrine between human utero-ovarian vessels, and of antipyrine between femoral vessels in the cat. *Acta Physiol. Scand.* 114:611–16.

Benziger, D.P., Edelson, J. 1983. Absorption from the vagina. *Drug Metab. Rev.* 14:137–68.

Borin, M.T., Powley, G., Tackwell, K., Batts, D.H. 1995. Absorption of clindamycin after intravaginal application of clindamycin phosphate 2% cream. *J. Antimicrob. Chemother.* 35:833–41.

Bowen-Simpkins, P., Hull, M.G.R. 1975. Intraepithelial vaginal neoplasia following immunosuppressive therapy treated with topical 5-FU. *Obstet. Gynecol.* 46:360–62.

Bulletti, C., Jasonni, V.M., Lubicz, S., Flamigni, C. Gurpide, E. 1986. Extracorporeal perfusion of the human uterus. *Am. J. Obstet. Gynecol.* 154: 683–88.

Bulletti, C., Jasonni, V.M., Tabanelli, S. 1988. Early human pregnancy *in vitro* utilizing an artificially perfused uterus. *Fertil. Steril.* 49: 991–96.

Bulletti, C., Ziegler, D., Flamigni, C., Giacomucci, E. 1997. Targeted drug delivery in gynecology: the first uterine pass effect. *Hum. Reprod.* 12: 1073–79.

Burgos, M.H., Roig de Vargas-Linares, C.E. 1978. Ultrastructure of the vaginal mucosa. In *The Human Vagina*, eds. Hafez, E.S.E., Evans, E.T. Amsterdam, the Netherlands: Elsevier.

Burton, F.G., Skiens, W.E., Gordon, N.R. 1978. Fabrication and testing of vaginal contraceptive devices designed for release of prespecified dose levels of steroids. *Contraception* 17:221–31.

Caglar, H., Hertzog, R.W., Hreshchyshyn, M.M. 1981. Topical 5-fluorouracil treatment of vaginal intraepithelial neoplasia. *Obstet. Gynecol.* 58: 580–83.

Casson, P.R., Straughn, A.B., Umstot, E.S., et al. 1996. Delivery of dehydroepiandrosterone to premenopausal women: effects of micronization and nonoral administration. *Am. J. Obstet. Gynecol.* 174:649–53.

Chakmakjian, Z.H., Zachariah, N.Y. 1987. Bioavailability of progesterone with different modes of administration. *J. Reprod. Med.* 32:443–48.

Cohen, M.S., Black, J.R., Proctor, R.A., Sparling, P.F. 1985. Host defense and vaginal mucosa: re-evaluation. *Scand. J. Urol. Nephrol. Suppl.* 86:13–24.

Creinin, M.D., Vittinghoff, E., Galbraith, S., Klaisle, C. 1995. A randomized trial comparing misoprostal three and seven days after methotrexate for early abortion. *Am. J. Obstet. Gynecol.* 173:1578–84.

Creinin, M.D., Vittinghoff, E., Keder, L., Darney, P.D., Tiller, G. 1996. Methotrexate and misoprostal for early abortion. A multicenter trial I. Safety and efficacy. *Contraception* 53:321–27.

Cunningham, F., Kraus, D., Brubaker, L., Fischer, J. 1994. Pharmacokinetics of intravaginal metronidazole gel. *J. Clin. Pharmacol.* 34:1060–65.

Dan-Axel Hallback, B.M., Hulten, L., Jodal, M., Lindhagen, J., Lundgren, O. 1978. Evidence for the existence of a countercurrent exchanger in the small intestine in man. *Gastroenterology* 74:683–90.

Del Priore, G., et al. 2009. A pilot safety and tolerability study of a nonhormonal vaginal contraceptive ring. *J. Reprod. Med.* 54(11–12):685–90.

Deutsch, S., Ossowski, R., Benjamin, I. 1981. Comparison between degree of systemic absorption of vaginally and orally administered estrogens at different dose levels in postmenopausal women. *Am. J. Obstet. Gynecol.* 39:967–70.

Devroey, P., Palermo, G., Bourgain, C. 1990. Progesterone administration in patients with absent ovaries. *Int. J. Fertil.* 34:188–93.

Dorr, R., Surwit, E., Meyskins, F.L. 1982. *In vitro* retinoid binding and release from a collagen sponge material in a simulated intravaginal environment. *J. Biomed. Mater. Res.* 16:839–50.

Edelman, D., North, B. 1989. Treatment of bacterial vaginosis with intravaginal sponges containing metronidazole. *J. Reprod. Med.* 34:341–44.

Einer-Jensen, N., McCracken, J.A., Schram, W., Bendz, A. 1989. Counter current transfer in the female adnexa. *Acta Physiol. Pol.* 40:3–11.

Embrey, M.P., Graham, N.B., McNeill, M.E. 1980. Induction of labour with sustained-release prostaglandin E2 vaginal pessary. *Br. Med. J.* 6245:901–2.

Embrey, M.P., Graham, N.B., Macneill, M.E., Hillier, K. 1986. In-vitro release characteristics and long-term stability of polyethylene oxide hydrogel vaginal pessaries containing prostaglandin E2. *J. Controlled Release* 3:39–45.

Eschenbach, D.A., Davick, P.R., Williams, B.L. 1989. Prevalence of hydrogen peroxide-producing lactobacillus species in normal women and women with bacterial vaginosis. *J. Clin. Microbiol.* 27:251–59.

Eschenbach, D.A., Hillier, S.L., Critchlow, C., et al. 1988. Diagnosis and clinical manifestations of bacterial vaginosis. *Am. J. Obstet. Gynecol.* 158:819–28.

Fihn, S.D., Lathan, R.H., Roberts, P. 1985. Association between diaphragm use and urinary tract infection. *JAMA* 253:240–45.

Forsberg, J. 1996. A morphologist's approach to the vagina. *Acta Obstet. Gynecol. Scand. Suppl.* 163:3–10.

Fujii, T., Naito, H., Kioka, H., et al. 1995. Effect of intravaginal administration of cisplatin (CDDP) suppositories to uterine cervical cancer—blood and tissue concentrations and the therapeutic effects. *Jpn. J. Cancer Chemother.* 22:99–103.

Gibaldi, M., Perrier, D. 2007. *Multicompartment Models in Pharmacokinetics*, 2nd ed. London: Informa Healthcare, 45–112.

Graham, N.B., McNeill, M.E. 1984. Hydrogels for controlled drug delivery. *Biomaterials* 5:27–36.

Gravett, M.G., Hummel, D., Eschenbach, Holmes, K.K. 1986a. Preterm labor associated with subclinical amniotic fluid infection and with bacterial vaginosis. *Obstet. Gynecol.* 67:229–37.

Gravett, M.G., Nelson, H., DeRouen, T. 1986b. Independent association of bacterial vaginosis and chlamydia trachomatis infection with adverse pregnancy outcome. *JAMA* 256:1899–903.

Hafez, E.S.E. 1975. In *Scanning Electron Microscopy Atlas of Mammalian Reproduction*. New York: Springer-Verlag.

Halket, J.M., Leidenberger, F., Einer-Jensen, N., Bendz, A. 1985. Determination of infused (13C)progesterone in ovarian arterial blood by selected ion monitoring. *Biomed. Mass Spectrom.* 12:429–31.

Heimer, G.M. 1987. Estriol in the postmenopause. *Acta Obstet. Gynecol. Scand. Suppl.* 139:5–23.

Heimer, G.M., Englund, D.E. 1984. Estriol absorption after long-term vaginal treatment and gastrointestinal absorption as influenced by a meal. *Acta Obstet. Gynecol. Scand.* 63:563–67.

Herbst, A.L., Daniel, R.M., Stenchever, M.A., Droegemueller, W., eds. *Comprehensive Gynecology*, 2nd ed. St. Louis, MO: Mosby, 43–77.

Hill, G.B. 1993. The microbiology of bacterial vaginosis. *Am. J. Obstet. Gynecol.* 169:450–54.

Hill, G.B., Eschenbach, D.A., Holmes, K.K. 1985. Bacteriology of the vagina. *J. Urol. Nephrol. Suppl.* 86:23–39.

Hill, G., Livengood, C.H. 1994. Bacterial vaginisos-associated microflora and effects of topical intravaginal clindamycin. *Am. J. Obstet. Gynecol.* 171:1198–204.

Hillier, S., Krohn, M., Watts, H., Wolner-Hanssen, P., Eschenbach, D. 1990. Microbiologic efficacy of intravaginal clindamycin cream for the treatment of bacterial vaginosis. *Obstet. Gynecol.* 76:407–13.

Hillier, S.L., Lipinski, C., Briselden, A., Eschenbach, D.A. 1993. Efficacy of intravaginal 0.75% metronidazole gel for the treatment of bacterial vaginosis. *Obstet. Gynecol.* 81:963–67.

Hillier, S.L., Martius, J., Krohn, M. 1988. A case-control study of chorioamniotic infection and histologic chorioamnionitis in prematurity. *N. Engl. J. Med.* 319:972–78.

Ho, N.F., Higuchi, W.I., Turi, J. 1972. Theoretical model studies of drug absorption and transport in the GI tract. 3. *J. Pharm. Sci.* 61:192–97.

Ho, N.F., Suhardja, L., Hwang, S., et al. 1976. Systems approach to vaginal delivery of drugs III: simulation studies interfacing steroid release from silicone matrix and vaginal absorption in rabbits. *J. Pharm. Sci.* 65:1578–85.

Houkkamaa, M., Stranden, P., Jousimies-Somer, H., Siitonen, A. 1986. Bacterial flora of the cervix in women using different contraceptive methods. *Am. J. Obstet. Gynecol.* 154:520–24.

Hsu, C.C., Park, J.Y., Ho, N.F., Higucho, W.I., Fox, J.L. 1983. Topical vaginal drug delivery I. Effect of estrous cycle on vaginal membrane permeability and diffusivity of vidarabine in mice. *J. Pharm. Sci.* 72:674–80.

Hwang, S., Owada, E., Suhardja, L. 1977a. Systems approach to vaginal delivery of drugs IV: methodology for determination of membrane surface pH. *J. Pharm. Sci.* 66:778–81.

Hwang, S., Owada, E., Suhardja, L. 1977b. Systems approach to vaginal delivery of drugs V: *in situ* absorption of 1-alkanoic acids. *J. Pharm. Sci.* 66:781–84.

Hwang, S., Owada, E., Yotsuyanagi, T., et al. 1976. Systems approach to vaginal delivery of drugs II: *in situ* vaginal absorption of unbranched aliphatic alcohols. *J. Pharm. Sci.* 65:1574–78.

Johnston, A. 1996. Estrogens-pharmacokinetics and pharmacodynamics with special reference to vaginal administration and the new estradiol formulation, Estring. *Acta Obstet. Gynecol. Scand. Suppl.* 163, 75:16–25.

Jollow, D.J., Brodie, B.B. 1972. Mechanisms of drug absorption and of drug solution. *Pharmacology* 8:21–32.

Kirwan, P. 1985. Topical 5-fluorouracil in the treatment of vaginal intraepithelial neoplasia. *Br. J. Obstet. Gynecol.* 92:287–91.

Krebs, H.B. 1986. Prophylactic topical 5-fluorouracil following treatment of human papillomavirus-associated lesions of the vulva and vagina. *Obstet. Gynecol.* 68:837–41.

Krebs, H.B. 1987. Treatment of vaginal condylomata acuminata by weekly topical application of 5-fluorouracil. *Obstet. Gynecol.* 70:68–71.

Krebs, H.B., Helmkamp, B.F. 1991. Chronic ulcerations following topical therapy with 5-fluorouracil for vaginal human papillomavirus-associated lesions. *Obstet. Gynecol.* 78:205–8.

Krieger, J.N., Tam, M.R., Stevens, C.R. 1988. Diagnosis of trichomoniasis. Comparison of confidential wet-mount preparations with cytologic studies, culture and monoclonal antibody staining of direct specimens. *JAMA* 259:1223–27.

Lamont, R.F., Taylor-Robinson, D., Newman, M., Wigglesworth, J., Elder, M.G. 1986. Spontaneous early preterm labour associated with abnormal genital bacterial colonization. *Br. J. Obstet. Gynecol.* 93:804–10.

Landgren, B., Aedo, A.R., Johannisson, E., Cekan, S.Z. 1994a. Pharmacokinetic and pharmacodynamic effects of vaginal rings releasing levonorgestrel at a rate of 27 micrograms/24 hours: a pilot study. *Contraception* 49:139–50.

Landgren, B., Aedo, A.R., Johannisson, E., Cekan, S.Z. 1994b. Studies on a vaginal ring releasing levonorgestrel at an initial rate of 27 micrograms/24 hours when used alone or in combination with a transdermal system releasing estradiol. *Contraception* 50:87–100.

Larsen, B. 1993. Vaginal flora in health and disease. *Clin. Obstet. Gynecol.* 36:107–22.

Larsen, B., Galask, R.P. 1980. Vaginal microbial flora: practical and theoretic relevance. *Obstet. Gynecol. Suppl.* 55:100s–13s.

Liggins, G.C. 1979. Controlled trial of induction of labor by vaginal suppositories containing prostaglandin E2. *Prostaglandins* 18:167–72.

Livengood, C., McCregor, J., Soper, D.E., et al. 1994. Bacterial vaginosis: efficacy and safety of intravaginal metronidazole. *Am. J. Obstet. Gynecol.* 170:759–64.
Livengood, C.H., Thomason, J., Hill, G. 1990. Bacterial vaginosis: treatment with topical intravaginal clindamycin phosphate. *Obstet. Gynecol.* 76:118–23.
Lossick, J.G., Muller, M., Gorrell, T.E. 1986. *In vitro* drug susceptibility and doses of metronidazole required for cure in cases of refractory vaginal trichomoniasis. *J. Infect. Dis.* 153:948–55.
Lundgren, O., Haglund, U. 1978. The pathophysiology of the intestinal countercurrent exchanger. *Life Sci.* 23:1411–22.
Lyons, J., Ito, J. 1995. Reducing the risk of chlamydia trachomatis genital tract infection by evaluating the prophylactic potential of vaginally applied chemicals. *Clin. Infect. Dis.* 21:s174–77.
Mackenzie, I.Z., Bradley, S., Embrey, M.P. 1981. A simpler approach to labor induction using lipid-based prostaglandin E2 vaginal suppository. *Am. J. Obstet. Gynecol.* 141:158–62.
McNeill, M.E., Graham, N.B. 1984. Vaginal pessaries from crystalline/rubbery hydrogels for the delivery of prostaglandin E2. *J. Controlled Release* 2:99–117.
Mardh, P.A. 1991. The vaginal ecosystem. *Am. J. Obstet. Gynecol.* 165:1163–68.
Martin, P.L., Yen, S.S.C., Burnier, A.M., Hermann, H. 1979. Systemic absorption and sustained effects of vaginal estrogen creams. *JAMA* 242:2699–700.
Meyskens, F.L., Graham, V., Chvapil, M. 1983. A phase I trial of beta-all-trans-retinoic acid for mild and moderate intraepithelial cervical neoplasia delivered via collagen sponge and cervical cap. *J. Natl. Cancer Inst.* 71:921–25.
Meyskens, F.L., Surwit, T., Moon, T., et al. 1994. Enhancement of regression of cervical intraepithelial neoplasia II (moderate dysplasia) with topically applied all-trans-retinoic acid: a randomized trial. *J. Natl. Cancer Inst.* 86:539–43.
Miles, R.A., Paulson, R.J., Lobo, R.A., et al. 1994. Pharmacokinetic and endometrial tissue levels of progesterone after administration by intramuscular and vaginal routes: a comparative study. *Fertil. Steril.* 62:485–90.
Mishell, D., Talas, M., Parlow, A. 1970. Contraception by means of a silastic vaginal ring impregnated with medroxyprogesterone acetate. *Am. J. Obstet. Gynecol.* 107:100–7.
Mizutani, T., Nishiyama, S., Amakawa, I., et al. 1995. Concentrations in ovary, uterus, and serum and their effect on the hypothalamic-pituitary-ovarian axis during vaginal administration of a danazol suppository. *Fertil. Steril.* 63:1184–89.
Mulders, T.M.T., et al. 2002. Ovarian function with a novel combined contraceptive vaginal ring. *Hum. Reprod.* 17:94–99.
Murphy, J.F., Krantz, K. 1994. Anatomic aspects of female pelvic infections. In *Obstetric and Gynecologic Infectious Disease*, ed. Pastorek, J.G., 27–36. New York: Raven Press.
Nachtigall, L.E. 1995. Clinical trial of the estradiol ring in the U.S. *Maturitas* 22:S43–47.
Nahoul, K., Dehennin, L., Jondet, M., Roger, M. 1993. Profiles of plasma estrogens, progesterone and their metabolites after oral or vaginal administration of estradiol or progesterone. *Maturitas* 16:185–202.
Nakayama, K., Shimizu, Y., Hasumi, K., Masubuchi, K. 1990. Intravaginal administration of CDDP in cervical cancer. *J. Jpn. Soc. Cancer Ther.* 25:826–29.
Nichols, D.H., Randall, C.L. 1996. Pelvic anatomy of the living. In *Vaginal Surgery*, 4th ed., 1–42. London: Williams & Wilkins.

Norchi, S., Zanini, A., Ragusa, A., Maccario, L., Valle, A. 1993. Induction of labor with intravaginal prostaglandin E2 gel. *Int. J. Gynecol. Obstet.* 42:103–7.

Pauwels, R., De Clercq, E. 1996. Development of vaginal microbicides for the prevention of heterosexual transmission of HIV. *J. Acquir. Immune Defic. Syndr. Hum. Retrovirol.* 11:211–21.

Pendergrass, P., Reeves, C., Belovicz, M., Molter, D., White, J. 1996. The shape and dimensions of the human vagina in three dimensional vinyl polysiloxane casts. *Gynecol. Obstet. Invest.* 42:178–82.

Piver, M.S., Barlow, J.J., Tsukada, S., Gamarra, M., Sandecki, A. 1979. Postirradiation squamous cell carcinoma *in situ* of the vagina: treatment of topical 20% 5-fluorouracil cream. *Am. J. Obstet. Gynecol.* 135:377–80.

Rigg, L.A., Hermann, H., Yen, S.S.C. 1978. Absorption of estrogens from vaginal creams. *N. Engl. J. Med.* 298:195–97.

Saxena, B.B., et al. 2004. Efficacy of nonhormonal vaginal contraceptives from a hydrogel delivery system. *Contraception* 70:13–19.

Schmidt, G., Anderson, S.B., Nordle, O., Johansson, C., Gunnarsson, P.O. 1994. Release of 17-beta-oestradiol from a vaginal ring in postmenopausal women: pharmacokinetic evaluation. *Gynecol. Obstet. Invest.* 38:253–60.

Schmitt, C., Pa., C., Sobel, J., Curtiz, M. 1992. Bacterial vaginosis: treatment with clindamycin cream versus oral metronidazole. *Obstet. Gynecol.* 79:1020–23.

Schneider, A., Grubert, T., Kirchmayr, R. 1995. Efficacy trial of topically administered interferon gamma-1 beta gel in comparison to laser treatment in cervical intraepithelial neoplasia. *Arch. Gynecol. Obstet.* 256:75–83.

Schuchner, E.B., Foix, A., Borenstein, C.A., Marchese, C. 1974. Electron microscopy of human vaginal epithelium under normal and experimental conditions. *J. Reprod. Fertil.* 36:231–38.

Shepherd, J., Pearce, J.M., Sims, C.D. 1979. Induction of labour using prostaglandin E 2 pessaries. *Br. Med. J.* 2:108–10.

Simon, J.A. 1995. Micronized progesterone: vaginal and oral uses. *Clin. Obstet. Gynecol.* 38:902–14.

Singer, Z., Beck, M., Jusic, D., Soos, E. 1990. The effect of vaginal administration of interferons on squamous intraepithelial cervical lesions. *Jugosl. Ginekol. Perinatol.* 30:27–29.

Smith, C.V., Miller, A., Livezey, G. 1996. Double-blind comparison of 2.5 and 5.0 mg of prostaglandin E2 gel for preinduction cervical ripening. *J. Reprod. Med.* 41:745–48.

Smith, C.V., Rayburn, W.F., Miller, A.M. 1994. Intravaginal prostaglandin E2 for cervical ripening and initiation of labor. *J. Reprod. Med.* 39:381–86.

Smith, P., Heimer, G., Lindskog, M., Ulmsten, U. 1993. Oestradiol-releasing vaginal ring for treatment of postmenopausal urogenital atrophy. *Maturitas* 16:145–54.

Smout, D.F.V., Jacoby, F., Lillie, E.W. 1969. In *Gynecological and Obstetrical Anatomy*. Baltimore: Williams & Wilkins.

Spence, M.R., Hollander, D.H., Smith, J. 1980. The clinical and laboratory diagnosis of *Trichomonas vaginalis* infection. *Sex. Transm. Dis.* 7:168–71.

Steger, R.W., Hafez, E.S.E. 1978. Aging changes in the vagina. In *The Human Vagina*, eds. Hafez, E.S.E., Evans, E.T. Amsterdam, the Netherlands: Elsevier.

Stehle, R.G., Higuchi, W.I. 1967. Diffusional model for transport rate studies across membranes. *J. Pharm. Sci.* 56:1367–68.

Stumpf, P.G. 1986. Selectin constant serum estradiol levels achieved by vaginal rings. *Obstet. Gynecol.* 67:91–94.

Stumpf, P.G., Maruca, J., Santen, R.J., Demers, L.M. 1982. Development of a vaginal ring for achieving physiologic levels of 17-estradiol in hypoestrogenic women. *J. Clin. Endocrinol. Metab.* 54:208–10.

Suzuki, A., Higuchi, W.I., Ho, N.F. 1970. Theoretical model studies of drug absorption and transport in the gastrointestinal tract, I. *J. Pharm. Sci.* 59:644–51.

Sweet, R.L. 1995. Clinical microbiology of the female genital tract. In *Infectious Diseases of the Female Genital Tract*, 3rd ed., eds. Sweet, R.L., Gibbs, R.S., 3–15. Baltimore: Williams & Wilkins.

Taylor, A.V.G., Boland, J., Mackenzie, I.Z. 1990. The concurrent *in vitro* and *in vivo* release of PGE2 from a controlled-release hydrogel polymer pessary for cervical ripening. *Prostaglandins* 40:89–98.

Vaughan, D.P., Trainor, A. 1975. Derivation of general equations for linear mammillary models when the drug is administered by different routes. *J. Pharmacokinet. Biopharm.* 3(3):203–18.

Villa, L., et al. 2006. High sustained efficacy of a prophylactic quadrivalent human papillomavirus types 6/11/16/18 L1 virus-like particle vaccine through 5 years of follow-up. *Br. J. Cancer* 95:1459–66.

von Peham, H., Americh, J. 1934. *Operative Gynecology*. Philadelphia: Lippincott.

Wang, K. 2007. Human papillomavirus and vaccination in cervical cancer. *Taiwan J. Obstet. Gynecol.* 46:4 352–62.

Weber, A., Walter, M., Schover, L., Mitchinson, A. 1995. Vaginal anatomy and sexual function. *Obstet. Gynecol.* 86:946–49.

Witkin, S.S. 1993. Immunology of the vagina. *Clin. Obstet. Gynecol.*36:122–28.

Woodruff, J.D., Parmley, T.H., Julian, C.G. 1975. Topical 5-fluorouracil in the treatment of vaginal carcinoma-in-situ. *Gynecol. Oncol.* 3:124–32.

World Health Organization. 1999. Sperm-cervical mucus interaction. In *WHO Laboratory Manual for the Examination of Human Semen and Sperm-Cervical Mucus Interaction*, 4th ed., 51–59. New York: Cambridge University Press.

Yotsuyanagi, T., Molokhia, A., Hwang, S., et al. 1975. Systems approach to vaginal delivery of drugs I: development of *in situ* vaginal drug absorption procedure. *J. Pharm. Sci.* 64:71–76.

9

Polymer-Based Scaffolds for Urinary Bladder Tissue Engineering

Srikanth Sivaraman and Jiro Nagatomi

CONTENTS

Introduction

Urinary Bladder

The urinary bladder is a hollow, distensible musculomembranous sac that lies in the pelvic cavity just posterior to the symphysis pubis (Gray and Howden 1916; Seeley, Stephens, and Tate 2000). It functions as a short-term reservoir for the urine produced by the kidneys. Under normal conditions, the human bladder has a capacity to store approximately 500 mL of urine, although a progressive sensation of fullness and a desire to void are experienced when the volume reaches around 300 mL. As it fills, the bladder expands up to 15 times its contracted size assuming an ovoid shape. During voluntary micturition, smooth muscle of the bladder contracts while sphincter muscles of the urethra relax to allow releasing of the content.

The bladder wall tissue is composed of four distinct layers: the urothelium, lamina propria, detrusor, and serosal (Figure 9.1). The mean bladder wall thickness measured from the urothelium to serosa in adult humans is approximately 3.3 ± 1.1 mm for males and 3.0 ± 1 mm for females (Hakenberg, Linne, Manseck, and Wirth 2000). The unique features of the bladder, the large capacity and high compliance, are due to the highly specialized properties of the urothelial lining and the smooth muscle wall of the bladder (Turner, Subramaniam, Thomas, and Southgate 2007).

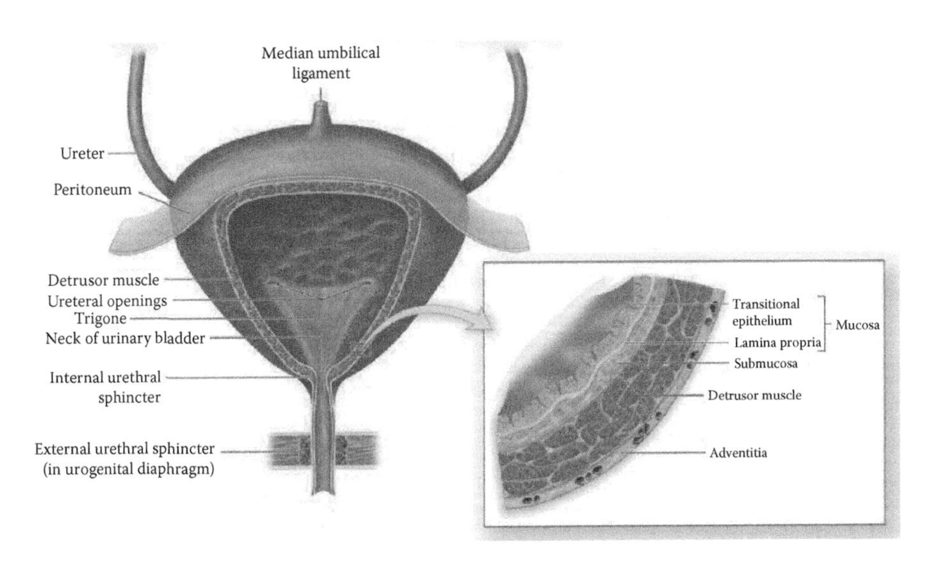

FIGURE 9.1
Tissue layers of the urinary bladder.

Urothelium

The urothelium is a specialized type of epithelium called transitional epithelium. The cells in the layer have the ability to slide past one another, and the number of cell layers decreases as the volume of the urinary bladder increases (Seeley, Stephens, and Tate 2000). The urothelium plays a major role in maintaining the composition of urine, akin to that generated by the kidneys. This is achieved via four unique features of the urothelium. First, the tissue offers a minimum surface area to urine for passive permeability of substances between blood and lumen. Second, the passive permeability of the tight junction between cells and apical cell membrane to electrolytes and nonelectrolytes is also very low. Third, the hormonally regulated absorptive system of the urothelium regulates sodium absorption to counter the passive movement of sodium from blood to urine. Last, all of these permeability properties of the urothelium are unaffected by most substances found in blood or urine; thus the composition of urine stays constant (Lewis 2000).

Lamina Propria

Lamina propria is a collagenous connective tissue (Turner, Subramaniam, Thomas, and Southgate 2007) that functions to maintain the shape of the bladder wall and to limit its overall compliance (ratio of maximum volume divided by pressure). This layer is approximately 1.3 mm thick in humans and supports various cell types, and the entire bundle of the capillary network is embedded in it (Turner, Subramaniam, Thomas, and Southgate 2007). The lamina propria is composed mainly of dense irregular connective tissue, fibroblasts, and a thin smooth muscle muscularis mucosa (Deveaud et al. 1998).

Detrusor and Serosal Layers

The detrusor muscle layer plays a major role in the voiding of urine by contraction (Korossis et al. 2006). Detrusor wall thickness in humans is approximately 1.4 mm for males and 1.2 mm for females (Oelke et al. 2006). This layer is mainly composed of coarse bundles of smooth muscle fibers (Koenig, Gonzalez, White, Lein, and Rajadhyaksha 1999; Shier, Butler, and Lewis 2007). The muscle fibers form branching, interlacing bundles loosely arranged into inner longitudinal, middle circular, and outer longitudinal layers (Brook 2007). However, in the upper aspect of the bladder, these layers are clearly not separable, and any one fiber can travel between each of the layers, change orientation, and branch into longitudinal and circular fibers. This meshwork of detrusor muscle is ideally suited for emptying the spherical bladder (Brook 2007). The individual smooth muscle fibers in these bundles run parallel to one another and are generally 1–2 μm in diameter. The muscle bundles have a diameter of 50–150 μm, and the interfascicular space between the bundles is usually between 20 and 50 μm. Within the interfascicular space, capillaries and larger blood vessels are observed (Koenig, Gonzalez, White, Lein, and Rajadhyaksha 1999).

The detrusor layer is surrounded by the serosal layer, which is a dense layer of fine collagen fibrils that are straight and uniform and are not interspersed with blood vessels (Turner, Subramaniam, Thomas, and Southgate 2007; Koenig, Gonzalez, White, Lein, and Rajadhyaksha 1999).

Pathological Conditions of the Urinary Bladder Requiring Repair and Reconstruction

Approximately 400 million people worldwide are affected by various diseases of the urinary bladder that require repair and reconstruction (Adelöw and Frey 2007). This figure includes, but is not limited to, congenital malformations of the lower urinary tract such as bladder exstrophy (part of the bladder is present outside the body and the pelvic bones are separated), myelomeningocele (spine does not close before birth), or posterior urethral valves (obstructing membrane in the posterior male urethra) (Atala, Bauer, Soker, Yoo, and Retik 2006). In addition, postnatally acquired diseases such as chronic interstitial cystitis (characterized by frequent and painful urination or pain in the bladder and pelvic region); neurogenic bladder (characterized by difficulty in storing or voiding urine); bladder fibrosis; and cancer (among the 10 most common cancers) cause a critical need for surgical replacement and repair (Adelöw and Frey 2007).

Current treatments of congenital malfunctions and bladder fibrosis involve surgical augmentation of the bladder, which often requires a second surgery to reconstruct surrounding bones and soft tissues (Brook 2007; Elder 2007; Gearhart and Mathews 2007; Kinsman and Johnston 2007; Warren, Pike, and Leonard 2004). In contrast, neurogenic bladders may be initially treated with medicines to activate or relax the bladders or through exercise to strengthen the pelvic muscles (Wein 2007; Shamliyan, Kane, Wyman, and Wilt 2008; Holroyd-Leduc, Tannenbaum, and Thorpe 2008). However, if the problem becomes severe neurogenic bladders are emptied by intermittent or permanent catheterization, and surgical approaches such as artificial sphincter, sling surgery, or electrical stimulation of the sacral nerve may be adopted (Wein 2007; Shamliyan, Kane, Wyman, and Wilt 2008; Holroyd-Leduc, Tannenbaum, and Thorpe 2008). Similarly, interstitial cystitis is treated mainly via medication, and surgical interventions (e.g., supratrigonal cystectomy and cystourethrectomy) are reserved as a last resort (Hanno 2007). Bladder cancer, on the other hand, is routinely treated surgically with a variety of techniques, such as partial or radical cystectomy in combination with radiation therapy, chemotherapy, or immunotherapy depending on the patient and the stage of the disease (Thrasher and Crawford 1993; Housset et al. 1993; Kachnic et al. 1997; Raghavan and Huben 1995).

While a number of urological complications are surgically treated, conventional modes of treatment for bladder repair suffer from several limitations.

Common risks for treatment of urinary bladder disorders are urinary tract infections (UTIs) and incontinence (Elder 2007; Gearhart and Mathews 2007; Kinsman and Johnston 2007; Warren, Pike, and Leonard 2004; Wein 2007; Shamliyan, Kane, Wyman, and Wilt 2008; Holroyd-Leduc, Tannenbaum, and Thorpe 2008; Hanno 2007). Apart from that, many treatment methods suffer from specific risks: sexual dysfunction in the case of surgery for exstrophy (Elder 2007; Gearhart and Mathews 2007); meningitis, hydrocephalus, and loss of bladder control in the case of surgery for myelomeningocele (Kinsman and Johnston 2007); renal failure and vesicoureteral reflex in the case of posterior urethral valve treatment (Warren, Pike, and Leonard 2004); and chronic urine leakage and kidney damage in the case of neurogenic bladders (Wein 2007; Shamliyan, Kane, Wyman, and Wilt 2008; Holroyd-Leduc, Tannenbaum, and Thorpe 2008). Treatment for bladder cancer also can lead to the risk of anemia, swelling of the ureters, and urethral strictures (Thrasher and Crawford 1993; Housset et al. 1993; Kachnic et al. 1997; Raghavan and Huben 1995; Thomas 1997).

Current Approaches in Bladder Repair

Currently, materials used in surgical repair to treat various complications of the urinary bladder include autografts, allografts, and xenografts, which have exhibited varying successes and problems as reviewed in the following sections.

Use of Autologous Tissues in Cystoplasty

Cystoplasty is one of the most common approaches to treat patients who lack adequate bladder capacity or detrusor compliance. Abnormal compliance or decreased bladder capacity may manifest as debilitating urgency, frequency, incontinence, recurrent UTIs, pyelonephritis, or progressive renal insufficiency. For many patients, augmentation cystoplasty can provide a safe functional reservoir that allows for urinary continence and prevention of upper tract deterioration (Rao, Iverson, Cespedes, and Sabanegh 2008). These problematic bladders have been conventionally treated using segments of autologous natural tissue, such as omentum, peritoneum, ureters, and most commonly a portion of the large intestine (enterocystoplasty) (Chun, Lim, Webster, and Haberstroh 2011). The procedure aims to improve bladder capacity in severely contracted bladders with compliant and vascularized tissues (Turner, Subramaniam, Thomas, and Southgate 2007). However, enterocystoplasty has been known to generate various long-term complications, including mucus production by the bowel epithelium, stone formation, bacteriuria, metabolic disturbances, malignancy, and intestinal complications (Turner, Subramaniam, Thomas, and Southgate 2007; Thomas 1997). These complications of enterocystoplasty may result from the fact that the intestinal epithelium is neither structurally nor physiologically adapted to prolonged exposure to urine (Cross, Thomas, and Southgate 2003).

Since the side effects of enterocystoplasty were considered due to the interaction of urine with the bowel mucosa, numerous animal model studies have been performed to expose the raw muscle surface to urine after the removal of the bowel epithelium and examine the effects of deepithelialization (Turner, Subramaniam, Thomas, and Southgate 2007). However, contrary to expectations, the results of these studies provided evidence of graft shrinkage and fibrosis, severe inflammation, infection, and ischemia (Lima, Araujo, Vilar, Kummer, and Lima 2004), all of which underscored the importance of epithelial tissue. Although complete elimination of these problems was not achieved, two major studies using a porcine model have demonstrated so far that fibrosis and shrinkage of the implanted grafts were minimized by covering the augmenting graft with autologous human urothelium (Hafez et al. 2005; Frazer et al. 2004).

The first study used autologous urothelial cells isolated at hemicystectomy and sprayed onto demucosalized colon, which was then incorporated into the remaining bladder. After 6 weeks, the presence of uroplakin-positive urothelium was observed on top of a bladder or colonic smooth muscle submucosa, and no inflammation was described (Hafez et al. 2005). In another study, *in vitro*-propagated autologous urothelial cells were implanted onto a vascularized, deepithelialized uterine tissue used as the augmenting segment in a "composite cystoplasty" (Frazer et al. 2004). However, there was evidence of stromal inflammation within both augmented and native segments along with incomplete urothelialization, leading to poor urinary barrier properties. Based on these findings, the authors hypothesized that implanting "differentiated" urothelium would lead to rapid establishment of an effective urinary barrier and would provide the stroma with immediate protection from urine-mediated damage (Frazer et al. 2004). However, enterocystoplasty as a technique still suffers from problems such as substantial graft shrinkage; thus alternatives are being sought to replace this technique.

Another approach to bladder repair using the patient's own tissue is ureterocystoplasty, which exploits the use of urothelium derived either from a grossly dilated ureter or from the bladder itself after excising the overlying detrusor muscle (Dewan and Anderson 2008). While it is a clinically proven concept and the use of autologous urothelial tissues can eliminate many, if not all, of the complications associated with enterocystoplasty, this approach is confined to a small minority of patients with gross ureteric dilation. Moreover, studies have demonstrated that it is not suited for small or trabeculated bladders, which are commonly encountered in neuropathic dysfunction (Dewan and Anderson 2008; Cross, Thomas, and Southgate 2003). These shortcomings of the currently available techniques of cystoplasty have led clinicians and researchers to turn to alternative biomaterials (e.g., free tissue grafts and decellularized matrices) for bladder repair.

Free Tissue Graft

A free tissue graft is a section of tissue detached from its blood supply, moved to another part of the body, and reattached by microsurgery to a new blood supply (*Gale Encyclopedia of Medicine* 2008). This is unlike cystoplasty, which retains the blood supply during transfer to the site of repair. A number of attempts have been made to incorporate various types of free human tissues, including muscle flaps, split skin grafts, placenta, peritoneum, and dural membrane, into the bladder in the form of patches (Turner, Subramaniam, Thomas, and Southgate 2007). The results to date have been mixed, ranging from graft contraction and stone formation to hair growth on grafts derived from skin (Turner, Subramaniam, and Thomas 2007).

Muscle Flap as Bladder Wall Substitute

An animal model study compared rectus abdominis and musculoperitoneal (rectus abdominis with overlying peritoneum) flaps used as urinary bladder wall substitutes in rats (Schwenke-konig, Hage, and Kon 2004). The quality of urothelium and smooth muscle layer regenerated with the detrusor myectomy (incorporation of skeletal muscle) was similar in both groups at the end of 6 and 90 days, indicating that the rectus abdominis muscle alone sufficed as a matrix for the bladder wall. Although both cases presented urolithiasis, this was attributed to the nonabsorbable sutures used in the surgery and to the rat model, which is prone to stone formation.

The efficacy of detrusor myectomy was also demonstrated by another study using a canine model of hematuria and stranguria, which revealed that when the rectus abdominis muscle flap was surgically sutured to the defective bladder, the dog maintained normal health and showed no signs of urinary incontinence even after a period of 2.5 years (Savicky and Jackson 2009). Neither caliculi nor stricture or scarring was visible in the abdominal radiographs (Savicky and Jackson 2009). Although the study was based on only one specimen, the study showed promise, and further research to confirm these findings would aid in the use of rectus abdominis muscle flap for bladder repair purposes.

Human Amniotic Membrane

The human amniotic membrane (hAM) is an avascular tissue that forms the inner layer of fetal membranes (Iijima et al. 2007). Since the hAM is normally disposed after parturition, it can be readily available for research use with few ethical concerns. To determine the efficacy, bladder augmentation in rats using hAM was performed, and the results were compared 3 and 6 months postoperatively (Iijima et al. 2007). Rats that received partial cystectomy with primary closure without an implant served as the control. The authors reported that the hAM-reconstructed bladder wall displayed all three major (mucosal, muscular, and serosal) layers of the bladder wall as well as nerve fibers, although nerve and smooth muscle bundles were sparser and smaller compared to control groups. In addition, very few inflammatory cells were observed after 3 months, suggesting the absence of rejection. While no obvious graft shrinkage was observed, bladder calculi were found in 8 of the 18 rats (44%) in the hAM group at 6 months (Iijima et al. 2007). When tested *in vitro*, regenerated bladder strips exhibited noticeable contractile responses to a muscarinic receptor agonist and to electrical field stimulation. The contractile responses by hAM bladder strips were, however, very low compared to those of the control bladder strips even after 6 months, indicating immature tissue development. Although hAM exhibits a number of positive features, the use of hAM as a bladder tissue substitute is limited since it cannot be mass produced or obtained in an off-the-shelf manner for all cases.

Decellularized Matrices

Small Intestinal Submucosa

Decellularized xenogeneic or allogeneic matrices prepared from the submucosa of small intestine and bladders have been tested in the surgical treatment of the urinary bladder and other tissues (Cross, Thomas, and Southgate 2003). Small intestinal submucosa (SIS; Figure 9.2) is a collagenous membrane derived from porcine small intestines that was first described by Badylak and coworkers (Badylak, Lantz, Coffey, and Geddes 1989). The

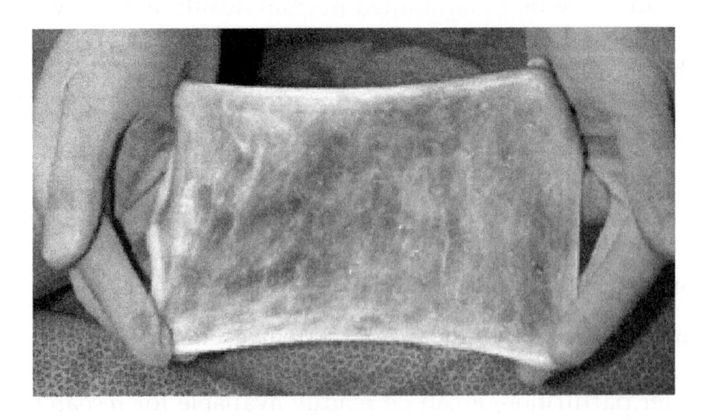

FIGURE 9.2
A sheet of small intestinal submucosal scaffold.

tunica mucosa, serosa, and tunica muscularis are mechanically removed from the inner and outer surfaces of the intestinal wall to leave a 0.1-mm collagen-rich membrane largely composed of the submucosal layer (Zhang et al. 2000). The early studies demonstrated that, when incorporated in the urinary bladder of rats, SIS allowed not only rapid cellular encroachment and infiltration but also vascularization and reinnervation (Vaught et al. 1996). SIS degrades completely in the body within a period of 4 to 8 weeks, and its by-products are excreted via the urine (Badylak, Kropp, McPherson, Liang, and Snyder 1998). Although the bladder-repairing approach using SIS allowed postsurgical regeneration of tissue that exhibited all three layers of the normal bladder (Badylak, Kropp, McPherson, Liang, and Snyder 1998), several unwanted outcomes were noted. For example, when implanted in dogs the regenerated bladders often exhibited a higher collagen-to-muscle ratio than normal bladders, and long-term clinical implications have not been fully understood (Badylak, Kropp, McPherson, Liang, and Snyder 1998). These SIS-based bladder grafts have also shown fibrosis and reduced smooth muscle contraction (Cross, Thomas, and Southgate 2003).

The regenerative potential of SIS was dependent on the age of the donor and the portion of the intestine from which the SIS matrices were derived (Turner, Subramaniam, Thomas, and Southgate 2007). An animal study provided evidence that SIS derived from pigs older than 3 years exhibited consistent bladder regenerative results compared to SIS derived from younger pigs (Kropp, Cheng, Lin, and Zhang 2004). In addition, the same study revealed that bladder regeneration is more reproducible with SIS from distal segments than from proximal segments of the ileum (Kropp, Cheng, Lin, and Zhang 2004).

While these studies have provided valuable information and demonstrated the feasibility of decellularized matrices as a bladder repair material, these limitations have prevented SIS from being considered an ideal implant to aid in effective bladder regeneration and remodeling.

Bladder Acellular Matrix

A bladder acellular matrix (BAM) graft is another type of decellularized tissue matrix that has been shown to support regeneration of the bladder *in vivo*. Following partial cystectomy and after 22 weeks of implantation, the BAM-augmented bladder exhibited urothelial and muscle layers with reinnervation and revascularization in porcine models (Brown et al. 2002). Histological analysis of excised BAM revealed that five major components of the extracellular matrix (ECM) (type I and type IV collagen, elastin, laminin, and fibronectin) were present in the matrix (Farhat et al. 2008; Brown et al. 2002), and similar results were seen in canine and murine models (Turner, Subramaniam, Thomas, and Southgate 2007).

Although many of the results have been positive, it has been reported that BAM also exhibited problems seen with SIS, namely lithogenesis, graft shrinkage, and incomplete and disorganized smooth muscle infiltration (Turner, Subramaniam, Thomas, and Southgate 2007). Moreover, despite the stringent decellularization process (with a series of hypotonic buffer solutions and various detergents), remnants of cellular components have been identified within BAM (Roth and Kropp 2009), which may lead to an immunogenic reaction when implanted into the body. Thus further improvement in processing and pretreatment may be necessary for BAM to be used successfully in bladder tissue regeneration.

Current Research in Bladder Tissue Engineering

Because of the various complications associated with auto-, allo-, and xenografts, alternative approaches are being sought in the direction of tissue engineering. This involves seeding appropriate autologous cells onto scaffolds to form live, implantable tissue constructs. The biomaterials used for scaffolds may be either synthetic polymers or naturally occurring materials. While synthetic polymer allows for controlling various parameters, such as mechanical properties and pore architecture, natural biomaterials have many inherent advantages, which include the presence of native growth factors, a naturally occurring architecture, and the presence of ubiquitous extracellular elements (Roth and Kropp 2009). The following sections review the current research in the field of bladder tissue engineering.

Clinical Success of Bladder Tissue Engineering

Since the advent of the term and concepts of tissue engineering in the early 1990s, the bladder has been one of the few organs synthesized *in vitro* and successfully implanted. Atala and colleagues were the first group to report such seminal work on tissue-engineered neobladders in both dogs and humans (Atala, Bauer, Soker, Yoo, and Retik 2006; Oberpenning, Meng, Yoo, and Atala 1998). The biomaterial used for the scaffolds was polyglycolic acid (PGA) coated with poly-DL-lactide-co-glycolide 50:50 (PLGA), and the implant was wrapped with the hosts' omentum (a fatty tissue layer under the peritoneum) in both cases (Atala, Bauer, Soker, Yoo, and Retik 2006; Oberpenning, Meng, Yoo, and Atala 1998). Briefly, after a trigone-sparing cystectomy, one group of beagle dogs underwent closure without a reconstructive procedure, the second group underwent reconstruction with cell-free scaffolds, and the third group received scaffolds seeded with autologous urothelial cells on the luminal surface and smooth muscle cells (SMCs) on the exterior surface. The results of this animal study clearly showed structural and functional differences among the three experimental groups 11 weeks postsurgery (Oberpenning, Meng, Yoo, and Atala 1998). The animals that received no implant gained a minimal increase, while the nonseeded bladders exhibited a slight increase in reservoir volume over time. Although these nonseeded scaffolds developed an intact urothelial layer, the smooth muscle layer was deficient and fibrotic, resulting in low compliance (Oberpenning, Meng, Yoo, and Atala 1998). In contrast, the cell-seeded neobladders exhibited capacities and compliance greater than the precystectomy level (Oberpenning, Meng, Yoo, and Atala 1998). The retrieved tissues displayed normal cellular organization, consisting of a trilayer of urothelium, submucosa, and muscle with innervations (Oberpenning, Meng, Yoo, and Atala 1998).

The group then investigated tissue-engineered bladder augmentation in humans with end-stage bladder diseases who needed cystoplasty (Atala, Bauer, Soker, Yoo, and Retik 2006). The study involved seven patients suffering from myelomeningocele, aged 4–19 years, with high pressure or poorly compliant bladders. Urothelial and SMCs were obtained from a bladder biopsy from each patient and expanded in culture for 7 weeks prior to seeding. The neobladder recipients were categorized based on three types of constructs: a homogeneous decellularized bladder submucosa scaffold, a cell-seeded collagen matrix implant wrapped with omentum, and a collagen-PGA composite implant wrapped with omentum (Figure 9.3).

While all three types of bladders displayed low intravesical pressure (below 40 cm H_2O) and stable renal functions postoperatively, the collagen-PGA composite scaffolds wrapped with omentum exhibited the greatest bladder capacity and compliance (Atala, Bauer, Soker, Yoo, and Retik 2006). Moreover, immunohistochemical analyses of biopsy tissues revealed that SMCs and urothelial cells within the regenerated bladder constructs were phenotypically normal.

The results of this seminal study demonstrated that the abnormally high bladder pressure before the operation clearly improved 10 months after implantation of the neobladder composed of cell-seeded collagen-PGA

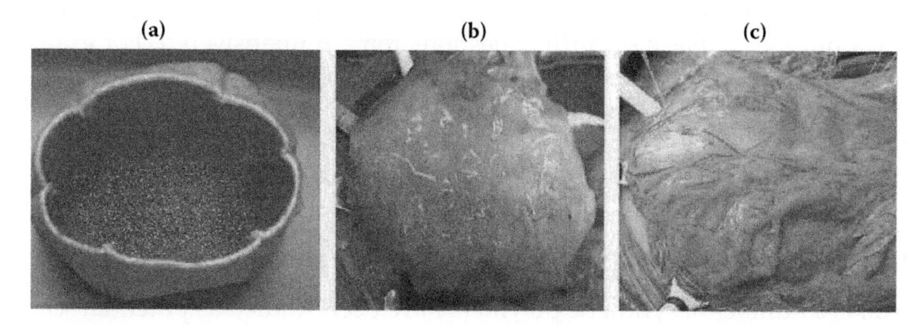

FIGURE 9.3 (see color insert)
Construction of engineered bladder: (a) scaffold seeded with cells; (b) engineered bladder anastomosed to native bladder with running 4-0 polyglycolic sutures; (c) implant covered with fibrin glue and omentum.

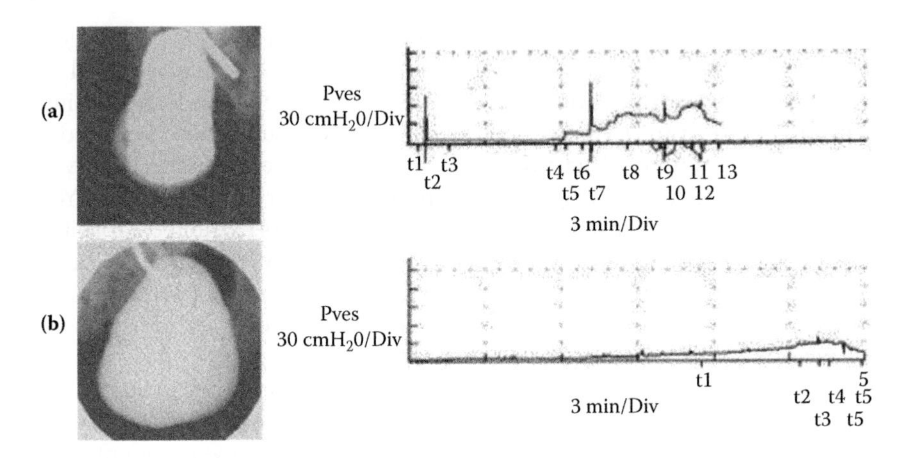

FIGURE 9.4
Cystograms and urodynamic findings in a patient with a collagen-PGA scaffold engineered bladder: (a) preoperative and (b) 10 months postoperative.

scaffold and the patient's omentum (Figure 9.4). Although these studies demonstrated the feasibility of bladder tissue engineering, several issues are still unresolved. For example, the success of bladder augmentation was limited and seemed to depend on the presence of omentum, which may or may not be available in all patients needing bladder replacement. Moreover, it is apparent from the report that the reinnervation of the organ was not entirely achieved, and muscle contraction necessary for voluntary voiding was absent.

In Vitro Cell Studies of Cell-Biomaterial Interactions

Although initial trials of bladder tissue engineering have met with some success, a number of basic scientific questions remain unanswered. For example, the choice and designs of scaffold materials are known to influence the behavior of seeded cells, which must be carefully examined and controlled prior to implantation of the engineered tissue constructs. The following sections review the current *in vitro* work on cell-biomaterial interactions.

Bladder Cell Interactions with Synthetic Polymers

To date, a number of synthetic polymers have been studied as potential scaffold materials for engineering of the urinary bladder. The advantages of these synthetic materials are that they can be manufactured rapidly in a large scale and can be processed to obtain desired levels of strength, microstructure, and degradation rate. In addition, some of the synthetic polymers (e.g.,

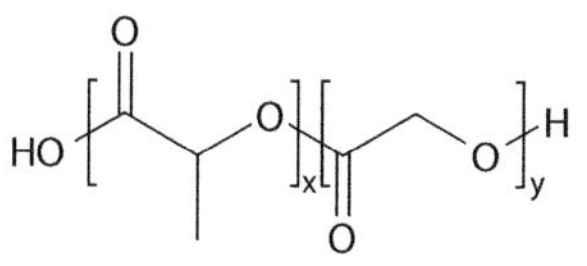

FIGURE 9.5
Basic structure of poly(lactic-co-glycolic acid) (PLGA). In this figure; 'X' represents the number of units of lactic acid and 'y' represents the number of units of glycolic acid.

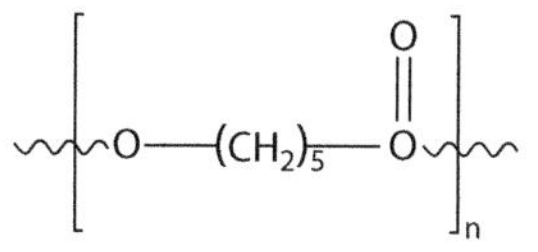

FIGURE 9.6
Basic structure of polycaprolactone (PCL).

polylactic acid [PLA], PGA, PLGA (Figure 9.5), and polycaprolactone [PCL]) (Figure 9.6) have been approved by the U.S. Food and Drug Administration (FDA) for use in medical devices and thus do not require additional regulatory compliance assessments prior to use in clinical applications.

Applicability of these polyesters to bladder tissue engineering was assessed by examining the influence of physical properties of PCL and PLGA films on the growth of normal human urothelial (NHU) cells and bladder SMCs *in vitro* (Rohman, Pettit, Isaure, Cameron, and Southgate 2007; Baker, Rohman, Southgate, and Cameron 2009). More specifically, two types (high and low elastic moduli) of PLGA and PCL films were compared with standard tissue culture plastic (control). The cell growth of both NHU cells and SMCs on the low-modulus PLGA films was greater than that on the high-modulus films at 24-, 48-, and 72-hour time points. A similar trend was observed for the SMC growth on PCL films; more cells were present on lower-modulus films at 72-hour and 7-day time points (Rohman, Pettit, Isaure, Cameron, and Southgate 2007). Together, these results demonstrated that the elastic modulus of the scaffold material is a critical parameter for the proliferative response by the seeded bladder cells.

The effect of mechanical properties of polyester scaffolds was further investigated in a three-dimensional (3D) environment by culturing human urinary tract stromal cells on PLGA and PCL foams prepared by emulsion freeze-drying (Baker, Rohman, Southgate, and Cameron 2009). The stromal cells on PCL scaffolds exhibited a 4.4-fold higher attachment and 2.4-fold higher rate of proliferation compared to the stromal cells cultured on PLGA scaffolds after a period of 7 days. Since the storage modulus of PCL (2 MPa) is half of that of PLGA and is closer to the storage moduli value for native bladder tissue (0.25 MPa) (Dahms, Piechota, Dahiya, Lue, and Tanagho 1998; Baker, Rohman, Southgate, and Cameron 2009), the authors concluded that cell attachment and proliferation were enhanced by the high-compliance nature of PCL (Baker, Rohman, Southgate, and Cameron 2009). Thus, based on the results from these two-dimensional (2D) and 3D studies, the PCL may be a better candidate material than PLGA in bladder tissue engineering applications, although a number of other parameters have yet to be examined.

Bladder Cell Interactions with SIS

To demonstrate the efficacy of SIS in use for bladder augmentation, Kropp and colleagues performed a series of studies using cell-seeded and non-seeded SIS (Kropp, Cheng, Lin, and Zhang 2004; Zhang et al. 2000; Zhang, Kropp, Ling, Cowan, and Cheng 2004). Specifically, SIS was evaluated *in vitro* after seeding it with human urothelial cells and SMCs (passages between 2 and 8) at a density of 1×10^5 cells/cm^2 in five different configurations (Zhang et al. 2000). The culture configurations that were evaluated were (a) urothelial cells seeded alone on the mucosal surface of SIS, (b) SMCs seeded alone on the mucosal surface, (c) layered coculture of SMCs seeded on the mucosal surface followed by urothelial cells 1 hour later, (d) sandwich coculture of SMCs seeded on the serosal surface followed by seeding of urothelial cells on the mucosal surface 24 hours later, and (e) mixed coculture of urothelial cells and SMCs seeded together on the mucosal surface. Four weeks after cell seeding, it was seen that layered and sandwich cocultures exhibited SMC invasion of SIS, organized cell sorting, and formation of well-defined urothelium, which were not seen with cultures of SMCs or urothelial cells alone (Zhang et al. 2000). The mixed coculture exhibited no evidence of cell sorting, although it exhibited smooth muscle penetration of the SIS matrix (Zhang et al. 2000). Their results suggest that establishment of cell-to-cell communications between identical cell types (i.e., SMC-SMC, urothelial-urothelial) seeded as separate layers may be a requisite for formation of distinct layers in neobladders engineered with SIS.

Application of Nanotechnology to Bladder Tissue Engineering

Among the limitations with use of synthetic materials in bladder tissue engineering are the mechanical property mismatch between the polymers and tissues as well as the lack of biological recognition of the polymer surface by the host cells. To address these issues, nanotechnology has been proposed as it has been shown to promote cell growth and tissue development through appropriate designing of the inner architecture of the scaffolds (Roth and Kropp 2009). For example, several groups (Thapa, Miller, Webster, and Haberstroh 2003; Pattison, Wurster, Webster, and Haberstroh 2005; Chun, Lim, Webster, and Haberstroh 2010) have studied nanostructured synthetic materials as bladder tissue replacements and demonstrated that increased surface roughness (at the nanometer and submicron levels) improved the adsorption of select proteins important for bladder cell functions. In theory, the surfaces of these nanomaterials offer a favorable environment for cell growth as they mimic the natural environment of the bladder. This is because it has been reported that the ECM proteins in bladder tissue are nanodimensional (Chun, Lim, Webster, and Haberstroh 2011).

This idea was tested in an *in vitro* study that examined human SMC function on PLGA, PCL, and polyurethane (PU) films with nanodimensional surface features in a range of 50–100 nm (created using chemical etching techniques via NaOH and HNO_3 soaking) (Thapa, Miller, Webster, and Haberstroh 2003). In comparison with the cells cultured on micron or submicron surfaces, bladder SMCs cultured on nanosurfaces exhibited greater elastin synthesis and collagen production, indicating that the difference in surface textures indeed influenced bladder cell behavior (Thapa, Miller, Webster, and Haberstroh 2003). This was further confirmed by a study using 3D nanotextured PLGA and PU scaffolds, which also demonstrated greater elastin and collagen production by bladder SMCs compared to conventional nanosmooth polymers (Pattison, Wurster, Webster, and Haberstroh 2005).

However, these results with bladder SMCs did not agree completely with other *in vitro* studies using rat PC12 adrenal medulla cells, which demonstrated that nanometer surface features alone did not influence cell proliferation unless serum proteins were present in the cell culture medium (Kleinman, Philp, and Hoffman 2003; Cooke et al. 2008). Taken together and applying this principle to bladder SMCs, it can be hypothesized that the adsorption of select soluble proteins to the substrate surface is essential for enhanced bladder SMC function (Chun, Lim, Webster, and Haberstroh 2010). To date, however, most of the studies using nanostructured materials have focused on *in vitro* assessment and not been subjected to *in vivo* testing for regeneration of bladder. Further study therefore is needed to evaluate the true efficacy of nanotechnology in bladder tissue engineering.

Effects of Mechanical Force Stimuli on Bladder Tissue Engineering

Since the urinary bladder is subjected to different mechanical forces during filling and emptying, it has been postulated that subjecting bladder cells and cell-seeded scaffolds to relevant mechanical forces *in vitro* may be beneficial for bladder tissue regeneration. For example, an *in vitro* study demonstrated penetration of rat bladder SMCs in SIS along with de novo synthesis of collagen and elastin by these seeded cells when the matrices were subjected to both chemical and mechanical stimuli for 2 weeks (Long-Heise, Ivanova, Parekh, and Sacks 2009). Briefly, the elastin synthesis by SMCs seeded on SIS was significantly greater when they were subjected to 15% cyclic stretch at a frequency of 0.1 Hz compared to the cells subjected to stretch at 0.5 Hz or maintained under static conditions. In addition, collagen synthesis, cell proliferation, and migration into SIS by SMCs were greater when exposed to cyclic stretch in the presence of vascular endothelial growth factor (VEGF) (10 ng/mL) compared to that in the absence of VEGF (Long-Heise, Ivanova, Parekh, and Sacks 2009). Although application of mechanical force and incorporation of growth factors enhanced the synthetic functions of SMCs, their effects on the contractile markers remain unknown.

This was addressed by another study that examined the effects of sustained tension on rat bladder SMCs in 3D collagen gel culture (Roby, Olsen, and Nagatomi 2008). More specifically, compared to the cells of no tension control, SMCs that were subjected to sustained tension inside the collagen gel exhibited significantly greater expression of α-smooth muscle actin and elongated cell morphology, both of which indicated enhanced contractile phenotype (Roby, Olsen, and Nagatomi 2008). Together, the results of these studies suggest that mechanical and chemical cues may be just as important as scaffold material selection for bladder tissue engineering.

In Vivo Animal Studies in Bladder Tissue Engineering

Application of SIS in Tissue Engineering

Motivated by the success of *in vitro* results, further studies were conducted to evaluate the performance of cell-seeded versus unseeded SIS *in vivo* (Zhang, Kropp, Ling, Cowan, and Cheng 2004). Human SMCs and urothelial cells were seeded on SIS in a layered coculture fashion and were implanted subcutaneously in nude mice (unseeded SIS was implanted as control). These grafts were then harvested at 4, 8, and 12 weeks after implantation. Evaluation of cell-seeded grafts at the 4-week time point indicated the presence of relatively fewer viable cells compared to the number of cells originally present at the time of implantation, indicating substantial cell death in the initial grafting process (Zhang, Kropp, Ling, Cowan, and Cheng 2004). However, the seeded SIS grafts exhibited progressively organized tissue regeneration at subsequent time points compared to unseeded SIS (Zhang, Kropp, Ling, Cowan, and Cheng 2004).

The feasibility of cell-seeded SIS for repairing bladder defects was further investigated in a canine model of subtotal cystectomy (90% partial cystectomy) with a control group that received no augmentation (Zhang, Frimberger, Cheng, Lin, and Kropp 2006). Unlike previous studies with smaller bladder defects, tissue regeneration was not achieved in this study, with no statistically significant difference in bladder capacity, function, or SMC regeneration among the three (seeded SIS, nonseeded SIS, and control) groups. This was mainly due to the inflammation and scarring of the remaining bladder from the cystectomy and the lack of neovascularization to the implanted grafts (Zhang, Frimberger, Cheng, Lin, and Kropp 2006). These results suggest that a cell-seeded SIS implant may be useful for repairing minor bladder defects, but methods to establish vascular networks into the implanted tissue rapidly would be an important requisite for improving its applicability to repairing larger bladder defects. The various advantages of SIS, including biocompatibility, degradability, and its ability to be used as an "off-the-shelf" bladder scaffold, make it an attractive option for bladder repair. However, there has not been an effective way to control graft shrinkage or encourage large-scale bladder regeneration. Overcoming these barriers would pave the way for SIS to be used as an effective scaffold for bladder tissue engineering.

Silk Fibroin Scaffold

Since 2000, silk fibroin has been investigated as potential scaffold material for diverse tissue engineering applications, such as bone, cartilage, ligament, and skin (Wang, Kim, Vunjak-Novakovic, and Kaplan 2006), mainly because of its exceptional combination of high tensile strength and elasticity (Lovett, Cannizzaro, Vunjak-Novakovic, and Kaplan 2008). Using a murine model of bladder augmentation, Mauney and coworkers investigated the utility of gel-spun silk fibroin scaffolds in bladder tissue engineering applications. After 70 days of implantation, the tubular shaped, non-cell-seeded, silk fibroin scaffolds showed regeneration of smooth muscle and urothelial layers along with evidence of substantial de novo ECM deposition with no signs of scaffold degradation. Cystometric analyses revealed that the voided urine volume and overall capacity of the augmented bladders were comparable with those of the nonsurgical control animals after 70 days. The augmented bladder, however, exhibited a mild, acute inflammatory reaction and high voiding frequency, which was presumably attributed to incomplete urothelial maturation (Mauney et al. 2011). Although silk fibroin has been known to elicit minimal inflammatory response due to its presence in the human body, the absence of scaffold degradation even after 70 days is a matter of concern. Further studies to characterize degradation of the scaffold would help in deciding the fate of the polymer in bladder tissue engineering studies.

Poly(lactic-co-glycolic acid)

Several *in vivo* studies have been performed to study the efficacy of cell-seeded PLGA scaffolds for bladder tissue engineering applications. For example, human adipose-derived stem cells (ASCs) were seeded on a PLGA scaffold designed to replicate the tissue architecture of the native bladder, and cell differentiation was examined *in vitro* and *in vivo* in a rat model (Jack et al. 2009). Specifically, the luminal surface of the construct was made from a thin layer of malleable and nonporous PLGA microfibers, which were tightly woven to keep the urine from permeating the graft yet strong enough to hold solid sutures without tearing. A thicker, 95% porous PLGA sponge was added to the outer surface of the composite to provide greater surface area for ASC seeding and to aid host cell penetration and vascularization when implanted in adult female Rnu athymic rats. Unseeded PLGA scaffolds and suture-closed scaffolds were prepared identically as controls. The authors reported that ASCs differentiated into SMCs within the cell-seeded bladder constructs after 12 weeks, which was evidenced by expression of molecular markers such as α-actin, calponin, caldesmon, and smooth muscle myosin heavy chain (MHC) (Jack et al. 2009). In addition, the ASC-seeded bladder constructs maintained viability *in vivo* and exhibited greater *ex vivo* contractility, compliance, and smooth muscle mass compared to the control bladder constructs after 12 weeks of implantation. However, the regenerated bladder in all the animals displayed signs of bladder calculi (Jack et al. 2009), which must be addressed and avoided in future studies. Moreover, the results that the acellular controls also formed a tissue structure similar to that of ASC-seeded constructs suggest that the contribution of ASCs to the regeneration of the bladder has to be carefully evaluated. These results are highly encouraging and demonstrated the potential of PLGA as an appropriate scaffold to support bladder regeneration and induce ASC differentiation into SMCs. However, further studies using larger animal models are necessary to demonstrate the true efficacy of the PLGA scaffolds in bladder tissue regeneration.

Hydrogel-Based Scaffolds

Hydrogels are a class of highly hydrated polymer materials (water content > 30% by weight) composed of hydrophilic polymer chains. Hydrogels that are used in biomedical applications such as tissue engineering can be either synthetic or natural in origin. The major advantages of using hydrogels are that they can be processed under relatively mild conditions (general absence of toxic chemicals in synthesis) and have structural and mechanical properties similar to the ECM (Drury and Mooney 2003). Hydrogel-based scaffolds have been studied for application for various organ systems, including the bladder.

Polyethylene Glycol

Polyethylene glycol (PEG) (Figure 9.7) is a synthetic hydrophilic polymer prepared by polymerization of ethylene oxide and is commercially available over a wide range of molecular weights, from 300 Da to 10,000 kDa (Drury and Mooney 2003; French, Thompson, and Davis 2009). Since PEG undergoes limited metabolism in the body, only PEGs with molecular weight less than 50 kDa are considered in tissue engineering applications as they can be completely eliminated from the body (via the liver and kidney) (Tessmar and Gopferich 2007).

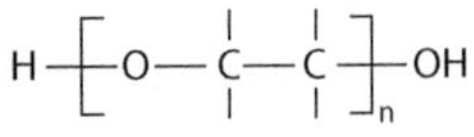

$$H{-}\left[O{-}C{-}C\right]_n{-}OH$$

FIGURE 9.7
Structure of polyethylene glycol (PEG).

PEGs have many advantageous characteristics essential for tissue engineering application. They are hydrolytically nondegradable polymers with excellent solubility in water and many other organic solvents. Melting points of the different PEG derivatives are dependent on the molecular weight of the chain, and this property can be exploited to manipulate the mechanical properties of polymers applied at room temperature. PEG can form highly hydrated polymer coils on the biomaterial surfaces, which can effectively be used to repel proteins. This property can be used to form inert polymer surfaces and nonfouling coatings to prevent bacterial growth or cellular adhesion on biomaterial surfaces. The terminal functional groups of PEG can be copolymerized with various polymers, and this property can also be used to manipulate its degradability (Tessmar and Gopferich 2007).

For bladder tissue engineering applications, the differentiation of human mesenchymal stem cells (MSCs) cultured on 3D PEG hydrogel scaffolds into SMC-like cells was examined by Adelöw and colleagues (Adelöw, Segura, Hubbell, and Frey 2008). More specifically, PEG hydrogel was modified with an adhesive peptide, arginine-glycine-aspartic acid (RGD) for stem cell attachment and matrix metalloproteinase- (MMP-) degradable peptides for enzymatic degradation of the matrix for cell infiltration. The human MSCs from bone marrow (300,000 cells per scaffold with 2.3 cm diameter) were seeded on the hydrogel scaffolds. Cell viability, spreading, and proliferation as well as key functional marker expression were assessed at various time points up to 21 days after hydrogel formation. The authors reported that after 2 weeks in culture both MSCs and SMCs within the 3D hydrogel exhibited the elongated, spindle-like morphology indicative of the contractile phenotype. The resulting cells in the 3D PEG hydrogels exhibited upregulation of markers associated with the less synthetic, but more contractile, phenotype of SMCs and increased cell proliferation compared to cells grown in 2D culture (Adelöw, Segura, Hubbell, and Frey 2008). These results demonstrated that strategic functional regulation of bladder SMCs can be achieved using PEG hydrogel, which may serve as an ideal scaffold to regenerate bladder tissue.

Collagen

Collagen (especially types I and IV) is one of the major components of the ECM and contains various cell adhesion domains important for maintaining native phenotype and activity of cells (Li 1995). It is readily purified from various animal tissue sources via enzyme treatment and salt/acid extraction; purified collagen products have been approved by the FDA for multiple medical applications (Engelhardt et al. 2010). Most collagen scaffolds used in bladder tissue engineering are in the form of hydrogels, and studies have shown cell compatibility, normal urothelium growth, and retention of the contractile phenotype of SMCs in collagen gels (Cen, Liu, and Cui 2008).

One of the major problems associated with collagen hydrogels, however, is its mechanical strength, which is not adequate for tissue wall reconstruction.

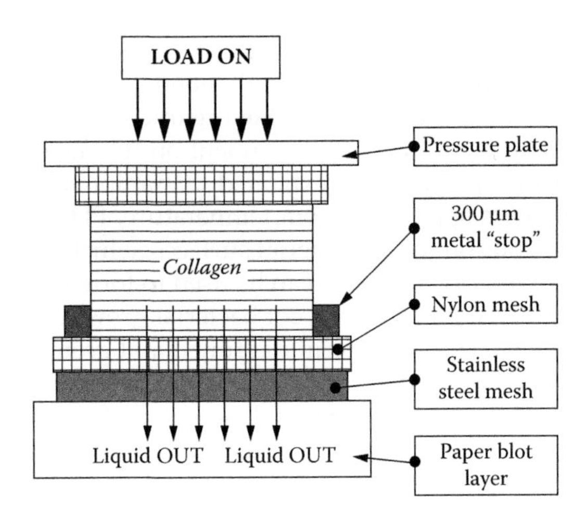

FIGURE 9.8
Routine assembly for plastic compression of preformed collagen gels.

For this reason, plastic compressed (PC) collagen gels have been proposed as a novel method to improve the mechanical properties of neotissues (Brown, Wiseman, Chuo, Cheema, and Nazhat 2005). PC collagen constructs were made by a simple and fast method and yielded controllable mesoscale structures. Briefly, collagen gel (preseeded with SMCs and urothelial cell [UC]) was sandwiched between two nylon meshes placed on top of a stainless steel mesh and filter paper and loaded with a 50-g flat plastic block for 5 minutes at room temperature (Figure 9.8).

The compression led to the expulsion of over 95% of the water contained within the gel and formation of a flat collagen sheet 20–40 μm thick with viable cells inside. Although PC collagen scaffolds supported cell growth for 2 weeks and exhibited greater tensile properties compared to uncompressed collagen gels, the gels were not strong enough to withstand suturing and handling in ultimate clinical use (Engelhardt et al. 2010).

It was thus necessary to improve on these limitations by combining PC collagen gels with biodegradable synthetic meshes composed of poly(lactic acid-co-ε-caprolactone) (PLAC) (Engelhardt et al. 2011). PLAC was chosen as it was a slow-degrading, elastic polymer and could provide the appropriate mechanical strength. The hybrid scaffolds were prepared by placing PLAC meshes between two layers of neutralized collagen gels, which were then subjected to plastic compression. The scaffolds were subjected to *in vitro* analysis to determine cell phenotype, distribution, and proliferation over a period of 14 days. Furthermore, the PC collagen-PLAC hybrid scaffolds were implanted subcutaneously in adult Swiss nude mice for up to 24 weeks to determine their biocompatibility. The results of the *in vitro* tests demonstrated that human SMCs and UCs embedded together in the hybrid scaffold proliferated well on the outer surface and interior of the scaffold by 14 days.

The specimens supported a maximum force of 33.62 ± 5.69 N before rupture. This force level corresponds to a pressure of 571 cm H_2O, indicating that the hybrid scaffold was strong enough to withstand internal bladder pressures (40–60 cm H_2O in adults during bladder contraction) (Engelhardt et al. 2011). The *in vivo* studies provided evidence of neutrophil and macrophage infiltration into the hybrid scaffold as early as 2 days after implantation, which subsided after 28 days, indicating a resolution of inflammation. However, a rise in the presence of immune cells such as macrophages and foreign body giant cells was noted in the PC collagen-PLAC hybrid scaffolds after 24 weeks of subcutaneous implantation. It was speculated that the degradation products of the PLAC mesh caused a rise in the inflammation reaction. The *in vivo* studies also indicated the near absence of SMC and UC activity in the hybrid scaffolds after 28 days (Engelhardt et al. 2011).

Although the *in vitro* results were highly promising, the hybrid scaffolds in the current form do not seem to support cell growth and are susceptible to inflammation *in vivo*. Addressing these long-term host response issues through strategic designing of polymer materials would certainly increase the utility of the hybrid scaffolds in bladder tissue engineering.

Conclusions

The urinary bladder is one of the few organs successfully engineered *in vitro* and implanted in humans (Atala, Bauer, Soker, Yoo, and Retik 2006). However, a number of functional criteria, such as innervation, vascularization, and retention of smooth muscle contractility, are still difficult to achieve. Both *in vitro* and *in vivo* studies using various natural, synthetic, and hybrid materials are being conducted to address these challenges and to optimize bladder regeneration. The limitations of the current tissue engineering protocols have been recognized, and further research is under way to better understand the nature of bladder tissue regeneration. Thanks to these advances, bladder tissue engineering is set to play a major role in alleviating and treating the various diseases of the bladder.

References

Adelöw C.A.M., Frey P. 2007. Synthetic hydrogel matrices for guided bladder tissue regeneration. *Methods in Molecular Medicine* 140:125–40.

Adelöw C., Segura T., Hubbell J.A., Frey P. 2008. The effect of enzymatically degradable poly(ethylene glycol) hydrogels on smooth muscle cell phenotype. *Biomaterials* 29:314–26.

Atala A., Bauer S.B., Soker S., Yoo J.J., Retik A.B. 2006. Tissue-engineered autologous bladders for patients needing cystoplasty. *The Lancet* 367:1241–46.

Badylak S., Kropp B., McPherson T., Liang H., Snyder P. 1998. Small intestinal submucosa: a rapidly resorbed bioscaffold for augmentation cystoplasty in a dog model. *Tissue Eng* 4:379–87.

Badylak S.F., Lantz G.C., Coffey A., Geddes L.A. 1989. Small intestinal submucosa as a large diameter vascular graft in the dog. *Journal of Surgical Research* 47:74–80.

Baker S.C., Rohman G., Southgate J., Cameron N.R. 2009. The relationship between the mechanical properties and cell behaviour on PLGA and PCL scaffolds for bladder tissue engineering. *Biomaterials* 30:1321–28.

Brown A.L., Farhat W., Merguerian P.A., et al. 2002. 22 week assessment of bladder acellular matrix as a bladder augmentation material in a porcine model. *Biomaterials* 23:2179–90.

Brown R.A., Wiseman M., Chuo C.B., Cheema U., Nazhat S.N. 2005. Ultrarapid engineering of biomimetic materials and tissues: fabrication of nano- and microstructures by plastic compression. *Advanced Functional Materials* 15:1762–70.

Cen L., Liu W., Cui L. 2008. Collagen tissue engineering: development of novel biomaterials and applications. *Pediatrics Research* 63:492–96.

Chun Y.W., Lim H., Webster T.J., Haberstroh K.M. 2010. Nanostructured bladder tissue replacements. *Nanomedicine and Nanotechnology* 3:134–45.

Chun Y.W., Lim H., Webster T.J., Haberstroh K.M. 2011. Nanostructured bladder tissue replacements. *Wiley Interdisciplinary Reviews: Nanomedicine and Nanobiotechnology* 3:134–45.

Cooke M.J., Philips S.R., Shah D.S.H., et al. 2008. Enhanced cell attachment using a novel cell culture surface presenting functional domains from extracellular matrix proteins. *Cytotechnology* 56:71–79.

Cross W.R., Thomas D.F.M., Southgate J. 2003. Tissue engineering and stem cell research in urology. *British Journal of Urology International* 92:165–71.

Dahms S.E., Piechota H.J., Dahiya R., Lue T.F., Tanagho E.A. 1998. Composition and biomechanical properties of the bladder acellular matrix graft: comparative analysis in rat, pig and human. *British Journal of Urology* 82:411–19.

Deveaud C.M., Macarak E.J., Kucich U., et al. 1998. Molecular analysis of collagens in bladder fibrosis. *Journal of Urology* 160:1518–27.

Dewan P.A., Anderson P. 2008. Ureterocystoplasty: the latest developments. *BJU International* 88:744–51.

Drury J.L., Mooney D.J. 2003. Hydrogels for tissue engineering: scaffold design variables and applications. *Biomaterials* 24:4337–51.

Elder J.S. 2004. Anomalies of the bladder. In: Kliegman R.M., Behrman R.E., Jenson H.B., Stanton B.F., editors. *Nelson Textbook of Pediatrics*. Philadelphia: Saunders.

Engelhardt E.M., Micol L.A., Houis S., et al. 2011. A collagen-poly (lactic acid-co-e-caprolactone) hybrid scaffold for application in bladder tissue regeneration. *Biomaterials* 32:3969–76.

Engelhardt E.M., Stegberg E., Brown R.A., et al. 2010. Compressed collagen gel: a novel scaffold for human bladder cells. *Journal of Tissue Engineering and Regenerative Medicine* 4:123–30.

Farhat W.A., Chen J., Haig J., et al. 2008. Porcine bladder acellular matrix (ACM): protein expression, mechanical properties. *Biomedical Materials* 3:025015.

Frazer M., Thomas D.F., Pitt E., et al. 2004. A surgical model of composite cystoplasty with cultured urothelial cells: a controlled study of gross outcome and urothelial phenotype. *BJU International* 93:609–16.

French A.C., Thompson A.L., Davis B.G. 2009. High-purity discrete PEG-oligomer crystals allow structural insight. *Angewandte Chemie (International Edition in English)* 48:1248–52.

Gale Encyclopedia of Medicine. Free tissue transfer (n.d.) http://medical-dictionary.thefreedictionary.com/Free+tissue+transfer.

Gearhart J.P., Mathews R. 2007. Exstrophy-epispadias complex: In: Brook J.D., editor, *Campbell-Walsh Urology*, 9th ed. Philadelphia: Saunders, ch. 119, pp. 3497–3498.

Gray H., Howden R. 1916. *Anatomy, Descriptive and Applied*. Longmans, Green.

Hafez A.T., Afshar K., Bagli D.J., et al. 2005. Aerosal transfer of bladder urothelial and smooth muscle cells onto demucosalized colonic segments for porcine bladder augmentation *in vivo*: a 6 week experimental study. *Journal of Urology* 174:1663–67, discussion 1667–68.

Hakenberg O.W., Linne, C., Manseck A., Wirth M.P. 2000. Bladder wall thickness in normal adults and men with mild lower urinary tract symptoms and benign prostatic enlargement. *Neurourology and Urodynamics* 19:585–93.

Hanno P.M. 2007. Painful bladder syndrome/intestinal cystitis and related disorders. In: Wein A.J., editor, *Campbell-Walsh Urology*, 9th ed. Philadelphia: Saunders.

Holroyd-Leduc J.M., Tannenbaum C., Thorpe K.E. 2008. What type of urinary incontinence does this woman have? *Journal of the American Medical Association* 299:1446–56.

Housset M., Maulard C., Chretien Y., et al. 1993. Combined radiation and chemotherapy for invasive transitional-cell carcinoma of the bladder: a prospective study. *Journal of Clinical Oncology* 11:2150–57.

Iijima K., Igawa Y., Imamura T., et al. 2007. Transplantation of preserved human amniotic membrane for bladder augmentation in rats. *Tissue Engineering* 13:513–24.

Jack G.S., Zhang R., Lee M., et al. 2009. Urinary bladder smooth muscle engineered from adipose stem cells and a three dimensional synthetic composite. *Biomaterials* 30:3259–70.

Kachnic L.A., Kaufman D.S., Heney N.M., et al. 1997. Bladder preservation by combined modality therapy for invasive bladder cancer. *Journal of Clinical Oncology* 15:1022–29.

Kinsman S.L., Johnston M.V. 2004. Congenital anomalies of the central nervous system. In: Kliegman R.M., Behrman R.E., Jenson H.B., Stanton B.F., editors, *Nelson Textbook of Pediatrics*. Philadelphia: Saunders, pp. 1983–1989.

Kleinman H.K., Philp D., Hoffman M.P. 2003. Role of the extracellular matrix in morphogenesis. *Current Opinions in Biotechnology* 30:526–32.

Koenig F., Gonzalez S., White W.M., Lein M., Rajadhyaksha M. 1999. Near-infrared confocal laser scanning microscopy of bladder tissue *in vivo*. *Urology* 53:853–57.

Korossis S., Bolland F., Ingham E., et al. 2006. Tissue engineering of the urinary bladder: considering structure-function relationships and the role of mechanotransduction. Review. *Tissue Engineering* 12:635–44.

Kropp B., Cheng E., Lin H., Zhang Y. 2004. Reliable and reproducible bladder regeneration using unseeded distal small intestinal submucosa. *Journal of Urology* 172(4 Pt 2):1710–13.

Lewis S.A. 2000. Everything you wanted to know about the bladder epithelium but were afraid to ask. *American Journal of Physiology Renal Physiology* 278:F687–74.

Li S.T., editor. 1995. *Biologic Biomaterials: Tissue Derived Biomaterials (Collagen). The Biomedical Engineering Handbook.* Boca Raton, FL: CRC Press.

Lima S.V.C., Araujo L.A.P., Vilar F.O., Kummer C.L., Lima E.C. 2004. Nonsecretory intestinocystoplasty: a 10-year experience. *Journal of Urology* 171:2636–39, discussion 2639–40.

Long-Heise R., Ivanova J., Parekh A., Sacks M.S. 2009. Generating elastin rich SIS-based smooth muscle constructs utilizing exogenous growth factors and cyclic mechanical stimulation. *Tissue Engineering Part A* 15:3951–60.

Lovett M.L., Cannizzaro C.M., Vunjak-Novakovic G., Kaplan D.L. 2008. Gel spinning of silk tubes for tissue engineering. *Biomaterials* 29:4650–57.

Mauney J.R., Cannon G.M., Lovett M.L., et al. 2011. Evaluation of gel spun silk-based biomaterials in a murine model of bladder augmentation. *Biomaterials* 32:808–18.

Oberpenning F., Meng J., Yoo J.J., Atala A. 1998. De novo reconstitution of a functional mammalian urinary bladder by tissue engineering. *Nature Biotechnology* 17:149–55.

Oelke M., Hafner K., Jonas U., et al. 2006. Ultrasound measurement of detrusor wall thickness in healthy adults. *Neurourology Urodynamics* 25:308–17.

Pattison M.A., Wurster S., Webster T.J., Haberstroh K.M. 2005. Three-dimensional, nano-structured PLGA scaffolds for bladder tissue replacement applications. *Biomaterials* 26:2491–500.

Raghavan D., Huben R. 1995. Management of bladder cancer. *Current Problems in Cancer* 19:1–64.

Rao P.K., Iverson A.J., Cespedes R.D., Sabanegh E.S., Jr. 2008. Augmentation cystoplasty. emedicine.medscape.com/article/443916

Roby T., Olsen S., Nagatomi J. 2008. Effect of sustained tension on bladder smooth muscle cells in three-dimensional culture. *Annals of Biomedical Engineering* 36:1744–51.

Rohman G., Pettit J.J., Isaure F., Cameron N.R., Southgate J. 2007. Influence of the physical properties of two-dimensional polyester substrates on the growth of normal human urothelial and urinary smooth muscle cells *in vitro*. *Biomaterials* 28:2264–74.

Roth C., Kropp B. 2009. Recent advances in urologic tissue engineering. *Current Urology Reports* 119–25.

Savicky R.S., Jackson A.H. 2009. Use of a rectus abdominis muscle flap to repair urinary bladder and urethral defects in a dog. *Journal of the American Veterinary Medicine Association* 234:1038–40.

Schwenke-Konig P.S.A., Hage J.J., Kon M. 2004. Comparison of rectus abdominis muscle and musculoperitoneal flap in closure of urinary bladder defects in a rat model. *European Journal of Plastic Surgery* 27:233–37.

Seeley R., Stephens T., Tate P., editors. 2000. *Anatomy and Physiology,* 5th ed. New York: McGraw-Hill Higher Education.

Shamliyan T.A., Kane R.L., Wyman J., Wilt T.J. 2008. Systematic review: randomized, controlled trials of nonsurgical treatments for urinary incontinence in women. *Annals of Internal Medicine* 148:459–73.

Shier D., Butler J., Lewis R., editors. 2007. *Hole's Human Anatomy and Physiology,* 11th ed. New York: McGraw-Hill Higher Education.

Tessmar J.K., Gopferich A.M. 2007. Customized PEG derived co-polymers for tissue engineering applications. *Macromolecular Biosciences* 7:23–39.

Thapa A., Miller D.C., Webster T.J., Haberstroh K.M. 2003. Nanostructured polymers enhance bladder smooth muscle cell function. *Biomaterials* 24:2915–26.

Thomas D.F. 1997. Surgical treatment of urinary incontinence. *Archives of Disease in Childhood* 76:377–80.

Thrasher J.B., Crawford E.D. 1993. Current management of invasive and metastatic transitional cell carcinoma of the bladder. *Journal of Urology* 149:957–72.

Turner A.M., Subramaniam R., Thomas D.F.M., Southgate J. 2007. Bladder tissue engineering. In: Boccaccini A.R., Grough J.E., eds., *Tissue Engineering Using Ceramics and Polymers*, London: CRC Press.

Vaught J.D., Kropp B.P., Sawyer B.D., et al. 1996. Detrusor regeneration in the rat using porcine small intestinal submucosal grafts: functional innervation and receptor expression. *Journal of Urology* 155:374–78.

Wang Y., Kim H.J., Vunjak-Novakovic G., Kaplan D.L. 2006. Stem cell-based tissue engineering with silk biomaterials. *Biomaterials* 27:6064–82.

Warren J., Pike J.G., Leonard M.P. 2004. Posterior urethral valves in eastern Ontario—a 30 year perspective. *Canadian Journal of Urology* 11:2210–15.

Wein A.J., editor. 2007. *Campbell-Walsh Urology*. 9th ed. Philadelphia: Saunders.

Wein A.J. 2007. Lower urinary tract dysfunction in neurologic injury and disease. In: Wein A.J., editor, *Campbell-Walsh Urology*, 9th ed. Philadelphia: Saunders, ch. 59, pp. 2011–2045.

Zhang Y., Frimberger D., Cheng E.Y., Lin H.K., Kropp B.P. 2006. Challenges in a larger bladder replacement with cell-seeded and unseeded small intestinal submucosa grafts in a subtotal cystectomy model. *BJU International* 98:1100–5.

Zhang Y., Kropp B.P., Ling H.K., Cowan R., Cheng E.Y. 2004. Bladder regeneration with cell-seeded small intestinal submucosa. *Tissue Engineering* 10:181–87.

Zhang Y., Kropp B.P., Moore P., et al. 2000. Coculture of bladder urothelial and smooth muscle cells on small intestinal submucosa: potential applications for tissue engineering technology. *Journal of Urology* 164:928–35.

10

Vascular and Urogenital Sealants and Blocks

M. Scott Taylor

CONTENTS

Introduction

Anatomy and Repair

Vascular and urogenital systems are in the most general sense conduits that are similar in form (Figure 10.1) and function; they are uniquely capable in their ability to transport materials within the body. The innermost layers, the intima in the vascular system and mucosa in the urogenital system, are

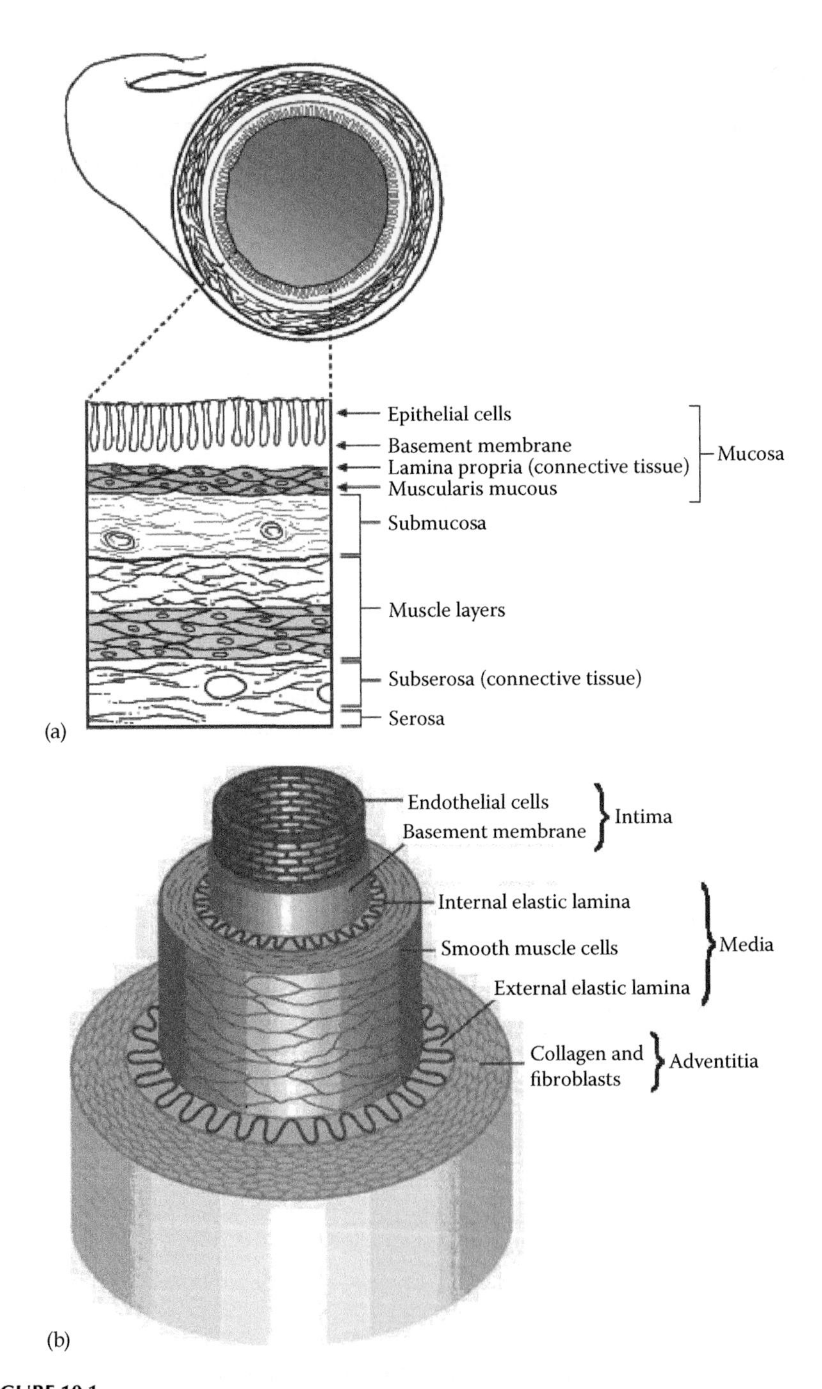

FIGURE 10.1
Anatomy in layers of the (a) colon and (b) artery. (Sarkar, S., Sales, K.M., Hamilton, G., and Seifalian, A.M. 2006. Addressing thrombogenicity in vascular graft construction. *J Biomed Mat Res B: Appl Biomat* 82B:100–8. With permission.)

internally lined with epithelial cells, which vary in form according to location and function. They are connected through the basement membrane to connective tissue, surrounded by smooth muscle cells, and ultimately encapsulated with layers composed of collagen and fibroblasts.

Although the vasculature has a much wider reach within the body, the urogenital system is of equal importance for the transport and excretion of waste, thereby contributing to the maintenance of a healthy physiology. As both systems perform similar functions, they also exhibit similar dysfunction and intervention for repair. Traumas through surgical incision or chronic disease states are primary causes of dysfunction, and the presence of comorbidities is typical. Often, sealants and blocks are required due directly to these comorbidities, which complicate the device design and require developers to view the mechanism of sealing and blockage in atypical environments. For instance, a patient requiring bypass surgery or the implantation of a replacement heart valve may require anticoagulation therapy, most often by the systemic administration of heparin or Coumadin, but the seal typically created through physiologically mediated blood coagulation at the anastomosis or access site is affected by the medication.

In vasculature, the efficacy of sealants is directly related to hemostasis and the ability of the closure mechanism to generate and maintain the seal quickly under physiologic pressures. Arterial pressures are greater than those found in veins, and smaller vessels exhibit reduced pressures compared to larger, although they require a more flexible device and are more difficult to access. Additional considerations must be taken into account to maintain patency of blood cells, which could be damaged as a result of direct contact with the seal or block or as a result of the mechanical or chemical characteristics of the device. In most patients, coagulation occurs through the basic mechanisms of (a) vascular spasms, (b) platelet aggregation or thrombosis, and (c) the formation of a fibrin plug, which can take up to 10 minutes (Stadelmann, Digenis, and Tobin 1998) or longer in patients with a compromised coagulation response due to medications or comorbidities. Failure to stop hemorrhage in a timely manner results in increased morbidity and mortality rates, and adjunct devices are often required to achieve improved patient outcomes.

Sealants and blocks are used surgically to affect closure, provide a seal where leakage is occurring, and temporarily or permanently create blockages to inhibit flow to and from desired areas. Injuries for which these types of intervention may be required are varied and are a result of trauma, surgical incision or intervention, or long-term tissue degeneration. Most often, these devices are not used to create the primary outcome but are used to improve patient outcomes adjuvant to the procedure and less often represent the sole purpose of the surgery. Surgical sealants are used to create a barrier between different cavities or conduits, and the focus of this review is those that are primarily indicated for prevention of the leakage of bodily fluids from the vasculature and urogenital conduits to the abdominal space. Blocks are herein defined as providing a barrier within the conduit and are used to chemically or mechanically partition an area.

Theories of "best practice" are widespread, and many products are available to meet the needs of each treatment modality. These include mechanical sealing, biologically mediated treatments, temporary and permanent devices, absorbable synthetic, nonabsorbable synthetic, and biologic materials. Implant locations cover the full spectrum as well, including intra-, trans-, or extrastructural deployment.

As with most advances in medical devices, newer products serve as an adjunct or replacement for existing technologies. Specialized devices are continually in development due to the desire to reduce or replace the use of sutures or simple compression, mainly due to the inefficiencies involved with traditional techniques, including lack of sustained closure; poor functionality, particularly in friable tissue; difficulty and slow speed associated with the techniques; and incomplete or inconsistent sealing.

Sealants

Sealants are described as a class of medical device designed to seal or partition one area from another. In the case of the vascular and urogenital systems, these devices are suited for stopping the flow of blood and waste fluids from leaving the respective conduits and entering the abdominal or other body cavities or exiting the body completely. While these devices must have adequate resilience to maintain a seal under the pressures exerted from either side of the treatment area, the devices typically do not support the surrounding tissue in any other modality.

Adhesive Sealants

Many surgical procedures require the approximation of body lumens, which is in large part supported through the use of traditional suture-based techniques. Adhesives, however, are becoming increasingly common alternatives for the provision of additional support or as the primary closure mechanism. These devices are particularly useful in friable areas, such as adipose tissue, or in small and delicate areas, such as in capillary vasculature, where the use of sutures is contraindicated. Adhesives create *in situ* bonds through chemical reactions at the implant site, including polymerization and cross-linking reactions, and are prepared from a wide variety of materials, including cyanoacrylate-based and naturally derived fibrin systems.

Prior to the mid-1990s, the nonabsorbable, hydrolytically stable n-butyl and isobutyl cyanoacrylates were acknowledged as the most effective type of tissue adhesives in terms of adhesive strength. They have been used as hemostatic sealants as well as for treating vascular aneurysms (Larrazabal, Pelz, and Findlay 2001). In spite of the availability of other tissue adhesives, such as gelatin-resorcinol, those cyanoacrylates retained their competitive edge because of their high adhesive joint strength. Their dominance was recently threatened by growing interest in biological or natural polymer-based systems. Studies, however, showed that none of those adhesives could create a full seal, particularly in hemorrhagic conditions, largely due to excessive bleeding that rendered the products incapable of adhering to the tissue interfaces or even cohering independently (Arnaud et al. 2009; Azadani et al. 2009; Fischer et al. 2004). To date, no commercially available products have gained broad adoption for multispecialty surgical application. As a result, hospitals are required to stock a suite of hemostatic products and sealants based on surgeon preference. The desired goal of new product development is ultimately to meet this need through the creation of a surgical sealant that can be used (a) in a multitude of clinical scenarios, (b) with little to no prep time, (c) to provide secure positional placement, (d) to seal quickly, (e) to absorb in a timely manner, and (f) regardless of comorbidities or adjunct therapies.

A common complication associated with the internal use of adhesives is the growth of adhesions, which create undesired attachments between organs or to the abdominal wall, resulting in pain and occasionally requiring secondary procedures to separate adhered organs. Additional procedural complexity is a result of the relatively low application viscosity of many adhesive sealants, particularly with cyanoacrylate-based systems, increasing the difficulty for precise and secure application.

Cyanoacrylate Adhesives

Cyanoacrylate-based tissue adhesives, initially developed in the 1950s, provide strong adhesive strength, although their use is predominantly limited to topical applications. Cyanoacrylates are supplied in a liquid form consisting of unreacted monomers that undergo rapid free radical polymerization in the presence of water and modifying agents such as stabilizers or copolymeric viscosity modifiers. The long chain polymer formed *in situ* is strong and relatively noncompliant. Primarily, cyanoacrylate tissue adhesives are prepared from methyl, ethyl, butyl, or octyl cyanoacrylate monomers. Each monomer type has a unique viscosity and curing time, and each resulting polymerized product has a different mechanical performance. The most common cyanoacrylate-based tissue adhesives and the associated monomer types can be seen in Table 10.1.

These devices exhibit a wide range of mechanical properties and as such have different indications. Dermabond™, for instance, is only indicated for low-tension or tension-free closure (Ethicon 2009), whereas Indermil™ can be used in areas requiring higher adhesive strength (Covidien 2005). The monomer type directly affects the joint strength, and, to a lesser extent, the mechanical compliance, with the smaller moledcular weight monomers (e.g., methyl and ethyl) providing higher strength compared to larger monomers (e.g., octyl). Larger molecular weight monomers increase polymerization time and exhibit reduced heat generation compared to smaller cyanoacrylates.

TABLE 10.1

Cyanoacrylate-Based Adhesive Summary

Device (Marketed by)	Cyanoacrylate Monomer(s)	T-Peel Strength, N
Dermabond™ (Ethicon)	2-Octyl	4.5
Indermil™ (Covidien)	n-Butyl	18
GluSeal90™ (GluStitch)	2-Octyl and n-butyl	11
TissueMend™ (VPL)	Methoxypropyl and ethyl	48

Source: Ingram and Garcia 2010.

Due to the inherent cytotoxicity of the monomeric constituents, high heat of polymerization, lack of mechanical compliance, and breakdown products, cyanoacrylates are primarily restricted for use internally. There are a few notable exceptions, and cyanoacrylate devices have shown efficacy as neurovascular aneurysm sealants (Raymond et al. 2002) and sealants for abdominal aortic aneurysms (Buckenham et al. 2009; Chiu et al. 2005). In these cases, aneurysms were filled with cyanoacrylate adhesives via a sponge or small microcatheter, respectively, resulting in the filling and sealing of the aneurysm and the formation of thicker neointimal formation compared to treatment with traditional coils.

There is currently no cyanoacrylate adhesive approved for internal use by the Food and Drug Administration (FDA), although there are several products in various stages of development. Neucrylate™, a novel cyanoacrylate-based device marketed by Valor Medical, has recently obtained CE marking (European clearance) for aneurysm treatment, which provides a path for other systems to enter the market. The Neucrylate system forms porous foam with increased mechanical compliance when cured, as opposed to standard cyanoacrylates, which form a stiff film (Pakbaz et al. 2010).

Naturally Derived Adhesives

While cyanoacrylates provide excellent strength, they lack compliance, and unreacted monomers are cytotoxic. As an alternative, several systems have been designed to provide a mechanism for tissue approximation and reinforcement. These systems typically form cross-linked networks *in situ* that bind to the surrounding tissue or form simple mechanical bonds, typically providing reinforcement with increased compliance (Azadani et al. 2009).

Bioglue™, marketed by CryoLife Europa Limited, is such an example. This device is supplied in a double-chamber syringe, with one barrel comprising bovine serum albumin (BSA) and the other glutaraldehyde. During injection, the components mix in the syringe tip, and a cross-linking reaction is initiated. Currently, Bioglue is indicated for use to reinforce friable tissue as well as for vascular anastomosis and other sealant applications. While Bioglue has been shown to be stiffer than human aortic tissue, 3,122 ± 1,640 KPa compared to 450 KPa, respectively, the increased strength compared to other naturally derived glues indicates its importance for the secure reinforcement and sealing of anastomosis sites (Azadani et al. 2009). Studies have also indicated the effectiveness of Bioglue for sealing urinary tracts (Louie et al. 2010), showing great improvement in hemostasis after a partial nephrectomy compared to saline irrigation. Similarly, Cardial™, a resorcinol formalin sealant marketed by Bard, has been successfully used to seal the anastomosis in thoracic aorta replacement (Apostolakis, Leivaditis, and Anagnostopoulos 2009).

Other naturally derived fibrin glues form cross-linked networks by reacting thrombin, particularly of bovine or human origin, and fibrinogen, which duplicates the final stage of the coagulation cascade (Park et al. 2002). These materials function primarily as a sealant, significantly reducing time for hemostasis, but do not provide immediate reinforcement strength compared to cyanoacrylates or surgical suture. Similarly, Baxter's Floseal™ is prepared from human-derived thrombin and gelatin cross-linked with glutaraldehyde and has been shown to decrease time to hemostasis in several treatment modalities. It is clear that thrombogenic glues combine an immediate hemostatic functionality, but they also rapidly absorb, which supports fast replacement of natural tissue (Park et al. 2002). This is diametrically opposed to cyanoacrylate systems, which only form a mechanical seal that degrades over an extended time.

Vascular Grafts

One method of mechanically sealing anastomoses, aneurysms, and other perforations to effect hemostasis involves the placement of vascular grafts. These implants are often viewed as a second option when less-aggressive treatment options, such as drug therapy, are not considered an adequate treatment course. Vascular grafts have been available for decades and have been dominated by systems based on ePTFE (expanded polytetrafluoroethylene) and Dacron (polyethylene terephthalate, PET), although alternative materials have been and are being developed to increase patency and provide superior long-term performance. These devices, because they are often in direct, permanent contact with blood, must prevent thrombogenesis within the vessel but provide a seal at the graft-tissue interface. The interior surface is often bound with active agents or other materials to prevent blood coagulation as well as reduce the proliferation of smooth muscle cells, the growth of which would result in intimal hyperplasia (IH) (Sarkar et al. 2006). To address the issue of IH, many studies have been performed to identify the effect of heparin bound into the graft to increase patency, and although early results indicated improved performance, there could be long-term effects similar to those seen in vascular stents, such as delayed thrombosis and slow vessel wall healing.

While graft materials provide the necessary barrier scaffold to create a secure seal, the materials often do not provide the structural support necessary to retain patency. One method of supporting the graft structure involves reinforcement provided by an internal stent or coil. In this case, the stent is a carrier for a patch-type seal, which can be prepared of Dacron knit (Mofidi et al. 2007), nonwoven felts, electrospun fabrics (Shalaby 2010), or other compliant fabrics or films (Shalaby 2008).

As vascular grafts, along with many other sealant materials, are considered permanent implants (meaning they dwell in the body for more than 30 days), they must provide long-term mechanical compatibility with the surrounding tissue. One of the major problems with many synthetic grafts is the mechanical compliance relative to the surrounding tissue. The graft is often stiffer than tissue, and this compliance mismatch can cause blood flow disturbances that result in IH near the graft interface (Sarkar et al. 2006).

Sealant Applications

Arterial Access Port Closure

Laparoscopic surgical procedures are increasingly common, and many involve accessing vasculature, particularly the femoral artery. These leave access ports that require postprocedure closure, which was traditionally effected with sutures or compression. The rising popularity of laparoscopically mediated vascular procedures, along with the slow and unreliable sealing provided by traditional techniques, has prompted the development of many specialized closure devices with unique functionality. These devices have reduced not only time to hemostasis but also ambulation, thereby improving patient wellness while reducing associated health care costs.

Traditional Closure Techniques

One of the most common, and the traditional standard, techniques for closing after vascular access involves simple manual compression. This technique requires approximately 8–10 minutes to effect closure after 6F to 8F femoral access, which represent the most common procedural sheath sizes. Compression can be applied through a device as simple as a sandbag, although more robust alternatives are available. Many of these devices are similar, comprising a tension strap with an inflatable area to provide further compressive force to the treatment area. An example device is the FemoStop™ Gold (St. Jude Medical Systems) (Figure 10.2).

Port closure after vascular access with catheters larger than 9F has been achieved using sutures, typically employing polypropylene suture in adults or Monocryl™ (Ethicon) absorbable suture for pediatric patients (Lin, Long, and Edlich 2005). Sutures, however, lead to a variety of complications, including constriction at the implant site. In addition, braided sutures are seldom

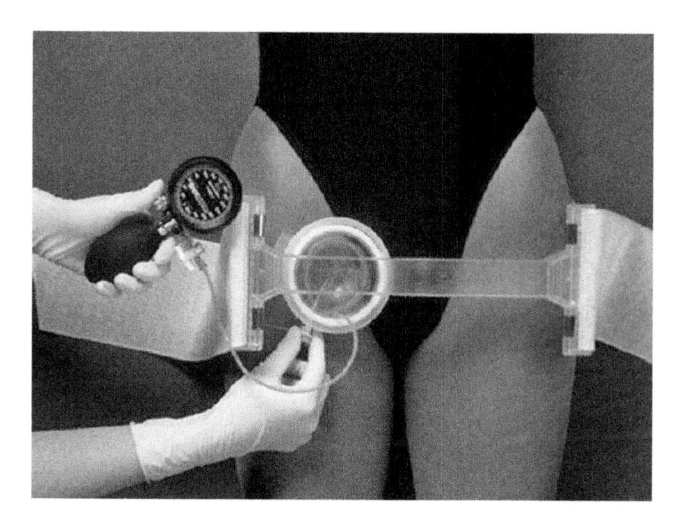

FIGURE 10.2
FemoStop™ Gold assisted compression device.

used due to the possibility of bacterial transport through the relatively open structure of the multifilament construct. Advances in medical materials and technology have paved the way for increasing options for sealing holes created by trauma or surgery.

Specialty Closure Products

Although new vascular closure devices (VCDs) have shown increased efficacy compared to simple compression, the adoption of these devices is low. In spite of the relatively low adoption rates compared to traditional standard compression, more than two million VCDs were sold worldwide in 2006 (Dauerman, Applegate, and Cohen 2007), and sales increased to an estimated \$500 to \$700 million in 2009 (Turi 2009). The market leader for most of the past decade was Angio-Seal™ (marketed by St. Jude), although newly developed technology is increasing competition in this space. The most common usage involves closure of the femoral artery, and to a much lesser extent radial artery closure, after catheterization for diagnostic and interventional procedures requiring vascular access. The goal of VCDs is to provide fast hemostasis and subsequent decreased time for patient ambulation and the ability to effect closure immediately postsurgery regardless of anticoagulation status. Generally, time to hemostasis is much faster than standard compression, less than 5 minutes compared to 15–30 minutes or more with manual compression (Dauerman, Applegate, and Cohen 2007).

Theories of femoral and radial port closure can be summarized as active or passive (Turi 2009), with example devices described in Table 10.2 and Figure 10.3. Active devices feature a primary closure effected by a mechanical

TABLE 10.2

Summary of Select Vascular Access Port Closure Devices

Device	Materials	Mechanism of Closure	Usage	Features
Angio-Seal™ (St. Jude Medical)	Suture Collagen Molded anchor	Mechanical seal with collagen as a thrombogenic agent	4F to 8F port closure	Fully resorbable in 90 days Intra- and extravascular
FemoSeal™ (St. Jude Medical)	Suture Molded sandwich	Mechanical seal	6F port closure	Fully resorbable
Perclose™ (Abbott Vascular)	Suture (polyester or polypropylene)	Mechanical cinch	5F to 8F port closure	Transvascular
StarClose™ (Abbott Vascular)	Nitinol	Mechanical clip	5F, 6F port closure	Transvascular Permanent implant
Mynx™ (Access Closure)	PEG-based hydrogel	Mechanical seal	5F to 7F port closure	Fully resorbable in 30 days Extravascular
ExoSeal™ (Cordis)	PGA felt tapenade	Coagulation bed	5F to 7F	Fully resorbable in 90 days Extravascular
Catalyst™ II (Cardiva Medical)	Nitinol disk Hemostatic coating	Provides area for clotting to occur	5F to 7F	Transient placement, removed after hemostasis
Duett Pro™ (Vascular Solutions Inc.)	Thrombin and collagen procoagulant	Expedites clotting cascade	5F to 9F	Transient intravascular balloon providing temporary seal during delivery of extravascular clotting aids

seal, often followed by a component that results in an increased rate of coagulation. A mechanical seal provides immediate hemostasis and ambulation, but this is often created using synthetic absorbable polymers, exemplified by the FemoSeal™ and ExoSeal™ devices. These rely on glycolide-based polymers to approximate the port closely and maintain closure. As the polymer is encapsulated and subsequently hydrolyzes, by-products such as glycolic acid are formed, which may lead to localized complications. Naturally derived materials like collagen do not share this risk and often will resorb faster, allowing for natural tissue ingrowth. While early devices primarily relied on mechanical (active) closure, newer devices have been designed to increase the rate of coagulation in much the same way as many *in situ* adhesive sealants. The Duett Pro™ and Mynx™ devices are recent examples and represent a more ideal treatment course due to the lack of any residual intravascular material.

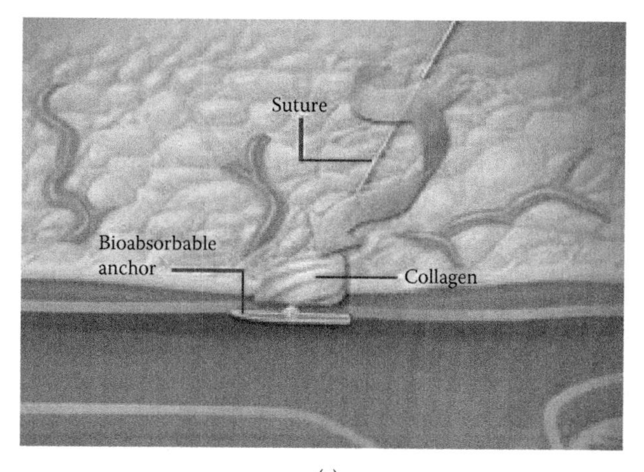

(a)

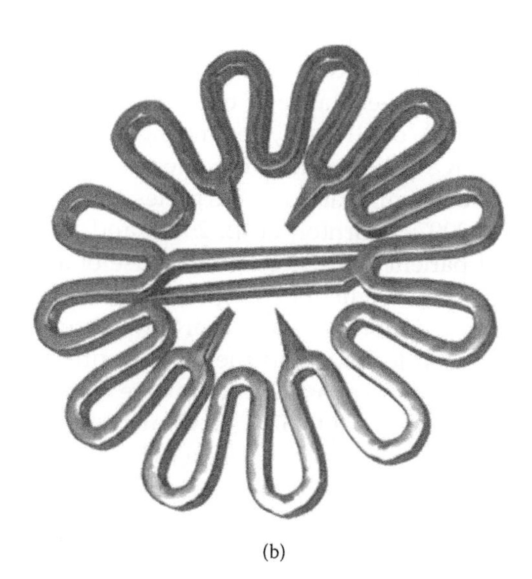

(b)

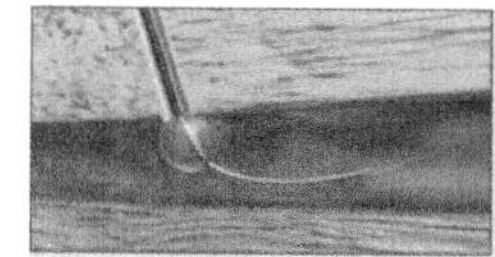

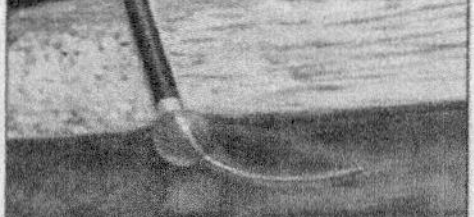

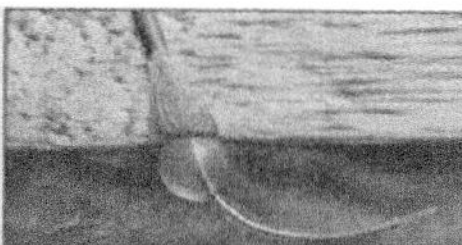

(c)

FIGURE 10.3 (see color insert)
(a) Angio-Seal™ after implantation; (b) StarClose™ clip; (c) steps involved with the implantation of the Mynx™ sealant system.

While there are myriad devices designed for closure postarterial access, there are surprisingly few options for puncture wounds within the urogenital tract. For instance, bowel surgery is commonly performed laparoscopically and more recently through robotic surgery. An uncommon, but possible, complication of these minimally invasive surgeries involves the perforation of the bowels, which immediately results in the transfer of the patient to open surgery to repair the area, followed by systemic antibiotics (Thomson et al. 2004). While urogenital perforations do not create the immediate dangers associated with vascular injuries, the risk of infection and sepsis is high, and the current lack of device alternatives provides an opportunity for new development.

Anastomosis Seal

Many surgical procedures, such as bypass surgery and radical prostatectomy, require the formation of an anastomotic juncture to provide biologic functionality and seal the conduit. Anastomoses can be end to end, end to side, or side to side, as indicated in Figure 10.4, and all require a securely sealed junction to reduce the chance of complications. Anastomotic leaks are reported in up to 30% of all cases, depending on inclusion criteria, and while other studies have indicated lower incidence rates, this is nonetheless a frequent and serious complication in surgeries such as colorectal resection (Veenhof et al. 2007; Thornton et al. 2011), and all studies reviewed identified improved patient outcomes with the use of adjuvant sealants at the anastomosis site. Improvement in surgically assisted anastomosis seals has resulted in decreased morbidity and mortality. One report highlighted the benefits of decreased leakage and the significantly higher 5-year survival rate for patients with no anastomotic leakage compared to those with leakage (76% survival compared to 57% survival rates) (Law et al. 2007).

A specific form of anastomosis is a fistula, which can form between an intestine and intestine (enteroenteric fistula), intestine and skin (enterocutaneous fistula), or an artery and vein (arteriovenous [AV] fistula), for example. Fistulas can be surgically produced or occur as a result of trauma. While often it is desired to close malformed fistulas, some AV fistulas are surgically created as an access point for hemodialysis treatments in patients with

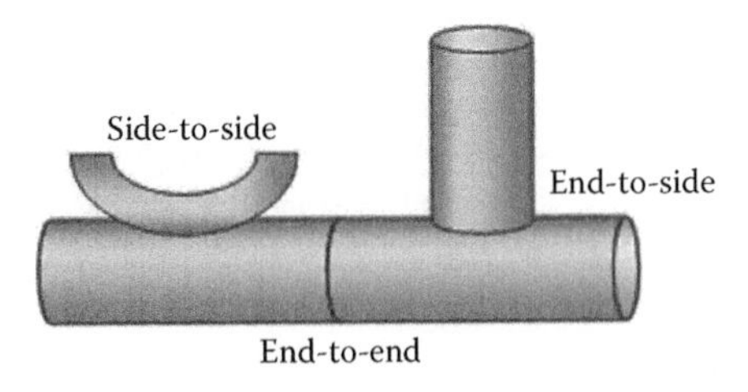

FIGURE 10.4
Three basic anastomotic configurations.

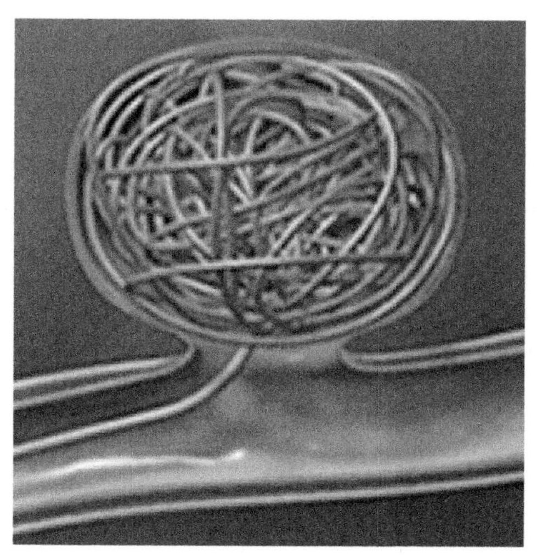

FIGURE 10.5
Treatment of aneurysm with detachable platinum coils.

end-stage renal failure. In these cases, the artery and vein are connected so that the vein is pressurized by the artery, thereby dilating the vein, allowing access with a larger cannula.

Aneurysm Closure

Vascular leakage, otherwise known as an aneurysm, is a complication that could occur throughout the body and has high morbidity and mortality rates. Treatment options are varied and represent a range of available technologies, but the gold standard of coil embolism involves placing flexible metallic coils, which are most often finely wound platinum threads, using a microcatheter within the aneurysm (Figure 10.5). Once the aneurysm is filled with the coils, the wound threads are detached using an electrical discharge.

Alternatives for sealing aneurysms are in development, including the use of gels and cyanoacrylate adhesives that form *in situ*. As described (Raymond et al. 2002; Buckenham et al. 2009; Chiu et al. 2005), cyanoacrylates are well suited for placement via microcatheters due to relatively low viscosity and poor tissue response to cytotoxicity; the exothermic polymerization is postulated actually to increase the efficacy of the treatment.

Nonspecific Area Closure

Most devices designed for hemostasis and closure of larger, nonspecific areas are indicated only for topical use. It can be difficult, however, to locate the source of leakage due to traumatic injury or tissue that may be otherwise compromised due to chronic conditions. Patients presenting nonlocalized bleeding or seepage of waste products are at high risk for morbidity. In addition, many sealants that form *in situ* are difficult to administer due to poor placement security and time required to prepare the devices. A "just-in-time" solution that can cover a wider area is desirable, and devices have been developed in the form of patches and foams. One such device, marketed by Nycomed as TachoSil™, is provided as a compliant collagen fleece coated with fibrinogen, thrombin, and aprotinin and has been cleared for use in vascular surgery for vein lacerations and kidney resections (Lattouf et al. 2007; Dregelid et al. 2008).

Blocks

Surgical blocks are specifically designed to temporarily or permanently prevent transport through an area within the same body lumen. In this way, they provide a different functionality from surgical sealants, which are designed to prevent transport from one body lumen to another. Often, blocks are used to occlude flow in an area to allow performance of a surgical procedure. As with sealants, blocks are commonly used to effect hemostasis during vascular procedures for interventional surgery or in a trauma situation.

Ligatures

The use of ligatures as blocking aids has been widespread for hundreds of years, particularly as a mechanism for effecting hemostasis as an alternative to cauterization (Selden 1917; Lattouf et al. 2007). A ligature consists of a length of suture that is tied around an anatomical structure (e.g., blood vessel or urethra) to create a blockage, as seen in Figure 10.6. Similarly, a tourniquet provides blockage, but without the use of knots, providing the

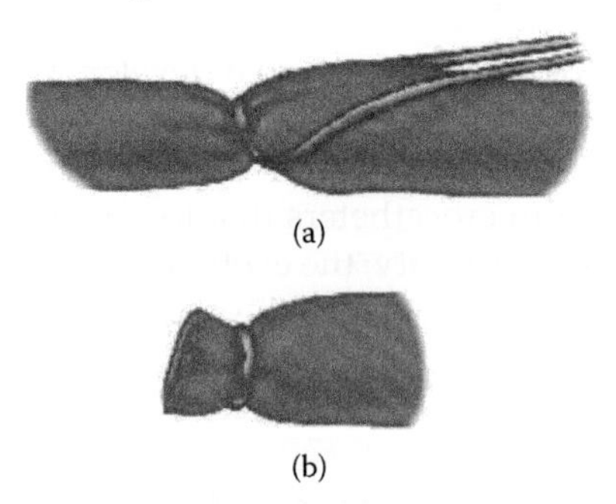

FIGURE 10.6
Filament ligature used to (a) block blood flow and (b) seal a vessel.

ability to tighten or loosen as needed. Typical ligatures are prepared of suture material, although specialty devices with similar functionality have been created.

Vascular Blocks

Occluding vasculature is necessary for a number of reasons, including (a) reduction of pressure on malformed (fistular), weakened (aneurysmal), or leaking blood vessels; (b) reduction of blood supply to tumors or growths in the body; (c) reduction of blood supply (and therefore overall size) of an organ or area prior to other therapies or procedures; and (d) rerouting of blood supply to a different blood vessel or part of the body ("Understanding Vascular Occlusion" n.d.). While occlusions have been historically created through ligatures, recent specialized devices have been developed to create occlusions quickly and reliably. One example is the AMPLATZER™ vascular plug (AGA Medical), which is a nitinol wire basket that is introduced through a sheath and expanded to fill the vessel and block blood flow, as seen in Figure 10.7. It provides a scaffold for blocking blood flow within several minutes for some placement sites (Abdel Aal et al. 2009).

Gel systems that form *in situ* are also of interest in the generation of blocks within vasculature. Poloxamer 407 is a water-soluble poloxamer prepared from 70% polyoxyethylene and 30% polyoxypropylene that is a thin liquid at room temperatures and gels into a hard plug at physiologic temperatures (Boodhwani et al. 2006). After several hours, the plug erodes in blood due to high water solubility. While there are many thermoresponsive gel systems based on poloxamers or polyethylene glycols, a novel system that gels in the presence of moisture was developed to provide increased gel stability for longer durations (Shalaby et al. 2009). Applications for these technologies include temporary vascular occlusion for surgical procedures, including

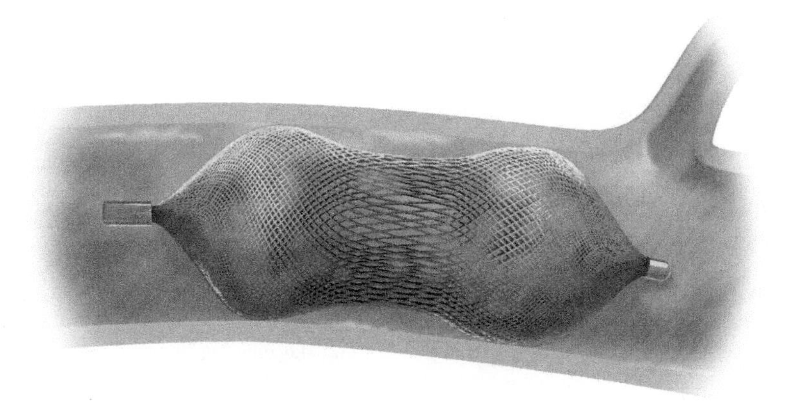

FIGURE 10.7
AMPLATZER™ vascular plug expanded to seal flow through a blood vessel.

vascular plugs and sclerotherapy (Bock 2008), and localized delivery of therapeutic agents.

Urinary Incontinence Repair

Urinary incontinence, particularly in older women, is a widespread disorder resulting in high health care costs and loss of patient comfort. Up to 35% of the total population over the age of 60 are estimated to be incontinent (Password and View 2001), and a portion of these patients do not respond to conservative treatment regimens through behavior management or medication. Surgical intervention provides a good treatment option with high rates of effectiveness. Most typically for stress incontinence, a "sling procedure" is performed, which involves the placement of natural tissue, mesh, or other synthetic materials to form a pelvic sling, or "hammock," around the neck of the bladder and urethra, as indicated in Figure 10.8. The sling serves as a block by maintaining closure of the urethra until the pelvis is tilted at a specific angle, thereby opening the urethra and allowing urine to pass.

Contraceptive Devices

An alternative to hormonal contraception involves the use of intrauterine devices (IUDs) as an effective "maintenance-free" therapy (Forthofer 2009). While these devices have low adoption rates in the United States (approximately 2% of U.S. women in 2008), IUDs are commonly prescribed worldwide (Forthofer 2009; Haimovich 2009). IUDs function by blocking the passage of functional sperm and creating a generally hostile environment to prevent ovum fertilization and inhibit implantation. There are two primary devices

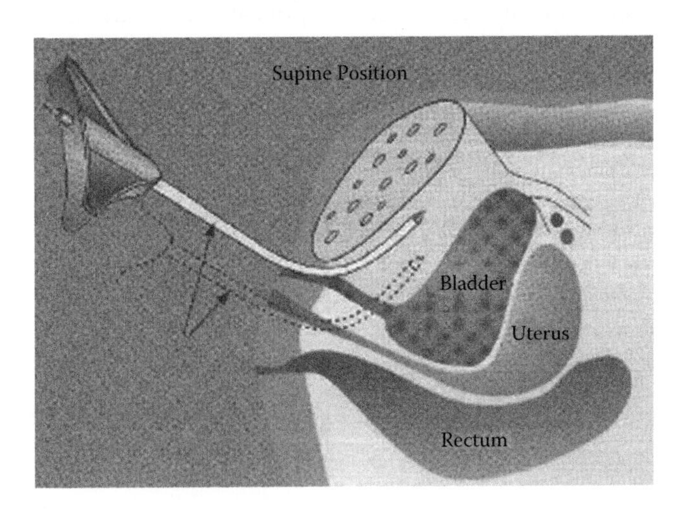

FIGURE 10.8
Location of sling to provide continence.

marketed in the United States, including the ParaGard copper-based contraceptive (Teva Women's Health) and Mirena system, which releases the hormone levonorgestrel. While the former relies on release of Cu^{+} ions (Alvarez et al. 1988), the latter involves standard hormonal therapy. The ParaGard is unique in that it does not contain hormones, thereby eliminating risks associated with their long-term use.

Other temporary blocks are also used as contraceptive devices, including condoms and diaphragms. Condoms, in particular, are useful not only for their prevention of contraception but also for their ability to reduce transmission rates of sexually transmitted diseases (STDs).

Materials

Mirroring the development history of many other medical devices, material selection to develop and manufacture devices for use in the vascular and urogenital system has evolved. These devices are prepared from standard metals, nonabsorbable synthetics, absorbable synthetics, and naturally derived materials. Common material selections include metals such as nitinol and stainless steel, nonabsorbable synthetics such as PET and ePTFE, and absorbable copolymers comprised of standard lactones such as glycolide, lactide, caprolactone, dioxanone, and trimethylene carbonate. Metals and nonabsorbable polymers are widely used, but they remain permanently after implantation. Many of the implanted sealant materials, such as the FemoSeal device, are prepared from absorbable materials. This allows implantation of the sealant inside the vascular wall or other tissues without requiring a second surgical procedure to remove the device.

More recently, interest in synthetic hydroswellables, gels that form *in situ*, and particularly naturally derived materials has resulted in the development of many specialized devices. This is in concert with a general shift toward minimally invasive surgical techniques, which require deployment of devices through small orifices, with the ultimate goal of generating the ability to treat ever-smaller arteries and veins in the peripheral vascular system.

Biologically generated materials (e.g., collagen, fibrinogen, gelatin, and thrombin) are generally produced from bovine or porcine origins, although this results in increased cost and inability to market the device in Europe due to the threat of bovine spongiform encephalopathy (mad cow disease). Thrombin is often derived from human plasma through chromatographic purification, calcium chloride activation, and nanofiltration (Omrix Biopharmaceuticals 2007). While these materials provide excellent functionality, device costs are high compared to synthetic counterparts. For instance, CoSeal™ and other biologic adhesive sealants can cost $1,000 or more per unit, while cyanoacrylate glues are generally less than $100.

Regulatory Considerations

The effects of a malfunctioning sealant or block in the vascular or urogenital system can be catastrophic. For this reason, these devices are often regulated by the FDA as class II or III medical devices, the latter of which is the most stringent regulatory classification, requiring devices to be approved through the Premarket Approval (PMA) process (FDA 2010). Class II devices may be cleared by the FDA through the 510(k) submission process, which significantly reduces time to market. In this process, documentation must be provided that the new device is "substantially equivalent" to a device that is already legally marketed for the same use (predicate device). *Substantial equivalency* refers to the indications for use of the new device and conformance to the predicate.

As with all FDA-regulated medical devices, submissions must prove device safety and efficacy. The former is partially proven through the application of standard biocompatibility testing, as outlined by International Organization for Standardization (ISO) 10993 or FDA guidance. Table 10.3 describes the biocompatibility test panel representing requirements for the majority of vascular and urogenital sealants and blocks. Devices for the urogenital system may be identified as surface devices unless they are placed within the tissue or subcutaneous spaces, and vascular products can generally be classified as tissue or blood contacting, which refers to the sustained contact with circulatory blood. In addition, biologically derived materials are reviewed under increased scrutiny due to the possible transmission of viruses or other diseases and are generally classified as class III devices. Other data expected to be included with the regulatory submission include (a) package labeling, (b) risk assessment and associated mitigation, (c) test method and standards description, and (d) a validated sterilization method.

Conclusions

The vascular and urogenital systems share many anatomical similarities and often require similar repair techniques when injured. Biologically mediated processes like the coagulation cascade are typically sufficient for the repair of minor injuries in a healthy physiology but are not able to self-repair many surgically induced or traumatic injuries. This, coupled with the rise of minimally invasive surgeries, has prompted the industry-wide development of innovative approaches for the sealing and blocking of the vascular and urogenital systems.

The goal of new device development is not to generate a new treatment—there is not currently a clinical need that is not at least partially

TABLE 10.3

Select Panel for Biocompatibility Testing for ISO 10993

Contact area		Duration[a]	Cytotoxicity	Sensitization	Irritation/Intracutaneous	Acute Systemic Toxicity	Subchronic Toxicity	Genotoxicity	Implantation	Hemocompatability	Chronic Toxicity	Carcinogenicity
Surface devices	Mucosal membrane	A	X	X	X							
		B	X	X	X	O	O		O			
		C	X	X	X	O	X	X	O		O	
	Breached or compromised surfaces	A	X	X	X	O						
		B	X	X	X	O	O		O			
		C	X	X	X	O	X	X	O		O	
Implant devices	Tissue/bone	A	X	X	X	O						
		B	X	X	X	X	X	X	X			
		C	X	X	X	X	X	X	X		O	O
	Blood	A	X	X	X	X	X		X	X		
		B	X	X	X	X	X	X	X	X		
		C	X	X	X	X	X	X	X	X	O	O

O, test may be applicable; X, test per ISO 10993-1.
[a] A, limited (<24 hours); B, prolonged (24 hours to 30 days); C, permanent (>30 days).
Source: Food and Drug Administration 2009.

addressed by one or more of the existing technologies—but to improve treatment efficacy, including (a) broadening the usage parameters (e.g., size limitations); (b) improving response time, biocompatibility, and resulting physiological responses (e.g., reduction of IH); (c) reducing surgical complexity and preparation time; (d) imparting device absorbability; and (e) improving patient outcomes by creating devices that meet specific clinical needs. The recent trend toward devices containing biologic materials has increased device costs significantly, but these costs are justified based on increased device efficacy. This trend is expected to continue along with the development of broad-based research in the use of cell signaling for the improved mediation of biologic responses, such as clot formation and tissue regrowth. Devices will continue to be designed for specific applications, like port closure after arterial access, but there is also a need for the development of multifunctional devices such as sealants for general use. These general use devices may result in widespread adoption, due not only to the vast and ever-increasing market, but also to the associated reduction in the number of products required for inventory at hospitals.

References

Abdel Aal, A.K., Hamed, M.F., Biosca, R.F., Saddekni, S., and Raghuram, K. 2009. Occlusion time for Amplatzer vascular plug in the management of pulmonary arteriovenous malformations. *Am J Roentgenol* 192:793–99.

Alvarez, F., et al. 1988. New insights on the mode of action of intrauterine contraceptive devices in women. *Fertil Steril* 49:768–73.

Apostolakis, E.E., Leviatidis, V.N., and Anagnostopoulos, C. 2009. Sutureless technique to support anastomosis during thoracic aorta replacement. *J Cardiothorac Surg* 4:66.

Arnaud, F., Teranishi, K., Tomori, T., Carr, W., and McCarron, R. 2009. Comparison of 10 hemostatic dressings in a groin puncture model in swine. *J Vasc Surg* 50:632–39.

Azadani, A.N., et al. 2009. Mechanical properties of surgical glues used in aortic root replacement. *Ann Thorac Surg* 87:1154–60.

Bock, R.W. 2008. Sclerotherapy for varicose veins. United States of America Patent 12/335,084. December 15.

Boodhwani, M., Feng, J., Mieno, S., et al. 2006. Effects of purified poloxamer 407 gel on vascular occlusion and the coronary endothelium. *Eur J Cardiothorac Surg* 29:736–41.

Buckenham, T., McKewen, M., Laing, A., et al. 2009. Cyanoacrylate embolization of endoleaks after abdominal aortic aneurysm repair. *ANZ J Surg* 79:841–43.

Chiu, C.-H., et al. 2005. Transcatheter arterial embolization with N-butyl 2-cyanoacrylate for ruptured pseudoaneurysm of gastroduodenal artery complicated by traumatic pancreatitis: report of a case. *Chin J Radiol* 30:41–45.

Covidien. 2005. Indermil tissue adhesive package label. Covidien Mansfield, MA.

Dauerman, H.L., Applegate R.J., and Cohen, D.J. 2007. Vascular closure devices: the second decade. *J Am Coll Cardiol* 50:1617–26.

Dregelid, E., Ramnefjell, M., Erichsen, C., et al. 2008. Effective hemostasis in severe mesenteric vein laceration with tachosil low- or non-thrombogenic patch to prevent tachosil. *Eur J Trauma Emerg Surg* 34:177–80.

Ethicon. 2009. High viscosity Dermabond package label. Ethicon, Somerville, NJ.

Fischer, T.H., Connolly, R., Thatte, H.S., and Schwaitzberg, S.S. 2004. Comparison of structural and hemostatic properties of the poly-N-acetyl glucosamine Syvek patch with products containing chitosan. *Microsc Res Tech* 63:168–74.

Food and Drug Administration (FDA). 2009. http://www.fda.gov/MedicalDevices/DeviceRegulationandGuidance/GuidanceDocuments/ucm080742.htm (accessed April 23, 2011).

Food and Drug Administration (FDA). 2010. http://www.fda.gov/medicaldevices/deviceregulationandguidance/howtomarketyourdevice/premarketsubmissions/premarketapprovalpma/default.htm#when (accessed April 23, 2011).

Forthofer, K.V. 2009. A clinical review of the intrauterine device as an effective method of contraception. *J Obstet Gynecol Neonatal Nurs* 38:693–98.

Haimovich, S. 2009. Profile of long-acting reversible contraception users in Europe. *Eur J Contracep Reprod Health Care* 14:187–95.

Ingram, D., and Garcia, K. 2010. *Tissue Adhesive Strength Comparisons.* Internal Memorandum, Poly-Med, Anderson, SC.

Johnston, L. 1999. *Colon and Rectal Cancer: A Comprehensive Guide for Patients and Families.* O'Reilly Media, Sebastopol, CA.

Larrazabal, R., Pelz, D., and Findlay, J.M. 2001. Endovascular treatment of a lenticulostriate artery aneurysm with N-butyl cyanoacrylate. *Can J Neurol Sci* 28:256–59.

Lattouf, J.B., Berri, A., Klinger, C., et al. 2007. Practical hints for hemostasis in laparoscopic surgery. *Min Inv Ther* 16:45–51.

Law, W.L., Choi, H.K., Lee Y.M., Ho, J.W.C., and Seto, C.L. 2007. Anastomotic leakage is associated with poor long-term outcome in patients after curative colorectal resection for malignancy. *J Gastrointest Surg* 11:8–15.

Lin, K.Y., Long, W.B., III, Edlich, R.F. 2005. Scientific basis for the selection of vascular suture closure. WoundClosures.com. March. http://www.woundclosures.com/Article4.pdf (accessed March 2011).

Louie, M.K., et al. 2010. Bovine serum albumin glutaraldehyde for completely sutureless laparoscopic heminephrectomy in a survival porcine model. *J Endourol* 24:451–55.

Mofidi, R., Flett, M., Milne, A., and Chakraverty, S. 2007. Endovascular repair of an anastomotic leak following open repair of abdominal aortic aneurysm. *Cardiovasc Intervent Radiol* 30:1013–15.

Omrix Biopharmaceuticals. 2007. Evithrom package insert. Omrix Biopharmaceuticals, Kiryat-Ono, Israel.

Pakbaz, R.S., Kerber C., Ghanaati H., Akhlaghpoor, S., and Shakoori, A. 2010. A new aneurysm therapy: neucrylate AN. *Neurosurgery* 66:E1030.

Park, W., Kim, W.H., Lee, C.H., et al. 2002. Comparison of two fibrin glues in anastomoses and skin closure. *J Vet Med A* 49:385–89.

Password, F., and View, I. 2001. How widespread are the symptoms of an overactive bladder and how are they managed? A population-based prevalence study. *BJU Int* 87:760–66.

Raymond, J., Berthelet, F., Desfaits, A.C., Salazkin, I., and Roy, D. 2002. Cyanoacrylate embolization of experimental aneurysms. *Am J Neuroradiol* 23:129–38.

Sarkar, S., Sales, K.M., Hamilton, G., and Seifalian, A.M. 2006. Addressing thrombogenicity in vascular graft construction. *J Biomed Mat Res B: Appl Biomat* 82B:100–8.

Selden, E. 1917. Sutures and ligatures. *Am J Nursing* 17:491–95.

Shalaby, S.W. 2008. Segmented copolyesters as compliant, absorbable coatings and sealants for vascular devices. United States of America Patent 7,348,364. March 25.

Shalaby, S.W. 2010. Micromantled drug-eluting stent. United States of America Patent 7,722,914. May 25.

Shalaby, S.W., Corbett, J.T., Ingram, D.R., and Vaughn, M.A. 2009. Hydroswellable, segmented, aliphatic polyurethanes and polyurethane ureas. United States of America Patent 12/380,391. September 17.

Stadelmann, W.K., Digenis, A.G., and Tobin, G.R. 1998. Physiology and healing dynamics of chronic cutaneous wounds. *Am J Surg* 176:26S–38S.

Thomson, S.R., Fraser, M., Stupp, C., and Baker, L.W. 2004. Iatrogenic and accidental colon injuries—what to do? *Dis Colon Rectum* 37:496–502.

Thornton, M., Joshi, H., Vimalachandran, C., et al. 2011. Management and outcome of colorectal anastomotic leaks. *Int J Colorectal Dis* 26:313–20.

Turi, Z.G. 2009. Overview of vascular closure. *Endovascular Today,* February, 24–32.

Understanding vascular occlusion. n.d. Kurt Amplatz Center for Patient Education. http://www.amplatzer.com/KurtAmplatzCenterforEducation/tabid/171/default.aspx (accessed March 21, 2011).

Veenhof, A.A.F.A., van der Pee, D.L., Sietses, C., and Cuesta, M.A. 2007. Pull-through procedure as treatment for coloanal anastomotic dehiscence following laparoscopic total mesorectal excision. *Int J Colorectal Dis* 22: 1413–14.

11

Materials and Polymers for Use in Surgical Simulation and Validation

David M. Kwartowitz

CONTENTS

Introduction

The history of medicine brings us back to the origin of humans, and their desire to prevent and rectify disease, disorder, and functional abnormality (Risse 1999). Early treatments for these ailments included the phenomenological use of medicinal agents, such as plants and herbs, as well as surgical practices. Over the years, while the understanding of the mechanism by which surgical practice affects maladies has improved, the training of surgeons has remained largely the same.

Medical practice has long used the apprenticeship model for training new practitioners. Students are provided general knowledge through teachings in medical school and learn a specific specialty (trade) through practicing it under the eyes of an attending physician (master craftsperson) during residency (apprenticeship) (Ellis 1963). This model relies on inexperienced practitioners to train on cadavers, living patients, or animals. Often, due to experiential and ethical concerns, these practitioners end up training on actual patients, progressively learning new parts of the procedure. While this model has worked for generations, modern advances in materials science, medicine, and computing have made it possible to develop simulations such that surgical practice can be learned in a pseudo-realistic environment.

These simulated tissue models or phantoms can provide a number of distinct advantages over their living counterparts. The major advantage of these materials is that they provide an artificial environment that can be used without regard for risk to a living patient or animal. This allows the development of new techniques and minimizes the potential for deleterious effects on patients. Further, these models allow for repeated creation of even rare medical conditions, allowing more thorough training, as well as the development of new medical techniques.

These phantoms can be divided into a number of classes depending on their function. In general, there are anthropomorphic, tissue-mimicking, imaging, and rigid phantoms. Anthropomorphic phantoms attempt to provide an analogue for the shape of tissue. Tissue-mimicking phantoms attempt to provide a material that has similar properties to tissue; this can be in a mechanical, visual, or chemical sense or any combination. Imaging phantoms attempt to provide certain properties under medical imaging, whether it is those similar to tissue or those that are at the boundaries of the imaging modality. Rigid phantoms have a definite shape that may or may not be an analogue to living tissue in shape, mechanics, or imaging qualities. These rigid phantoms are most often used for system validation. A phantom may fall into any one category or multiple categories.

This chapter examines the different materials used for the construction of these phantoms, as well as some of the applications for which these phantoms are used. Highlighted are some of the desirable properties of these materials and the rationale for their use, as well as some of the ongoing research efforts to improve these materials to mimic human or animal tissues more closely, thus becoming better surrogates for their living counterparts.

Indeed, polymer use in vascular and urogenital surgery is not limited to the clinical realm, but also is present in the preclinical or research phases for design of new devices and procedures. Materials such as rubbers, plastics, ceramics, and synthetics can be used to act as surrogates for the actual tissues, acting to reduce patient risk and animal use. Phantoms are designed to match the properties, morphology, or both of a patient's native tissues. Currently, there are many commonly used materials for vascular phantom design, including natural rubbers and other rubbery polymers. There are far fewer documented materials as surrogates for urogenital tissue; there is therefore a need for development of good materials for phantom design.

Tissue Models

Probably the simplest case of a tissue-mimicking material is the use of some surrogate tissue with similar properties as the tissue of interest. The concept of using a model such as an animal or cadaver in place of a patient for the development and validation of surgical and imaging techniques is well established and frequently used. These techniques will naturally provide the best coupling between the tissue of interest and the chosen surrogate, but introduce confounds not present in artificial tissue and anatomic phantoms.

The use of cadaveric tissue as a surrogate for living tissues provides similar morphology and material properties as those found in living organisms. The use of postmortem surgical study dates to antiquity, when cadavers were used for the earliest anatomic exploration (Risse 1999). In modern medicine, the use of cadavers is well documented in the scientific literature, popular literature, and arts. This form of study introduces ethical, biological, and mechanical confounds.

The acquisition of cadaveric samples is fraught with both ethical and logistic challenges (Catalano 1994). The ethical concerns regarding the use of human remains for science and teaching have been raised in the popular media and have led to many institutions distancing themselves from this type of work (Schwartz and Vogel 1993; Warren 1985a, 1985b, 1999; Jacobs 2005; "Surgeons Use" 1999; Charles and Alan 2004; Folmar 1999). Beyond the ethical concerns, the cause of death, stillness, and the preservation of tissues make cadavers far from an ideal surrogate for normal living tissues.

In addition to using cadaveric specimens, there is a long history of the use of animals as substitutes for human tissues. Animal models are well established and characterized and can often be an excellent step between *in vitro* and *in situ* experiments. In many cases, animal tissue provides similar anatomic and physiologic structure to human tissues. It is important to realize, however, that animal tissues are not human, and whereas one organ in a particular species may closely mimic its human counterpart, other tissues within the same species often will not have the same morphology or function. Further confounding animal models is that many animal systems function differently from their human counterparts. Further, in humans there can be a large intrasubject variation in the shape and position of tissues. While the use of *ex vivo* animal tissues is common, they often have the same scientific confounds due to tissue hemolysis; Figure 11.1 shows an experiment conducted using animal suet for medical image analysis.

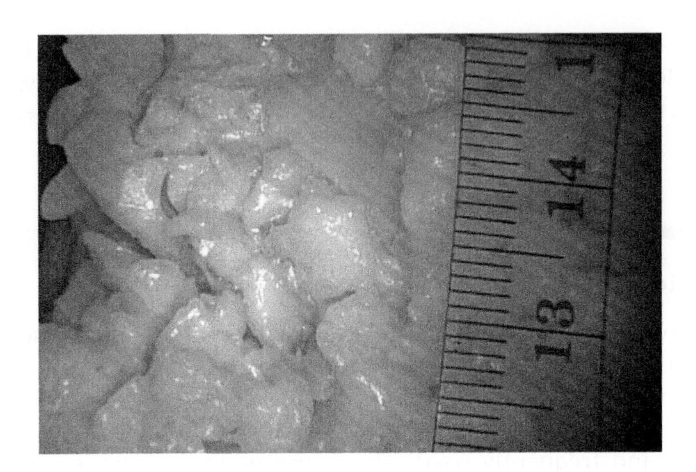

FIGURE 11.1
Phantom constructed from animal suet for medical imaging. (Image from research conducted under the direction of Dr. Richard Robb and Dr. David R. Holmes, Mayo Clinic.)

In addition to the experimental confounds present in animal models, there are regulatory and ethical concerns in the use of animals. As animals cannot provide informed consent or assent, their participation in studies is not voluntary. Further, as many studies cause serious injury, these studies will often require sacrifice of the animal, which has obvious ethical implications. Because of these implications, a high level of protection and supervision is provided in animal studies. These protections become increasingly rigid with species more similar to humans.

While cadaveric and animal studies provide some of the best models for anatomy and morphology, they are not ideal, especially for use in tests in which a high level of repeatability is required. Animal and cadaver studies are excellent methods for final validation; however, they add confounds to basic science, which in many cases can be eliminated using tissue-mimicking materials.

In the next sections, I review some of the common phantom models currently used and describe their benefits and drawbacks, as well as provide some sample applications for each phantom design material.

Rigid Phantoms

From its original meaning as "a ghost" (McKean 2005), the term *phantom* has come to mean a nonliving surrogate for tissues that can be used in the place of natural tissue. The use of phantoms for both medical imaging and image guidance research and validation is both well established and widespread due to the relative simplicity of the design and use of different phantom devices. Design of phantom devices is often application specific; a device is optimized for the specific goal or test it is designed to accomplish. This application-specific design motif allows for maximal flexibility, with direct characterization of the problem being queried.

In designing phantoms, the simplest schema is a phantom that does not attempt to match the anatomic structure or tissue properties of human or animal flesh. Often these phantoms fit into the category of "rigid phantoms." This classification means that the phantoms do not change in morphology under mechanical load. For many applications, this form of phantom is advantageous as repeated validation experiments can be performed with well-defined expected results.

Another important application for these rigid phantoms is in the form of registration phantoms, such as the "checkerboard" phantoms. This type of phantom has the advantage that homologous point pairs are guaranteed to align with a high level of precision. This type of phantom also allows for validation of measurement devices, as the geometry is often known and can be compared to the sampled points. This style, however, can be restrictive in its application as the points are rigidly defined and do not fit the geometry or morphology present in natural organs.

Anthropomorphic Phantoms

While the classic rigid checkerboard, registration, or geometric-style phantoms provide some advantage, the lack of the resemblance to organ structure acts to limit the applications of such devices. The next level of complexity appears with the anthropomorphic phantoms, which attempt to mimic tissue shape, but not necessarily material properties. This type of phantom has many uses, ranging from exam room model in a physician's office, to research on shape for medical technique development, to physician training. This type of phantom is functional primarily because its shape closely resembles the shape of the target anatomy.

The design of an anthropomorphic phantom is often based directly on an anatomic specimen, illustration, or image. These phantoms can be molded, carved, extruded, modeled, or printed using a rapid prototyping machine. Because in a purely anthropomorphic phantom shape is the primary concern, the material used for its construction does not necessarily have to resemble the tissue of interest. This leads to flexibility in manufacturing method but limits the applications within the surgical simulation and planning realm.

While purely anthropomorphic phantoms have a limited application in the realm of soft tissue simulation, work has been done to bring this type of phantom into the clinic. One such example is the use of three-dimensional

(3D) printed spine phantoms for application in scoliosis surgery (Augustine et al. 2010). Beyond orthopedics, rigid phantoms can be used for the design and development of maxillofacial implants (Eggers, Muehling, and Marmulla 2006; Ewers et al. 2005, 2010; Hassfeld and Muhling 2001; Jayaratne et al. 2010; Korb et al. 2004; Olszewski et al. 2008; Widmann and Bale 2006), as well as validation of computer-assisted surgery systems for direct patient interaction (Mozer et al. 2005).

Natural Tissues

Basing tissue-mimicking phantoms on natural tissue requires a fundamental understanding of the properties of the tissue of interest. Broadly, tissues can be divided into two categories, hard tissue and soft tissue. Hard tissues are those such as bone that exhibit primarily rigid mechanical properties and in many cases can be mimicked using rigid materials. Soft tissues exhibit more complex behavior, including viscoelasticity and plasticity, as well as more traditional material properties.

The properties of bone were measured in the 1970s by Yamada and coworkers and were summarized by Fung and colleagues (Yamada and Evans 1970; Fung 1997). The values for human femur and Grade 1 titanium are summarized in Table 11.1. The inclusion of titanium is for comparison between a common rigid metal used in biomedical applications and the natural tissues it interfaces. It is obvious that while more ductile than the bone, the titanium is also stiffer.

Soft tissues, however, follow more complex and often nonlinear behaviors, making creation of a true tissue-mimicking device difficult, if not impossible. These properties include deformability, relaxation, viscoelasticity,

TABLE 11.1

Mechanical Properties of Bone for Human Femur of Subjects 20–39 Years of Age

Property	Bone (Fung 1993; Yamada and Evans 1970)	Titanium, ASTM F67, Grade 1 (Niinomi 1998)
Ultimate tensile strength (UTS), MPa	124 ± 1.1	240
Ultimate elongation, %	1.41	24
Modulus of elasticity E, GPa	17.6	102.7
Ultimate shear strength (USS)	54 ± 0.6 MPa	
Torsional modulus of elasticity, GPa	3.2	45

Source: Adapted from Fung, Y.C. 1993. *Biomechanics: Mechanical Properties of Living Tissues*. 2nd ed. New York: Springer-Verlag; and Yamada, H., and Evans, F.G. 1970. *Strength of Biological Materials*: Baltimore: Williams & Wilkins.

TABLE 11.2

Selected Mechanical Properties of Human Tissues

Tissue	Density, g/cm³ (Hubbell and Seltzer 2004)	Young's Modulus E, kPa	
Skin		20–850	Serup, Jemec, and Grove 2006; Agache et al. 1980; Sanders 1973; Koene, Id-Boufker, and Papy 2008
Breast	1.040	1.8	Samani et al. 2003
Muscle	1.050	0.675×106	Grimal, Naili, and Watzky 2005
Brain	1.020	28–41	Walsh and Schettini 1976

and perfusion as well as others. Different soft tissues can vary greatly in their mechanical properties and thus require different materials to act as surrogates.

Soft tissues can be further categorized by the cell types constructing them, the function, or the general tissue structure. One such classification is from histology, which divides all tissues by cell type and general function. This classifies all tissues as muscle, connective tissue, nervous tissue, or epithelium. This is useful in the stratification of tissue, although the histologic makeup of tissues is only part of the explanation of tissue mechanical properties. Additional factors including tissue density, water content, fat content, and the source (person or animal) all play a part in determining the properties of tissues.

Because of the general structure of tissue, a directional anisotropy in material properties exists, and aging of tissue changes properties; thus tissue properties are particular not only to access but also to patient. A general table of mechanical tissue properties was summarized by Koene and colleagues (Koene, Id-Boufker, and Papy 2008) (Table 11.2).

Each tissue type exhibits different mechanical behavior, which translates to different feel in palpation, rigidity, and cutting characteristics. For this reason, much research has gone into a variety of materials for use as tissue-mimicking surrogates.

For medical imaging, it is important that a material have similar acoustic or attenuation properties to the tissues being mimicked. For this reason, an understanding of the imaging modalities being used and of the specific tissue of interest is important. Table 11.3 shows some significant properties for tissues for use in medical imaging; for x-ray, 60 keV was chosen for beam energy as it is similar to the mean energy of a 120-kvP x-ray tube.

Tissue-Mimicking Phantoms

There are obvious limitations of "rigid" and non-tissue-mimicking phantoms as they will not necessarily resemble the viscoelasticity, shear, or

TABLE 11.3

Imaging Properties of Selected Tissues

Tissue	X-Ray Attenuation at 60 keV, cm^3/g[a]	Speed of Sound,[b] m/s	Acoustic Impedance,[b] rayls
Breast	0.2006	1430–1570[a]	1.42×10^6 to 1.66×10^6[b]
Fat	0.1974	1450	1.34×10^6
Lung	0.2053	600	0.18×10^6
Skeletal muscle	0.2048	1600	1.71×10^6

[a] Hubbell, JH and Seltzer, SM. 2011. *Tables of X-Ray Mass Attenuation Coefficients and Mass Energy-Absorption Coefficients* (1.4). National Institutes of Standards and Technology (NIST), July 12 2004 [cited May 30 2011]. Available from http://physics.nist.gov/xaamdi

[b] Zell, K., Sperl, J.I., Vogel, M.W., Niessner, R., and Haisch C. 2007. Acoustical properties of selected tissue phantom materials for ultrasound imaging. *Physics in Medicine and Biology* 52:N475–84. With permission.

cutting properties of natural tissue. This lack of similarity can provide confounds for use in surgical simulation or exploration. Much work has been performed in both image-guided surgery and surgical simulation into the development of tissue-mimicking materials, such that a better analogue for tissue may be constructed.

Desirable Material Properties

When examining materials for tissue surrogates, it is important to realize that no material will be a perfect analogue in all properties. For this reason, there is a range of materials commonly used, which are selected based on application and desirable properties. It is also important to realize that most materials will have some deleterious aspects. Finding a favorable balance between the benefits and drawbacks of a specific material is an important part of the selection and adoption of a material for a specific application.

When looking at medical imaging, for example, one would like modality-specific contrast to match the tissue being investigated closely. Specifically in x-ray, this means similar material density and photon attenuation as compared to living tissues. In ultrasound, however, the desirable properties are similar acoustic impedances, speeds of sound, and impedance boundaries. In magnetic resonance imaging (MRI), similar T_1, T_2, and spin density might be desirable or flow rate of fluid. It is easy to see in even these few cases that no one material would be ideal for all cases.

Another important application for tissue-mimicking phantoms is surgical simulation. In this case, desirable properties tend to be mechanical, as it is desired for materials to feel, palpate, and cut like natural tissues. These properties translate to shear tolerance, density, Young's modulus, and viscoelasticity. Each of these properties varies by tissue type and composition, meaning that construction of tissue-mimicking phantoms for surgical simulation may require the use of multiple materials, each simulating different tissues.

Various materials have been investigated for use in phantom construction. Materials used for phantom construction include both organic and inorganic polymers, including gelatins, plastics, and rubbers. While each material has benefits and drawbacks, judicious selection of materials for tissue-mimicking phantoms can provide for both realistic and repeatable scenarios for the development and validation of medical techniques.

Considerations in the Design of a Phantom Material

Beyond the material properties, there are a number of considerations in the choice of a material for tissue-mimicking phantoms. These considerations include concepts such as longevity and viability of the material. Some materials will break down quickly when exposed to the environment, while others are stable indefinitely. Some materials involve the use of carcinogenic media, solvents, or stabilizers, while others use materials that are innocuous. Other materials require complicated methods or long curing or setting times, and these methods may take a long time for material production; others are relatively fast. One property that is ubiquitously desirable is the ability to be shaped, molded, or carved into a material with relevant morphology.

It is important to be aware of the various materials available and their benefits and drawbacks to determine the one that is best for a given application. While there is no perfect material for all cases, the trade-offs can be mitigated using combinations of materials. As naturally occurring tissues are a combination of materials with different material properties, tissue-mimicking phantoms are also often constructed using multiple materials, optimizing both the properties of each material and the interactions between the materials.

Materials Used

Because no one material provides an ideal surrogate for natural tissue, a range of materials is used, including organic media, such as gelatins and rubbers, and inorganics, such as plastics and synthetic rubbers. The properties of each tissue-mimicking material are a function of not only material type but also material formulation environment and composition. For this reason, a single material can exhibit a range of properties. This range can allow the same basic material to act as a range of tissues. This is much the same as cells of similar type providing different bulk properties.

The materials used can be broken into three general classes: organic polymers, such as gelatin; rubbers; and other materials, such as synthetic gels. Each of these categories can be further broken down by specific material type and properties. In the following sections, I provide a survey of these materials and key properties of each.

Organic Polymers

Gelatin

One material that has long been used for tissue mimicking is gelatin, which is an organic polymer derived from natural collagenous tissues. Gelatins have been used since the early 1980s for forensic science in ordinance or ballistics gelatins (Fackler 1987; Jussila 2004). These gelatins are chosen because under impulse they behave in the same way as natural tissues. Gelatins can have a range of properties based on average molecular weight; Bloom, a measure of stiffness under specific conditions (Phillips and Williams 2009); water content at manufacture; added plasticizers; and manufacturing conditions.

Gelatin is widely accepted as a tissue-mimicking material because it is inexpensive, safe, and easy to manufacture. Simple gelatin phantoms can be constructed by adding boiling water to gelatin powder, followed by adding cold water, then cooling the solution. Laboratory-grade gelatin is manufactured in a range of molecular weights and Bloom strengths.

When gelling using the simple water-and-cooling method, Bloom strength will dictate the stiffness of the gel under compression, while average molecular weight will dictate gel viscosity (Phillips and Williams 2009). Gelatins are roughly broken into three ranges: high (200–300 g), medium (100–200 g), and low (50–100 g). Gelatin purity is rated as type A and type B; Type A directly derives from the parent media, while type B is modified by the boiling process, causing breakdown of some of the proteins (Phillips and Williams 2009). In addition to the innate properties of the gelatin, the rate of cooling (Jussila 2004) and composition of the gelatin mixture can have an impact on the properties of the resulting gel.

A reference for the elasticity of gelatin was provided by Samani and Plews using a type B gelatin from bovine skin in a 0.14-g/mL concentration (Samani and Plewes 2007). This gel was measured as having an elastic modulus of 14.89 kPa. The manufacturer stated the gelatin had a Bloom strength of 225 g and was thereby a high-Bloom gel. Ballistics gel has been assessed as having an elastic modulus of 100–150 kPa when made from a 20% 250 Bloom type A gelatin (Juliano et al. 2006; Amato et al. 1970; Fackler 1988).

It is apparent that gelatins can provide a wide range of mechanical properties and can be used to mimic a wide range of soft tissues. As a hydrocolloid derived from animal skin, many of the properties of the parent tissue are retained. Gelatin, however, presents a number of drawbacks, one of which is temperature dependency, that is, the mechanical properties, such as modulus, change as temperature changes (Phillips and Williams 2009). Further, gelatin tears within strain rates much lower than tissue and will not cut the same as natural tissues (Miller 1899). To mitigate these factors, plasticizers and cross-linkers such as formaldehyde may be used; however, these often are dangerous chemicals and still may not ultimately provide long-term stability.

Rubbers and Elastomers

Gelatins not only provide many benefits but also present drawbacks, such as temperature stability and long-term stability. Rubbers, however, have excellent longevity and, depending on the specific material, may have good temperature stability. Rubbers can be broken down into two general categories, natural rubber and synthetic rubber or elastomers. Synthetic rubbers contain a number of specific compounds. These materials can provide a range of beneficial properties; however, they also bring their own drawbacks. In this section, I discuss natural rubber as well as the synthetic rubber silicone, which has gained popularity for phantom construction.

Natural Rubber

Latex is a naturally occurring elastomer produced by numerous plants and fungi, primarily those found in tropical regions. Latex is then processed to form a natural rubber, which can be shaped, molded, cast, or carved. Natural rubber is frequently made into products such as tubing, gloves, or sheets. Natural rubbers are supple and flexible with a viscoelastic stress-strain profile. Natural rubbers are tear resistant and will expand 650% before failure (Harris and Piersol 2002). This property is ideal when large strains are placed on a device.

Natural rubbers, however, are impacted by environmental factors and will degrade relatively quickly. Beyond the degradation from environmental sources, natural rubber is affected by solvents and biological factors (Steinbüchel and Hofrichter 2001). This degradation causes cracks in the material. In the case of using latex tubing for flow phantoms, care must be taken to use a fluid that does not cause rapid degradation of the tubing.

Latex has gained some popularity in tissue-mimicking phantoms used for vasculature in ultrasound. This popularity is due to the acoustic properties of natural rubbers when compared to other tubing materials. The speed of sound C in natural rubber is 1,549 m/s, and acoustic impedance Z is 1.74 (NDT Systems Incorporated 2011) compared to silicone at 940 m/s and 1.4 (NDT Systems Incorporated 2011).

Contrast in ultrasound is achieved by having differences in acoustic impedance. Reflected pressure is expressed as (Bushberg 2002)

$$R_p = \frac{P_r}{P_i} = \frac{Z_2 - Z_1}{Z_2 + Z_1}$$

It is apparent that a difference in acoustic impedance between a liquid flowing within the material and the material itself is desirable. In many cases, natural rubber tubing is used in invisible wall flow phantoms (Dabrowski et al. 1997; Rickey et al. 1995).

Inorganic Polymers

In addition to the use of naturally occurring polymers, such as gelatin and natural rubbers, the use of inorganic polymers, elastomers, and plastics is well established in the area of tissue-mimicking phantoms. These materials are often preferable because the mechanical properties of the media can be more easily controlled and repeated. Probably the most commonly used elastomer from the synthetics is silicone, which can be modified through changes in the curing media. In addition to silicone, polyurethane foams and poly(vinyl) alcohol cryogel (PVA-C) have gained some popularity.

Silicone

Polydimethylsiloxane or silicone rubber is a material that is synthetically produced and has many properties similar to rubber. Silicone can be produced in a liquid form that, when introduced to a catalyst, will cure into a solid rubberlike material. This catalyst is often either tin or platinum based. In the case of most silicones used for tissue-mimicking phantoms, they are room temperature vulcanizing (RTV), meaning that they cure without production of heat. This allows for a range of applications for which exothermic curing reactions would cause damage.

Tin-cured silicones are produced as a two-part mixture, which is mixed immediately before pouring into a mold. Oomoo™ (Smooth-on, Easton, PA), a popular silicone rubber for tissue-mimicking phantoms, has a pot life of less than 30 minutes and a curing time of less than 6 hours (Smooth-On Inc. 2011). This allows for rapid casting and production of phantom materials. This material has a shore hardness of 25–30 A depending on the chosen formulation and an elastic modulus of 1–5 MPa (Matbase). It is apparent that this material is less elastic than natural tissue. In addition, tin-cured silicones have a short "library time," meaning that the final phantom will shrink over time, and thus material properties will change. Because of these limitations, there has been a shift toward platinum-cured silicone and polyurethane foams.

Platinum-cured silicone, like tin-cured silicone, is produced as a two-part mixture using a platinum-based catalyst, as opposed to the tin-based catalyst used previously. One popular platinum-cured silicone is Dragon Skin (Smooth-On Inc.). This material comes in a number of variations with a pot life ranging from 8 to 45 minutes and cure time ranging from 40 minutes to 16 hours. These materials range in shore hardness from 2 A to 30 A and have a range of ultimate elongation of 364% to 1,000% (Smooth-On Inc. 2011). This allows for a range of material properties to be generated with a generally similar material.

This material has gained wide acceptance in a range of medical disciplines (Davis et al. 2011; Rost et al. 2004; Vosburgh and EstÈpar 2003; Miller 2010; Benincasa et al. 2008). This is largely because of the ease of manufacture, as well as the relatively quick preparation and cure time. Platinum-cured silicone can be cast into molds that are applicable to most body parts and has an excellent library time.

One of the largest problems with platinum-cured silicone is the relative expense due to the platinum-based enzyme. Further, this material is natively somewhat stiffer than natural tissue, making it behave somewhat differently from the tissue it is mimicking. Because of the relative expense, repeated validation studies are often not practical. Dragon Skin is subject to bubbles and other artifacts when not molded in a vacuum.

A softer silicone material called Ecoflex, based on Dragon Skin, has been developed. This material is softer and more pliable, with a shore hardness of 00–5 A, ultimate elongation of 800% to 1,000%, pot life ranging from 1 to 30 minutes, and cure time ranging from 5 minutes to 4 hours depending on specific formulation. This material eliminates many of the stiffness concerns present in Dragon Skin and because of a lower working viscosity (3,000–13000 cPs as opposed to 18,000–30,000 cPs) is less susceptible to bubbles. One of the largest limitations of Ecoflex™ is the relative expense associated with all platinum-cured silicones. This material also is subject to shrinkage over time and thus has a limited library time. A comparison of computed tomographic (CT) images of an Oomoo and Ecoflex phantom is provided in Figure 11.2. This material has found wide acceptance among biomedical engineers and medical scientists due to its desirable properties (Gwilliam et al. 2009; Yamamoto et al. 2009; Leskovsky, Harders, and Szeekely 2006; Ong et al. 2010).

Other Polymers

Of materials that have gained some acceptance in the field of tissue-mimicking phantoms that do not fall into the previously specified categories, one particular material of interest is PVA-C, which is a cross-linked gel formed from hydrolyzed poly(vinyl) alcohol (PVA). Other materials that would fall into this category would be urethane foams and rubbers, as well as plastics and other inorganics.

Poly(Vinyl) Alcohol Cryogel

PVA-C was first introduced for imaging and flow in 1997 by Chu and coworkers (Chu and Rutt 1997) and further popularized by Surry and Fenster in 2004 (Surry et al. 2004). The formulation of this material starts with a PVA hydrolate, and repeated freezing and thawing cycles cause increasing levels of cross-linking.

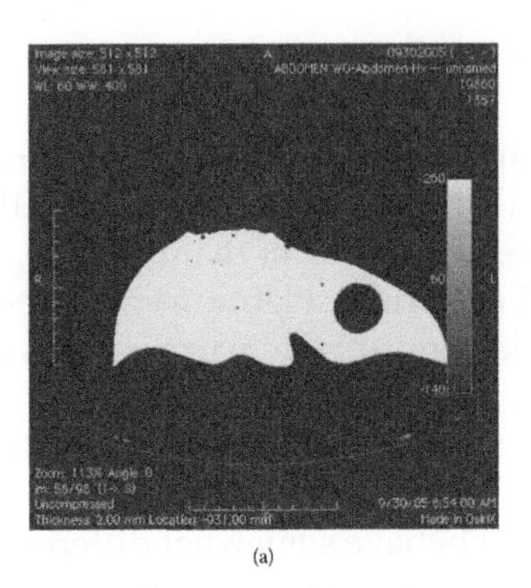

(a)

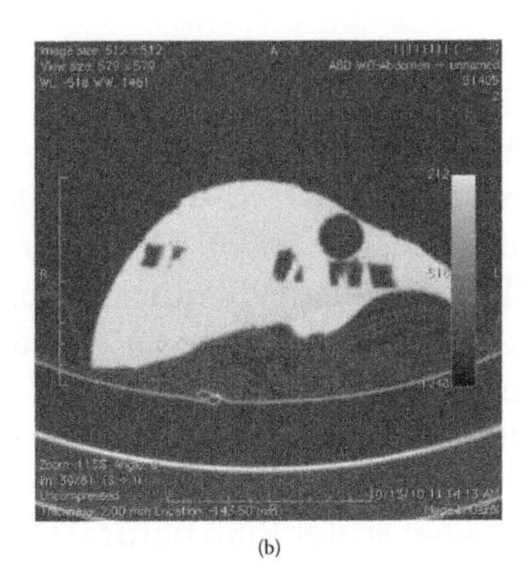

(b)

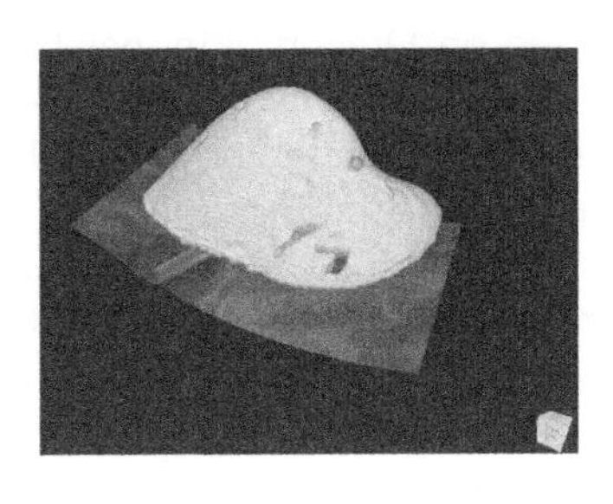

(c)

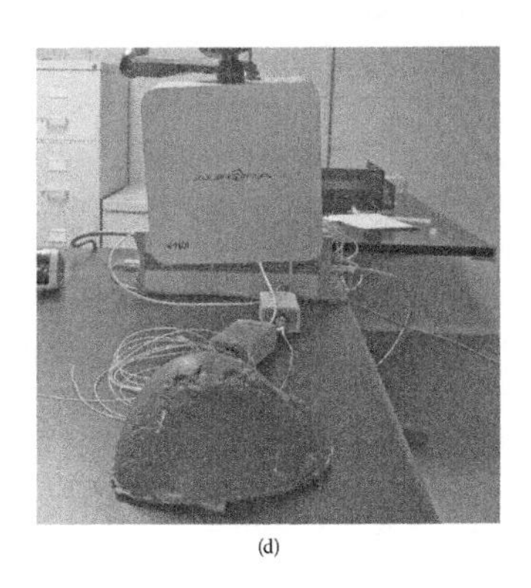

(d)

FIGURE 11.2
Images of liver phantoms made of platinum-cured silicone: (a) CT slice of Oomoo25™ phantom, with intensity approximately 500 HU; void shown is Styrofoam ball representing tumor. (b) CT slice of EcoFlex™ phantom, with intensity approximately 200 HU. (c) Volume rendering of 3D volume of EcoFlex phantom. (d) Photograph of EcoFlex phantom. (Phantoms courtesy of Dr. Bob Galloway. With permission.)

Preparing PVA phantoms begins with water and PVA, which are mixed to blend. The mixture is slowly heated until the PVA goes into solution. The solution is allowed to cool into a supersaturated state. Once the solution has reached room temperature, it is frozen until solid and then thawed. Repeating the freeze-thaw cycles acts to stiffen the cryogel. The material properties are dictated by the concentration of hydrolate and number of freeze-thaw cycles. Other chemicals, such as surfactants, dies, and the like, can be added to the mixture to affect crystallization and material shelf life. This process was patented by Ku in 1999 (Ku, Braddon, and Wootton 1999), although it is commonly used in many laboratories and companies (Herrell et al. 2009; Ou et al. 2008; Comeau et al. 2000; Surry et al. 2004; Chu and Rutt 1997; Gobbi, Comeau, and Peters 2000).

This material is inexpensive and relatively easy to formulate. At the time of writing, 500 g of PVA hydrolyte was approximately $20(USD), which is

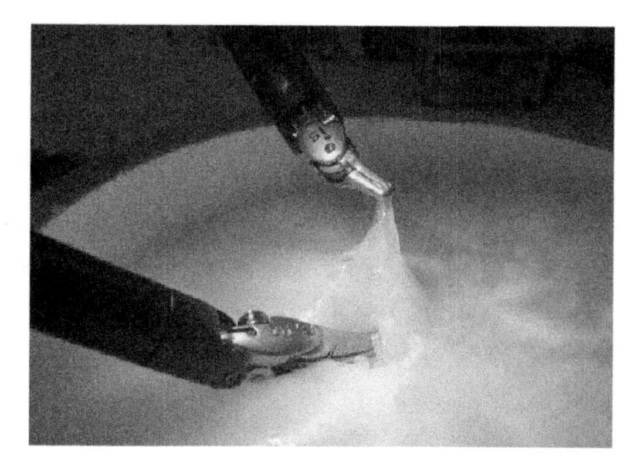

FIGURE 11.3
Poly(vinyl) alcohol phantom made from 6% stock solution. Phantom material being dissected using a daVinci™ surgical robotic system. Image demonstrates the natural retraction and cutting present in this material. (Image from unpublished work by Kwartowitz, D.M., Ou, J., and Galloway, R.L. 2007.)

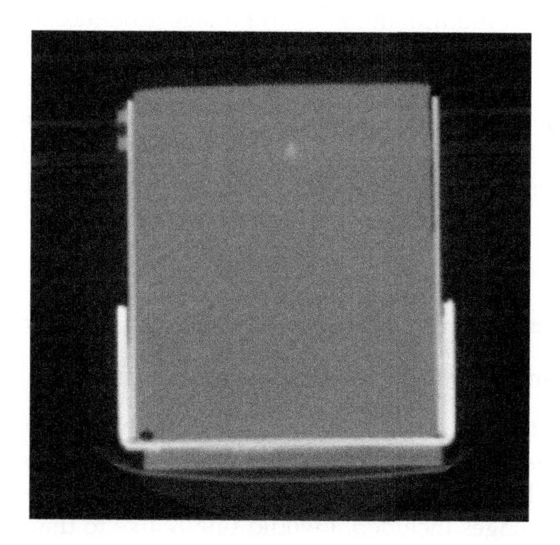

FIGURE 11.4
CT slice of phantom shown in Figure 11.2; this demonstrates the uniform x-ray attenuation created by the PVA material. The bright enhancement is a bolus of iodinated contrast agent that has a higher attenuation rate than the surrounding gel.

enough to make 6.25 L of an 8% PVA stock solution, compared to $300(USD) for an equivalent amount of platinum-cured silicone. Beyond the cost considerations, PVA-C cuts and tears very much like natural tissue, as is shown in Figure 11.3, and has the feel of natural tissue. In medical imaging, PVA-C will appear much the same as water, and modulation in material density can be seen. Unlike the silicone counterparts, this material will appear clearly in

MRI due to the water in the gel matrix. An example of the imaging properties of a sample of PVA cryogel is shown in Figure 11.4.

PVA-C, however, has many limitations not seen in other materials; the library time is extremely short, about days. Because the cryogel has a water-encapsulated matrix structure, it is susceptible to rapid drying as well as mold growth when not stored in water. Further, as PVA-C is cold worked, there is risk due to water expansion and contraction that the final gel will always be smaller than the mold in which it was formed, and there is risk of damage to the mold if it is not properly vented.

Conclusions

This chapter has presented a number of materials that can be used for development of tissue-mimicking phantoms. We have examined the properties of natural tissues, as well as the properties of a range of different tissue surrogates often used for medical imaging and image guidance applications. The materials studied ranged from hard plastics, to organic polymers, to inorganic polymers. It is important to look into the specific application that is being studied before choosing a material to mimic tissue. Each material not only has benefits and applications for which it excels but also has drawbacks, which may hinder its use in certain applications. Understanding the various materials will aid in the development of an ideal tissue-mimicking device.

Acknowledgments

I would like to thank Dr. Bob Galloway, Dr. Cynthia Paschal, Dr. Richard Robb, and Dr. David R. Holmes III for all of the assistance, knowledge, and background for the writing of this chapter. Further, I would like to thank each of them for the images included. I would finally like to thank the members of the Clemson University of Department of Bioengineering for help with materials background, as well as support during the writing of this chapter.

References

Agache, P.G., Monneur, C., Leveque, J.L., and Rigal, J. 1980. Mechanical properties and Young's modulus of human skin *in vivo*. *Archives of Dermatological Research* 269:221–32.

Amato, J.J., Billy, L.J., Gruber, R.P., Lawson, N.S., and Rich. N.M. 1970. Vascular injuries. An experimental study of high and low velocity missile wounds. *Archives of Surgery* 101(2):167–74.
Augustine, K.E., Stans, A.A., Morris, J.M., et al. 2010. Plan to procedure: combining 3D templating with rapid prototyping to enhance pedicle screw placement, at San Diego, CA.
Benincasa, A.B., Clements, L.W., Herrell, S.D., and Galloway R.L. 2008. Feasibility study for image-guided kidney surgery: assessment of required intraoperative surface for accurate physical to image space registrations. *Medical Physics* 35:4251.
Bushberg, J.T. 2002. *The Essential Physics of Medical Imaging*. 2nd ed. Philadelphia: Lippincott Williams & Wilkins.
Catalano, J.T. 1994. The ethics of cadaver experimentation. *Critical Care Nurse* 14:82.
Charles, O., and Zarembo, A. 2004. The UCLA body parts scandal; UCLA suspends body-donor program after alleged abuses; medical school's actions follow accusations that cadavers have been sold illegally to outsiders. *Los Angeles Times*, A.1.
Chu, K.C., and Rutt, B.K. 1997. Polyvinyl alcohol cryogel: an ideal phantom material for MR studies of arterial flow and elasticity. *Magnetic Resonance in Medicine* 37:314–19.
Comeau, R.M., Sadikot, A.F., Fenster, A., and Peters, T.M. 2000. Intraoperative ultrasound for guidance and tissue shift correction in image-guided neurosurgery. *Medical Physics* 27:787.
Dabrowski, W., Dunmore-Buyze, J., Rankin, R.N., Holdsworth, D.W., and Fenster, A. 1997. A real vessel phantom for imaging experimentation. *Medical Physics* 24:687.
Davis, C.A., Mittura, K.L., Copeland, G.E., and Hawkins, E.M. 2011. Feasibility of a touch sensitive breast phantom for use in the training of physicians in clinical breast examination.
Eggers, G., Muehling, J., and Marmulla, R. 2006. Image-to-patient registration techniques in head surgery. *International Journal of Oral and Maxillofacial Surgery* 35:1081–95.
Ellis, J.R. 1963. Apprenticeship in medicine. *Academic Medicine* 38(8).
Ewers, R., Schicho, G., Undt, F., et al. 2005. Basic research and 12 years of clinical experience in computer-assisted navigation technology: a review. *International Journal of Oral and Maxillofacial Surgery* 34:1–8.
Ewers, R., Seemann, R., Krennmair, G., Schicho, K., Kurdi, A.O., Kirsch, A., and Reichwein, A. 2010. Planning implants crown down—a systematic quality control for proof of concept. *Journal of Oral and Maxillofacial Surgery* 68 (11):2868–78.
Fackler, M.L. 1987. *Ordnance Gelatin for Ballistic Studies: Detrimental Effect of Excess Heat Used in Gelatin Preparation*. DTIC Document.
Fackler, M.L. 1988. Wound ballistics. A review of common misconceptions. *JAMA: The Journal of the American Medical Association* 259:2730–36.
Folmar, K. 1999. Use of cadaver slipped by official; UCI anatomy chairman says he didn't pursue matter now investigated. *Los Angeles Times*, 1-1.
Fung, Y.C. 1993. *Biomechanics: Mechanical Properties of Living Tissues*. 2nd ed. New York: Springer-Verlag.
Fung, Y.C. 1997. *Selected Works on Biomechanics and Aeroelasticity*. 2 vol. *Advanced Series in Biomechanics*. Singapore: World Scientific.
Gobbi, D., Comeau, R., and Peters, T. 2000. Ultrasound/MRI overlay with image warping for neurosurgery.

Grimal, Q., Naili, S., and Watzky, A. 2005. A high-frequency lung injury mechanism in blunt thoracic impact. *Journal of Biomechanics* 38:1247–54.

Gwilliam, J.C., Mahvash, B., Vagvolgyi, A., et al. 2009. Effects of haptic and graphical force feedback on teleoperated palpation.

Harris, C.M., and Piersol, A.G. 2002. *Harris' Shock and Vibration Handbook*. 5th ed. New York: McGraw-Hill.

Hassfeld, S., and Muhling, J. 2001. Computer assisted oral and maxillofacial surgery—a review and an assessment of technology. *International Journal of Oral and Maxillofacial Surgery* 30:2–13.

Herrell, S.D., Kwartowitz, D.M., Milhoua, P.M., and Galloway, R.L. 2009. Toward image guided robotic surgery: system validation. *The Journal of Urology* 181:783–89; discussion 789–90.

Hubbell, J.H., and Seltzer, S.M. 2004. Tables of x-ray mass attenuation coefficients and mass energy-absorption coefficients (1.4). National Institutes of Standards and Technology (NIST). July 12.http://physics.nist.gov/xaamdi.

Jacobs, A. 2005. Cadaver exhibition raises questions beyond taste. *New York Times*, B.1.

Jayaratne, Y.S.N., Zwahlen, R.A., Lo, J., Tam, S.C., and Cheung, L.K. 2010. Computer-aided maxillofacial surgery: an update. *Surgical Innovation* 17:217–25.

Juliano, T.F., Moy, P., Forster, A.M., et al. 2006. *Multiscale Mechanical Characterization of Biometric Gels for Army Applications*. U.S. Army Research Laboratory, Weapons and Materials Research Directorate, Aberdeen Proving Ground, MD.

Jussila, J. 2004. Preparing ballistic gelatine—review and proposal for a standard method. *Forensic Science International* 141(2–3):91–98.

Koene, L., Id-Boufker, F., and Papy, A. 2008. Kinetic non-lethal weapons. *Netherlands Annual Review of Military Studies* 9–24.

Korb, W., Marmulla, R., Raczkowsky, J., Muhling, J., and Hassfeld, S. 2004. Robots in the operating theatre—chances and challenges. *International Journal of Oral and Maxillofacial Surgery* 33:721–32.

Ku, D.N., Braddon, L.G., and Wootton, D.M. 1999. Poly (vinyl alcohol) cryogel. Google Patents.

Leskovsky, P., Harders, M., and Szeekely, G. 2006. Assessing the fidelity of haptically rendered deformable objects. Matbase.

McKean, E., editor. 2005. *The New Oxford American Dictionary*. 2nd ed. New York: Oxford University Press.

Miller, A. 1899. On the manufacture of artificial silk from gelatin and a method for ascertaining the relative merits of different samples of gelatin for that manufacture. *Journal of the Society of Chemical Industry* 18:16–20.

Miller, R.J. 2010. *Artificial Skin Tactile Sensor for Prosthetic and Robotic Applications*. San Luis Obispo: California Polytechnic State University.

Mozer, P., Leroy, A. Payan, Y., et al. 2005. Computer-assisted access to the kidney. *The International Journal of Medical Robotics and Computer Assisted Surgery* 1:58–66.

NDT Systems Incorporated. 2011. Acoustical properties of common materials. http://www.ndtsystems.com/Reference/Velocity_Table/velocity_table.html.

Niinomi, M. 1998. Mechanical properties of biomedical titanium alloys. *Materials Science and Engineering A* 243(1–2):231–36.

Olszewski, R., Tran Duy, K., Raucent, B., Hebda, A., and Reychler, H. 2008. Communicating a clinical problem to the engineers: towards a common methodology. *International Journal of Oral and Maxillofacial Surgery* 37:269–74.

Ong, R.E., Glisson, C., Altamar, H., Viprakasit, D., Clark, P., Herrell, S.D., and Galloway, R.L. 2010. Intraprocedural registration for image-guided kidney surgery. *IEEE/ASME Transactions on Mechatronics* 15(6):847–52.

Ou, J.J., Ong, R.E., Yankeelov, T.E., and Miga, M. 2008. Evaluation of 3D modality-independent elastography for breast imaging: a simulation study. *Physics in Medicine and Biology* 53:147.

Phillips, G.O., and Williams, P.A. 2009. *Handbook of Hydrocolloids*. Boca Raton, FL: CRC Press.

Rickey, D.W., Picot, P.A., Christopher, D.A., and Fenster, A. 1995. A wall-less vessel phantom for Doppler ultrasound studies. *Ultrasound in Medicine and Biology* 21:1163–76.

Risse, G.B. 1999. *Mending Bodies, Saving Souls: A History of Hospitals*. New York: Oxford University Press.

Rost, J., Harris, S.S., Stefansic, J.D., Sillay, K., and Galloway, R.L., Jr. 2004. Comparison between skin-mounted fiducials and bone-implanted fiducials for image-guided neurosurgery.

Samani, A., Bishop, J., Luginbuhl, C., and Plewes. D.B. 2003. Measuring the elastic modulus of *ex vivo* small tissue samples. *Physics in Medicine and Biology* 48:2183–98.

Samani, A., and Plewes, D. 2007. An inverse problem solution for measuring the elastic modulus of intact *ex vivo* breast tissue tumours. *Physics in Medicine and Biology* 52:1247–60.

Sanders, R. 1973. Torsional elasticity of human skin *in vivo*. *Pflugers Archiv European Journal of Physiology* 342:255–60.

Schwartz, J., and Vogel, S. 1993. Amid German uproar, U.S. auto researchers defend use of corpses. *The Washington Post* A.39.

Serup, J., Jemec, B.E., and Grove, G.L. 2006. *Handbook of Non-invasive Methods and the Skin*. 2nd ed. Boca Raton, FL: CRC/Taylor & Francis.

Smooth-On Incorporated. 2011. http://www.smooth-on.com.

Steinbüchel, A., and Hofrichter, M. 2001. *Biopolymers*. Chichester, UK: Wiley-VCH.

Surgeons use bone of cadaver to save boy's cancerous arm. 1999. *Los Angeles Times*, 4-4.

Surry, K.J.M., Austin, H.J.B., Fenster, A., and Peters, T.M. 2004. Poly(vinyl alcohol) cryogel phantoms for use in ultrasound and MR imaging. *Physics in Medicine and Biology* 49:5529.

Vosburgh, K.G., and EstÈpar, R.S.J. 2003. Abdominal and laparoscopic surgery. *Therapy* 10:176–79.

Walsh, E.K., and Schettini, A. 1976. Elastic behavior of brain tissue *in vivo*. *American Journal of Physiology—Legacy Content* 230(4):1058–62.

Warren, J. 1985a. Cadaver class in San Marcos frustrated by balky insurer. *Los Angeles Times* 1-1.

Warren, J. 1985b. "More impact" than a textbook: teacher plans to use cadaver in high school. *Los Angeles Times* 1-1.

Warren, P.M. 1999. Records lost, UCI can't use willed bodies; medical school: because of computer virus, dean says he can't be sure cadavers are free of disease. Officials scramble to replace them for student labs. *Los Angeles Times* 1-1.

Widmann, G., and Bale, R.J. 2006. Accuracy in computer-aided implant surgery—a review. *International Journal of Oral and Maxillofacial Implants* 21:305–13.

Yamada, H., and Evans, F.G. 1970. *Strength of Biological Materials*: Baltimore: Williams & Wilkins.

Yamamoto, T., Vagvolgyi, B., Balaji, K., Whitcomb, L.L., and Okamura, A.M. 2009. Tissue property estimation and graphical display for teleoperated robot-assisted surgery.
Zell, K., Sperl, J.I., Vogel, M.W., Niessner, R., and Haisch C. 2007. Acoustical properties of selected tissue phantom materials for ultrasound imaging. *Physics in Medicine and Biology* 52:N475–84.

Index

E

I

P

Q

R

W

X

Y

For Product Safety Concerns and Information please contact our EU representative GPSR@taylorandfrancis.com Taylor & Francis Verlag GmbH, Kaufingerstraße 24, 80331 München, Germany

Printed and bound by CPI Group (UK) Ltd, Croydon, CR0 4YY

01/05/2025

01858528-0001